HISTORIES OF SEXUALLY TRANSMITTED DISEASES AND HIV/AIDS IN SUB-SAHARAN AFRICA

Recent Titles in
Contributions in Medical Studies

Health Care Patterns and Planning in Developing Countries
Rais Akhtar, editor

Fertility Control: New Techniques, New Policy Issues
Robert H. Blank

A Community Approach to AIDS Intervention: Exploring the Miami
Outreach Project for Injecting Drug Users and Other High Risk Groups
Dale D. Chitwood, James A. Inciardi, Duane C. McBride, Clyde B. McCoy,
H. Virginia McCoy, and Edward Trapido

Beyond Flexner: Medical Education in the Twentieth Century
Barbara Barzansky and Norman Gevitz, editors

Mother and Fetus: Changing Notions of Maternal Responsibility
Robert H. Blank

The Golden Wand of Medicine: A History of the Caduceus Symbol in Medicine
Walter J. Friedlander

Cancer Factories: America's Tragic Quest for Uranium Self-Sufficiency
Howard Ball

The AIDS Pandemic: Social Perspectives
Howard Ball

Childbed Fever: A Scientific Biography of Ignaz Semmelweis
K. Codell Carter and Barbara R. Carter

James Cook and the Conquest of Scurvy
Francis E. Cuppage

Romance, Poetry, and Surgical Sleep: Literature Influences Medicine
E. M. Papper

Sex, Disease, and Society
Milton Lewis, Scott Bamber, and M. Waugh, editors

HISTORIES OF SEXUALLY TRANSMITTED DISEASES AND HIV/AIDS IN SUB-SAHARAN AFRICA

Edited by
Philip W. Setel, Milton Lewis, and
Maryinez Lyons

Contributions in Medical Studies, No. 44

GREENWOOD PRESS
Westport, Connecticut
London

Library of Congress Cataloging-in-Publication Data

Histories of sexually transmitted diseases and HIV/AIDS in Sub-Saharan
    Africa / edited by Philip Setel, Milton Lewis, and Maryinez Lyons.
        p.   cm. — (Contributions in medical studies, ISSN 0886–8220 ;
    no. 44)
    Includes bibliographical references and index.
    ISBN 0–313–29715–0 (alk. paper)
    1. Sexually transmitted diseases—Africa, Sub-Saharan—History.
    2. AIDS (Disease)—Africa–Sub–Saharan—History. I. Setel, Philip.
    II. Lewis, Milton James. III. Lyons, Maryinez. IV. Series.
    RA644.V4H55   1999
    616.95'1'00967—dc21   98–38207

British Library Cataloguing in Publication Data is available.

Library of Congress Catalog Card Number: 98–38207
ISBN: 0–313–29715–0
ISSN: 0886–8220

First published in 1999

Greenwood Press, 88 Post Road West, Westport, CT 06881
An imprint of Greenwood Publishing Group, Inc.

Printed in the United States of America

The paper used in this book complies with the
Permanent Paper Standard issued by the National
Information Standards Organization (Z39.48–1984).

10 9 8 7 6 5 4 3 2 1

Contents

HISTORIES OF SEXUALLY TRANSMITTED DISEASES AND HIV/AIDS IN SUB-SAHARAN AFRICA

1

Comparative Histories of Sexually Transmitted Diseases and HIV/AIDS in Africa: An Introduction

Philip W. Setel

This book is the second in a two-volume set of comparative histories of sexually transmitted diseases (STDs) and human immunodeficiency virus/acquired immune deficiency syndrome (HIV/AIDS) in the non-Western world. The contributions in this volume, like those of the companion book, *Sex, Disease, and Society: A Comparative History of Sexually Transmitted Diseases and HIV/AIDS in Asia and the Pacific*,[1] comprise a series of case studies that focus on the social, cultural, and politicoeconomic bases of past and present epidemics. The cases are drawn from anglophone and francophone countries in West, East, Central, and Southern Africa (see Figure 1.1).

As many authors have noted, the global HIV/AIDS pandemic is largely responsible for stimulating the scholarly attention now being paid to STDs in the developing world — in both the past and present. It has also opened up a lively critical inquiry into topics (sex and sexuality) once anathema to mainstream scholarly inquiry.[2] The epidemic has also prompted a reevaluation of theory and praxis in branches and subfields of the social sciences concerned with health. Theory-oriented scholars have been challenged to imbue more of their work with practical insight, and applied researchers have been pressed to remove their gaze from the immediacy of the epidemic and reflect in more abstract terms upon the ways in which AIDS must be comprehended, analyzed, and combatted.

This volume contributes to this discussion by presenting several cases from around the African continent. To foster a comparative set of case studies in both the Asia and Africa volumes, contributors were asked to

FIGURE 1.1
Geographic Scope of the Book

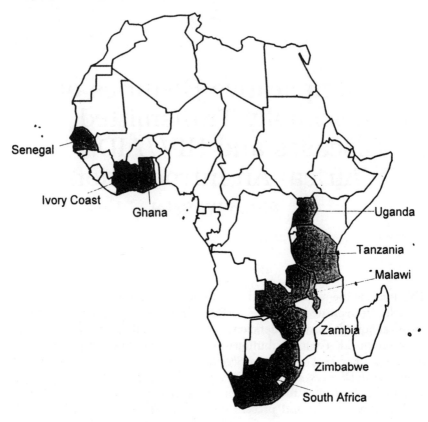

consider how particular constellations of cultural, social, political, and economic factors in different countries have affected the historical patterns of disease and collective (official and community) response to them. The cases presented here transcend the particular national and regional contexts with which they are concerned. In doing so, certain common issues have emerged that provide insight into the conjunctions and disjunctions between the histories of STDs and the AIDS pandemic as it has developed in sub-Saharan Africa.

The contributors to this book have probed present and past epidemics for continuities and disjunctures in a number of key related areas. These include gender relations and sexuality, patterns of population mobility (particularly with regard to labor migration), and official and popular responses to STDs and HIV/AIDS. The data available to historians and anthropologists seeking to explore these issues range from archival and medical records to more recent sources such as population-based epidemiologic studies, press reports, and other more direct observational and interview techniques. Particularly for the retrospective picture, however, there are severe constraints on the depth of knowledge. As the following chapters indicate, data for analyzing STDs in historical perspective vary greatly in quality and quantity across the continent. In general, however, it appears that where colonial anxieties about the impact of STDs upon the vitality and reproductive abilities of African labor forces were greatest, more archival materials are to be found.

There are few, if any, instances in which a proper historical epidemiology of STDs can be constructed for sub-Saharan Africa. There were few enough accurate censuses, let alone community-based prevalence studies of major STDs that would permit such an exercise. Furthermore, given the dearth of clinical health services for Africans into the late twentieth century, it cannot be assumed that the quantity of documentation from health facilities reflects the severity of infection in any given area. Often the most that can be quantified are point prevalence rates among certain categories of male laborers, among the sub-set of African men and women who had contact with Western clinical services, or among some groups of women who sold sex in major colonial towns and cities.

In the Asia volume, the contributors identified ten factors that significantly influenced the spread of STDs and HIV/AIDS and helped to shape the character of local and official responses. These factors were: colonialism (including the internal colonization of ethnic minorities); economic growth; urbanization; migration of labor; gender and economic inequality; religion and sexual morality; war; permeability of borders; nationalism and xenophobia; and economic and political barriers to effective health services.[3] The chapters in this collection touch on many of the same themes, but also point to the divergent manifestations of these forces in African contexts. It is also clear that in Africa these forces are inextricably bound up with one another. The historical and social anatomies of STDs including HIV/AIDS are "joined at the hip," as it were, to the colonial legacy and the post-colonial political economies in Africa. The following interconnected themes, in particular, recur throughout the book: ambiguity and diversity; cultural change; racism; gender; labor migration and economic instability; and the practice of biomedicine and epidemiology in African contexts.

AMBIGUITY AND DIVERSITY

Of all the hallmark themes of the histories of STDs and AIDS in Africa, ambiguity is perhaps the most dogged and, from a public health perspective, the most pernicious. Ambiguity has both stood in the way of clear

understanding as a basis for effective action and permitted the perpetua-
tion of pejorative stereotypes of African cultures, bodies, and persons.
During the colonial era venereal syphilis was typically confused with
yaws, a non-sexually transmitted illness caused, like syphilis, by a spirochete. This often led to wild overestimates of the prevalence of the venereal form. Even when perceptions of disease were clinically sound (as
among restricted populations of migrant workers), the community epidemiology of the disease was usually a product of highly biased guess-
work. In the AIDS era, simply identifying the international scope of the
epidemic has proved an intractable task, despite the vast resources
deployed to confront it. Sources such as the HIV/AIDS Surveillance Database maintained by the U.S. Bureau of the Census[4] highlight the continued lack of high quality data about the status of the epidemic in many
countries of sub-Saharan Africa. For several of the countries covered in
this book, no epidemiologic data that allow estimates of HIV prevalence
among healthy adults and are considered to meet high scientific standards have been published since 1995. The uncertainties about how to
measure the epidemic and how to estimate rates of transmission led the
United Nations AIDS Organization (UNAIDS) and the World Health
Organization (WHO) in 1997 to increase sharply the estimates of the numbers of infected individuals around the world and in Africa in particular
(Table 1.1).[5] The 1997 UNAIDS/WHO report estimated that 90 percent of
those infected with HIV were living in developing countries, with more
than two-thirds (20.8 million) in sub-Saharan Africa.

Although the UNAIDS/WHO Surveillance Unit provided a single estimate of 7.4 percent of all African adults living with HIV/AIDS, another
leitmotif of the pandemic lies behind such global figures: diversity. Table
1.1 gives an immediate impression of diversity in the global pandemic.
Yet within regions there are also enormous variations. By 1997, Southern
Africa had become the most severely affected part of the continent. The
South African government estimated a 33 percent increase in HIV prevalence between 1996 and 1997. Prevalence rates among adults in some
urban areas of Southern Africa doubled over the five years between 1992
and 1997. In Botswana, 43 percent of pregnant women tested in Francis-
town were HIV positive in 1997, while in Beit Bridge, Zimbabwe the percentage rose from 32 to 59 percent in a single year (from 1995 to 1996). In
at least one East African country, however, signs were more positive, with
a 20 percent drop in prevalence estimates between 1996 and 1997 for several populations in Uganda. In general, rates of HIV-1 in West Africa have
been much lower than in East and Southern Africa, although HIV-2 has
been more prevalent there than in other regions of sub-Saharan Africa.[6]
As the chapter on Tanzania points out, diversity is not only a regional
issue but also a factor of the national experience of STDs and HIV/AIDS.

TABLE 1.1
Global HIV/AIDS Statistics, December 1997

Region	Adults and Children Living with HIV/AIDS (millions)	Adult Prevalence (percent)	HIV-Positive Adults Who Are Female (percent)
Sub-Saharan Africa	20.80	7.40	50
North Africa & Middle East	0.21	0.13	20
South & Southeast Asia	6.00	0.60	25
East Asia & Pacific	0.44	0.05	11
Latin America	1.30	0.50	19
Caribbean	0.31	1.90	33
Eastern Europe & Central Asia	0.15	0.07	25
Western Europe	0.53	0.30	20
North America	0.86	0.60	20
Australia & New Zealand	0.01	0.10	5
Total	30.60	1.00	41

Source: UNAIDS/WHO Global HIV/AIDS and STD Surveillance Unit, *Report on the Global HIV/AIDS Epidemic*, 3.

CULTURAL CHANGE

Another overriding conclusion to be drawn from the case studies of STDs and AIDS in the Greenwood series is that much of the newness of HIV is illusory. Its roots can be traced to long processes of cultural change that have been fundamentally shaped through the colonial experience. As Karen Jochelson and colleagues so succinctly put it for South Africa, many aspects of the AIDS epidemic for developing countries in Africa and Asia can be summed up in the idea of "old crisis, new virus."[7] In Asia, the conditions that fostered the rapid spread of STDs "began to come into being from about the sixteenth century when trade and commerce expanded and when large urban centers began to develop."[8] In Africa, the conditions favorable to the epidemic spread of STDs were more a product of conditions that emerged from the mid- to late-nineteenth century up until shortly before the present: the colonial era. Thus, if one truly wishes to comprehend the motive forces behind the epidemic, one must begin by examining the constellation of forces that gave rise to conditions of risk and contagion in which HIV has so devastatingly thrived. The appropriate starting point for research is not the year in which the first case of AIDS was diagnosed in Africa but lies further in the past. Although very little can be said about STDs in the pre-colonial era, colonialism had a clearly discernible impact upon the disease ecologies of populations across the continent and the means by which these diseases were addressed. As Lewis and Bamber aver for Asia, "the economics and politics of colonization influenced both the spread of STDs and the manner in which official policy on STDs developed."[9]

Our knowledge about African subjectivities in relation to STDs before the AIDS era, however, is very limited. For those interested in narrowing the focus of inquiry to African perceptions of sexual disorders that can be understood according to Western clinical categories and attributed to specific pathogens, the picture is yet more indistinct. Records of cultural belief and ritual related to sexuality and the consequences of sexual transgression are not adequate to reconstruct a model of the day-to-day historical or cultural consciousness about these topics. In contrast, the ethnographic literature does contain examples of long-standing local disease categories that relate somatic, psychological, or spiritual disorder to misdeeds such as extramarital sex or sexual precocity.[10] Where evidence about African sentiments does exist, it often comes to us either through the filter of colonial presumption or through highly synthesized and depersonalized cultural representations, such as songs or recorded beliefs about sickness linked to sexual indiscipline or misdeed.[11] More mundane and interpersonal aspects of the subjective experience of STDs in Africa before the age of AIDS are difficult to ascertain. The pleas from local political leaders and elites for assistance in combatting STDs are among the

African perspectives on STDs that have survived the historical record. As Maryinez Lyons points out for Uganda, these calls have often been for a law-and-order approach to disease control. In many cases, these reactions were prompted by the kinds of rights and freedoms (including sexual and nuptial) that young men and especially women began to assert under colonialism. In Eastern and Southern Africa, the pursuit of such unprecedented opportunities was perceived as a direct threat to clan- and lineage-based partriarchal and gerontocratic power structures.[12]

The law-and-order approach has been revitalized since the advent of AIDS. Many of those who have researched AIDS in Africa are familiar with calls to close guest houses, ban discos, conduct compulsory testing, redouble efforts to stamp out commercial sex trade, and even outlaw polygyny.[13] However, these are by no means the only African perspectives on how to confront AIDS within communities. AIDS has yielded up a host of cultural representations that give insight into the meaning that various groups attach to this new disease. As Bryan T. Callahan and Virginia Bond state for Zambia, "HIV/AIDS provides a potent metaphor for the dangers of modern life." This issue of "competing"[14] or parallel discourses about health and control that AIDS has prompted throughout Africa is not addressed substantially in this volume. It should, however, prompt future researchers to consider how an illness like AIDS bears upon variation in concepts of individual rights and obligations and which social actors are empowered to determine these.

RACISM

The racism intrinsic in European conceptions of Africans and their bodies that was so much a part of the colonial medical enterprise and late nineteenth century cultural representations of the continent[15] is abundantly evident in the historical record with regard to STDs. That STDs were perceived to be so rampant in sub-Saharan populations led to the direct inference that Africans were by nature promiscuous, hence constitutionally predisposed to immorality. The relative sexual permissiveness and frank methods of sexual initiation among young adults found in many places did nothing to dispel such perceptions.[16] Even African behavior toward the treatment of illness seemed an outward indication of their supposed inferiority. The frequency with which Africans abandoned treatment with antibiotics after the alleviation of symptoms (a practice that can lead to resistance of microorganisms to antibiotic agents) was seen to demonstrate to colonial medical authorities in Senegal the "'native's incredible carelessness about disease," as Charles Becker and René Collignon note in Chapter 4.

Colonial Zimbabwe provides an extreme example of the phenomenon of Western stereotypes of African bodies and persons. As Jock McCulloch illustrates in Chapter 9, the myth of the sexually uncontrollable African male reached a zenith there. Such Black Peril panic was bound up with the morbid fear of STD infection through the rape of white women (a fear all the more ironic and irrational given the frequency of white male sexual relations with African women). Similar fears were found elsewhere but seldom reached the same fevered pitch as in colonial Zimbabwe. A colonial fixation on what, in Chapter 10, Jochelson calls the "peculiarities of the African body" reemerged in the early days of the AIDS epidemic. As Lyons points out in Chapter 5, there was a construction of a "definition for African AIDS distinct from that of the epidemic in the West."[17] As in the pre-AIDS era, it was a definition concocted by Western medical experts based on notions of the peculiarity of African bodies and practices.[18]

GENDER, LABOR MIGRATION, AND ECONOMIC INSTABILITY

Although the range of African experiences of STDs may remain obscure, much can be deduced about the social conditions (and attitudes toward them) in which women and men experienced risk, opportunity, and hardship in sexual and reproductive life. The cases of Malawi, Zambia, and South Africa (Chapters 7, 8, and 10) demonstrate that gender relations and cultural changes in the organization of reproductive and non-reproductive sexuality were inextricably linked to the movement and organization of African men's labor in the colonial era. In Zambia and other parts of Southern Africa, colonial officials worked with the mines to redirect regional migration patterns. The links between the movement of labor and disease in general have been well documented,[19] and STDs were no exception. Although married women were encouraged in some areas to relocate to mines (and help absorb some of the costs of reproducing the labor force), unmarried women were subject to controls on their movements and efforts to ensure their continued participation in agricultural production. As Wiseman Chijere Chirwa shows for Malawi, there were also many consequences for local women in the vicinity of the destinations of male migration (plantations and estates in this case). A competitive and status-oriented sexual microculture emerged in these locations among migrant men and, thus, "it can be argued that STDs derived more from the social conditions on the estates than the natural moral behavior of the African people."[20] In all of these cases, explicit and multi-layered moral discourses emerged in which sex, traditional belief systems, Christianity, intra- and cross-cultural authority, and STDs were all enrolled. In Senegal and Côte d'Ivoire, the movement of large cohorts of young people has also been related to long-standing seasonal patterns of mobility and urbanization.[21] Although migrants have often been men, this is not exclusively the case as has been demonstrated for the Wahaya in Tanzania,[22] among the Sereer in Senegal,[23] and for some of the main migration routes between Ghana and Abidjan, Côte d'Ivoire.[24]

As Deborah Pellow notes in Chapter 2 on Ghana, "the social and economic reality resulting from culture change is that men have greater earning power than women." This economic advantage is tied to other shifts in the balance of power between men and women within marital and non-marital sexual relationships, most of which have resolved in favor of men.[25] Students of gender and power in Africa have correctly pointed out the dangers of oversimplifying the day-to-day realities of men's power over women[26] and overstating the degree of powerlessness that women have in the initiation and negotiation of sexual relationships, whether commercial or not.[27] Indeed, some studies suggest that even in cultures with powerful ideologies of male superiority, mundane behavior related to gender and health may contradict stated norms.[28]

Nevertheless, this should not obscure the fact that all observers concur that on the whole women are at particular risk in the AIDS pandemic. Not only does the virus appear to be transmitted more efficiently from men to women but also the reality of male power and the fact that the condom is the only effective method for preventing HIV transmission clearly put enhanced responsibility on men to respond. This is also not to deny the weight of contextual forces and risks that have shaped the contours of the AIDS epidemic for both sexes[29] and the previous patterns of spread of STDs. Rather, it is to acknowledge that opportunities for prevention exist on many levels simultaneously and that all of these levels are affected by historical, social, and politicoeconomic processes. As Pellow puts it, "Social and economic change facilitated the movement of people and the spread of venereal disease. Social and economic disappointments have facilitated the spread of AIDS."

THE PRACTICE OF BIOMEDICINE AND EPIDEMIOLOGY IN AFRICAN CONTEXTS

Although health services for Africans during the colonial era were universally inadequate, the demographic fears prompted by STDs often led to comparatively large and focussed allocations of resources. In Uganda, as Lyons points out, the campaign against STDs was matched in scope only by that against sleeping sickness. The perception that McCulloch records for Zimbabwe that "the African laborer '. . . was often nothing less than a walking reservoir of disease'" was common among Europeans. Such concerns for keeping a hygienic distance between Africans and Europeans influenced urban planning in West Africa.[30] The organization of services for Africans in Zimbabwe, as elsewhere, was often influenced by the concerns of white settler communities to simultaneously stamp out epidemics that were seen to threaten them and to ensure the ability of African labor to reproduce itself and pay rates. These concerns are brought out dramatically by Becker and Collignon, who write of the pronatalist colonial policy of *faire du noire* (produce Blackies).

It should be noted, though, that there were some strong voices within the colonial services for what (in hindsight) were more enlightened approaches to the treatment of Africans with STDs. Measures aimed at reducing stigma and conducting preventive education were launched in both French and British colonies. In colonial Zambia, Callahan and Bond argue, labor policies that permitted men to move to the mines with their wives and an elaborate system of medical surveillance account for why STDs were not nearly such serious worries to the administration as in Southern Rhodesia and South Africa. Ultimately, however, the vigorousness with which colonial authorities pursued policies of offering services to Africans was subject to a shifting climate of opinion from within the white community. Even when curative services have been available, a number of mediating forces have affected the degree to which they have been taken up. These include practical and institutional obstacles (such as stigmatization of STD patients in clinics and the lack of drug availability) to cultural preferences for using local therapeutic techniques to treat STDs.

There are other layers to the issue of medical practice in Africa. These concern the use of biomedicine as a tool of cultural domination, as an extension of racist and imperialist projects, and the use of Africa as a safe place to conduct experiments and engage in coercive action that would have been considered unethical and unenforcable in Europe.[31] In *Curing Their Ills*, Vaughan likened colonial Africa to a laboratory for the new microbiology. In the AIDS era, by analogy, it has become the laboratory for the new immunology. Cutting edge medical science takes place in countries that live in relative denial and ignorance of the epidemic, and virtual wars are fought over the ethics of HIV vaccine trials among people who might never be able to afford the product of research.

The continued epidemiological focus on heterosexual versus homosexual intercourse (or more accurately, men who have sex with men) as a route of transmission[32] is a holdover from the earliest days of sectoral thinking[33] in the AIDS epidemic. It cloaks social judgments of personal conduct in notions of biological risk. In this regard, too, there are continuities between past and present. In the North and West, for example, dominant social values are encoded in the fact that AIDS has been seen to move along networks of those who are viewed as unproductive and unreproductive members of society (drug addicts and homosexuals). In Africa, by contrast, the disease was slotted early on into two dominant narrative genres about illness. These genres tended to stigmatize those who were both productive and reproductive, (African elites and heterosexual men and women), a recapitulation of major themes in medical discourse on STDs among Africans. One of these themes, that of the peculiar African body, was taken to an extreme in sociobiological and evolutionary arguments about the inherent susceptibility of Africans to sexual excess and, hence, to infection with HIV.[34] Although this particular line of argument failed to gain ground, it nevertheless rendered explicit an early line of thinking that suggested that the scope of the African epidemic might at least be partly due to something innate in the African body.

The second line of argument about African vulnerabilities to AIDS has been much more embedded in the epidemiologic literature and also has a distinct genealogy. In this line of argument, Africans have been thought to be vulnerable to AIDS primarily because of the loss of traditions that enforced sexual discipline.[35] These losses have taken place through the influences of modernization and urbanization. According to the narrative formulations of colonial medical writings, Vaughan concludes, Africans became sick essentially because they forgot who they were.[36] This topic returns us once again to the question of how to interpret risk in light of the sweeping social and cultural change people in Africa have passed through in the past century and all that lies before them. Without abandoning the notion that many individuals are in a position to protect themselves given adequate knowledge and the means to effect preventive action, the chapters in this book point strongly to the conclusion that structural risks exist that place individuals in a vulnerable state. The forces that create these conditions of risk operate at a level far beyond the influence of health education or motivated change on the part of individual women and men.

PROVISIONAL CONCLUSIONS

As many of the contributors acknowledge, the chapters in this book represent a preliminary attempt to unravel a topic that touches upon core themes and values of any social system: sexuality and the conditions of social reproduction. These histories are certainly limited vertically to the very late pre-colonial and early colonial eras because of the limits placed upon retrospective views by a lack of historical materials. However, much wider scope can be given to the horizontal view. Future studies of STDs and society in Africa will draw upon perspectives of historical demography, epidemiology, medical and social history, and historical anthropology and will expand upon or refute many of the core themes identified here. Nothing more than provisional conclusions can be offered about the history of AIDS in Africa. The regional character of the epidemic has changed enormously in the past 15 years and, aside from massive mortality and hardship, no one can predict what the next 15 years will bring.

Clearly, though, the impact of the epidemic upon communities and social systems will be one feature of these future histories.

Most of the preliminary conclusions that can be reached in this enterprise have been discussed above and are summarized here:

The historical manifestations of STDs and HIV/AIDS in Africa are often both ambiguous and diverse, and knowledge of them has been and continues to be limited by reliable epidemiologic data.

Despite the rapidity of sweeping cultural change in sexual and reproductive life and values across the continent, the general shape of change reveals structural similarities between past and present epidemics.

Assumptions about the inherent difference of Africans from Europeans are imbedded in colonial medical discourse about STDs.

In African contexts, vulnerability and risk increase in situations where women are less empowered and have fewer social and material resources at their disposal and for men and women subject to geographic mobility and economic insecurity.

In both the pre- and post-independence eras, access to curative health services for STDs has been limited, and uptake has often not been strong.

Medical practice, epidemiology, and health education have often been informed by long-standing, oversimplified, and highly individualized assumptions about the nature and origin of risk among Africans.

The editors believe that the significance of this comparative history of STDs and HIV/AIDS should not be limited to that of an intellectually gratifying solution to complex puzzles about the relationship between people and pathogens over time. It should also contain lessons learned that may influence how these diseases are confronted by whatever means, and so lessen the suffering they cause. It is also our hope that this book will continue to blur the arbitrarily drawn lines between basic and applied research.[37]

NOTES

1. Milton Lewis, Scott Bamber, and Michael Waugh, *Sex, Disease, and Society: A Comparative History of Sexually Transmitted Diseases and HIV/AIDS in Asia and the Pacific* (Westport, Conn.: Greenwood Press, 1997).

2. Carol S. Vance, "Anthropology Rediscovers Sexuality: A Theoretical Comment," *Social Science and Medicine* 33 (1991): 875–84.

3. Milton Lewis and Scott Bamber, "Introduction," in *Sex, Disease, and Society: A Comparative History of Sexually Transmitted Diseases and HIV/AIDS in Asia and the Pacific*, edited by Milton Lewis, Scott Bamber, and Michael Waugh (Westport, Conn.: Greenwood Press, 1997), p. 2.

4. U.S. Bureau of the Census, *HIV/AIDS Surveillance Database* (Washington, D.C.: International Programs Center, Population Division, 1998). Of the countries

represented in this book, since 1995 high quality data about pregnant women, normally healthy adults, and blood donors have been published for Ghana, South Africa, Tanzania, and Zimbabwe. No high-grade data at all have been published since 1995 for Côte d'Ivoire, Senegal, Uganda, and Malawi.

5. UNAIDS/WHO Global HIV/AIDS and STD Surveillance Unit, *Report on the Global HIV/AIDS Epidemic — December 1997* (Geneva: UNAIDS and the World Health Organization, 1997), pp. 3, 12. According to the report, the estimates of the scope of the epidemic have increased markedly because new infections have been occurring at "an alarming rate" and previous calculations greatly underestimated the rate of transmission, particularly in sub-Saharan Africa.

6. Ibid., p. 4.

7. Karen Jochelson, K. M. Mothibeli, and Jean-Patrick Leger, "Human Immunodeficiency Virus and Migrant Labor in South Africa," *International Journal of Health Services* 21 (1991): 158.

8. Lewis and Bamber, "Introduction," p. 13.

9. Ibid., p. 3.

10. In East and Southern Africa, some of these categories have been redefined to encompass HIV/AIDS. See Christine Obbo, "Is AIDS Just Another Disease?" in *AIDS 1988: Symposia Papers, American Association for the Advancement of Science*, edited by Ruth Kulstad (Washington, D.C.: American Association for the Advancement of Science, 1988), pp. 191–98; Hanne Overgaard Mogensen, "The Narrative of AIDS among the Tonga of Zambia," *Social Science and Medicine* 44 (1997): 431–39.

11. Agnes Odinga, "Syphilis, Infertility, and Compulsory Treatment: Control of Women's Reproduction and Sexuality in South Nyanza, Kenya, 1920–1945," paper presented at African Studies Association Annual Meetings, Columbus, Ohio, November 13–16, 1997.

12. Diana Jeater, *Marriage, Perversion, and Power: The Construction of Moral Discourse in Southern Rhodesia 1894–1930* (Oxford: Clarendon Press, 1993).

13. It is worth noting that polygyny has not been consistently associated with increased risk of infection with HIV, and some studies have found it to be protective.

14. See Gill Seidel, "The Competing Discourses of HIV/AIDS in Sub-Saharan Africa: Discourses of Rights and Empowerment vs. Discourses of Control and Exclusion," *Social Science and Medicine* 36 (1993): 175–94.

15. Sander L. Gilman, *Difference and Pathology: Stereotypes of Sexuality, Race and Madness* (Ithaca, N.Y.: Cornell University Press, 1985); Philip Setel, "'A Good Moral Tone': Victorian Ideals of Health and the Judgement of Persons in Nineteenth Century Travel and Mission Accounts from East Africa," Working Papers in African Studies No. 150 (Boston, Mass.: Boston University African Studies Center, 1991); Megan Vaughan, 1990, *Curing Their Ills: Colonial Power and African Illness* (Stanford, Calif.: Stanford University Press, 1991); Jean Comaroff, "The Diseased Heart of Africa: Medicine, Colonialism and the Black Body," in *Knowledge, Power & Practice: The Anthropology of Medicine and Everyday Life*, edited by Shirley Lindenbaum and Margaret Lock (Berkeley: University of California Press, 1993), pp. 305–29.

16. See, for example, John C. Caldwell, Pat Caldwell, and Pat Quiggen, "The Social Context of AIDS in Sub-Saharan Africa," *Population and Development Review*

15 (1989): 185–235; Beth Maina Ahlberg, "Is There a Distinct African Sexuality? A Critical Response to Caldwell, " *Africa* 64 (1994): 220–42.

17.   Maryinez Lyons, this volume.

18.   See, for example, Randall M. Packard and Paul Epstein, "Epidemiologists, Social Scientists, and the Structure of Medical Research on AIDS in Africa," *Social Science and Medicine* 33 (1991): 771–94.

19.   As others have pointed out, the history of African labor under colonialism is fundamental to the overall contemporary disease ecology, not just the manifestations of STDs. See, for example, Meredith Turshen, *The Political Ecology of Disease in Tanzania* (New Brunswick, N.J.: Rutgers University Press, 1984); Randall Packard, *White Plague, Black Labor* (Berkeley: University of California Press, 1989).

20.   Wiseman Chijere Chirwa, this volume.

21.   Michel Garenne, Charles Becker, and Rosario Cardenas, "Heterogeneity, Life Cycle, and the Potential Demographic Impact of AIDS in a Rural Area of Africa," in *Sexual Behaviour and Networking: Anthropological and Socio-Cultural Studies on the Transmission of HIV*, edited by Tim Dyson (Liège: Editions Derouaux Ordina, 1992), pp. 269–82; Jeanne-Marie Amat-Roze, this volume.

22.   See Philip W. Setel, this volume; Brad Weiss, "'Buying Her Grave': Money, Movement, and AIDS in North-West Tanzania," *Africa* 63 (1993): 19–35.

23.   Garenne, Becker, and Cardenas, "Heterogeneity, Life Cycle, and the Potential Demographic Impact of AIDS," p. 272; Amat-Roze, this volume.

24.   John Anarfi, "Sexual Networking in Selected Communities in Ghana and the Sexual Behavior of Ghanaian Female Migrants in Abidjan, Côte d'Ivoire," in *Sexual Behavior and Networking. Anthropological and Socio-Cultural Studies on the Transmission of HIV*, edited by Tim Dyson (Liège: Editions Derouaux Ordina, 1992), pp. 233–47.

25.   N. Thomas Håkansson, "Why Do Gusii Women Get Married? A Study of Cultural Constraints and Women's Strategies in a Rural Community in Kenya," *Folk* 27 (1985): 89–114; Margarethe Silberschmidt, "Have Men Become the Weaker Sex? Changing Life Situations in Kisii District, Kenya," *Journal of Modern African Studies* 30 (1992): 237–53.

26.   Henrietta L. Moore, *Space, Text, and Gender: An Anthropological Study of the Marakwet in Kenya* (New York: Guilford Press, 1996); Silberschmidt, "Have Men Become the Weaker Sex?"

27.   Hellen Pickering and H. A. Wilkins, "Do Unmarried Women in African Towns Have To Sell Sex, or Is It a Matter of Choice?" *Health Transition Review* 3 supplement (1993): 17–27; Soori Nnko and Robert Pool, "Sexual Discourse in the Context of AIDS: Dominant Themes on Sexual Relations among School Children in Mwanza, Tanzania," *Health Transition Review* 7 supplement (1997): 85–90.

28.   Lee Cronk, "Intention versus Behaviour in Parental Sex Preferences among the Mukogodo of Kenya," *Journal of Biosocial Science* 23 (1991): 229–40.

29.   Peter Lurie, Percy Hintzen, and Robert A. Lowe, "Socioeconomic Obstacles to HIV Prevention and Treatment in Developing Countries: The Roles of the International Monetary Fund and the World Bank," *AIDS* 9 (1995): 539–46; Michael Sweat and Julie A. Denison, "Reducing HIV Incidence in Developing Countries with Structural and Environmental Interventions," *AIDS* 9 supplement (1995): S251–57; Philip Setel, "AIDS as a Paradox of Manhood and Development in Kilimanjaro, Tanzania," *Social Science and Medicine* 43 (1996): 1169–78.

30.   Philip Curtin, "Medical Knowledge and Urban Planning in Colonial Tropical Africa," *American Historical Review* 90 (1985): 594–613.

31.   Comaroff, "The Diseased Heart of Africa"; Vaughan, *Curing Their Ills.*

32.   UNAIDS/WHO Global HIV/AIDS and STD Surveillance Unit, *Report on the Global HIV/AIDS Epidemic,* p. 3.

33.   Philip Setel, "Upside-down and Backwards: Epistemologies of AIDS in the West as Applied to Africa," unpublished manuscript, 1991.

34.   J. Philippe Rushton and Anthony F. Bogaert, "Population Differences in Susceptibility to AIDS: An Evolutionary Analysis," *Social Science and Medicine* 28 (1989): 1211–20.

35.   It should be noted that Africans were also thought to be vulnerable to AIDS because they were so tradition bound. Customs such as female circumcision and the practice of traditional medicine were proposed as cultural risk factors from early on.

36.   Vaughan, *Curing Their Ills,* p. 202.

37.   This dichotomy is seldom challenged. For an exception see Frants Staugård, "Anthropological and Public Health Research: An Issue of Academic Excellence or of Pragmatic Relevance," in *AIDS and the Grassroots: Problems, Challenges, and Opportunities,* edited by C. Cabrera, D. Pitt, and F. Staugård (Gaborone: Ipelegeng, 1996).

2

Sex, Disease, and Culture Change in Ghana

Deborah Pellow

In Ghana,[1] epidemiologists worry that they are seeing the tip of the ice-berg in the Acquired Immune Deficiency Syndrome (AIDS) pandemic. This situation has resulted from the combination of cultural, economic, and political factors with the trajectory of diseases. Until the first cases of AIDS were diagnosed in Ghana in 1986, little attention was paid to sexu-ally transmitted diseases (STDs). It was the other communicable diseases, such as malaria, tuberculosis, diarrhea, and respiratory diseases that were the major killers and, thus, of greater concern to the medical and epi-demiological establishment. However, the data on STDs in combination with the inadequacy of health facilities point to an enormous health prob-lem. Moreover, it is well established that in Africa STDs (especially those improperly treated) assist the transmission of the AIDS-causing human immunodeficiency virus (HIV).[2]

There is a specific cultural and economic context to sexuality in Ghana and, thus, to the incidence of STDs and AIDS. It has been said that to understand AIDS, we must come to terms with major problems of cultur-al change.[3] I submit that the same is true of STDs. STDs have a long his-tory in Ghana. AIDS displays a striking parallel to STDs not only in its sexual mode of transmission but also in that its spread has been driven by social, political, and economic change brought by colonialism and mod-ernization, which facilitated travel and exposure to new modes of behav-ior. There are similarities, too, in problems with medical management and record keeping, lack of facilities for treatment, and the fear of stigma that causes the larger part of the iceberg to remain hidden.

THE CULTURAL CONTEXT OF SEX

In these post-colonial times, for a European to speak of a kind of sexual license in Ghana, of an ease of sexuality that flavors all interactions between men and women, is to invite censure. However, in my comments, I do not have in mind old myths about the sexual excesses of Africans, of carnal feats, or of uncivilized behavior that Victorians used to justify colonial control.[4] I am not criticizing. I am simply making observations about behavior.

There is in contemporary Ghanaian society a sexual permissiveness. Although promiscuity itself does not cause STDs, it is instrumental to their transmission and as such provokes concern. In the early 1970s a Ghanaian doctor noted the casualness of sex among all ages of schoolgoers.[5] In a 1992 study of 250 out-of-school youth aged 10–24 years surveyed in Accra,[6] the majority of both sexes were sexually active. Males reported more sexual partners at any time than females — in the three months prior to being interviewed, for males 2.4 partners, for females 2.3; and in the previous year, 3.2 versus 2.3.

A study[7] in 1993 of 2,116 respondents from the ten regions of Ghana, aged 15–49, of varying educational backgrounds, indicates that two-thirds of the men reported that in the last 12 months they had sex with at least one partner, 42 percent with only one partner, 25 percent with more than one, 26 percent with none, and 6 percent did not respond or did not know. Of the unmarried women, two-thirds reported they had one or more partners during the same period, 38 percent had one partner, 27 percent had more than one, 20 percent had none, and 15 percent either did not respond or did not remember. The results of this study in combination with one done in 1988 "suggest that a large share of Ghanaian women become sexually active with men while they are in their teens, whether they are married or not."[8]

One contemporary anthropologist working on STDs and AIDS in Africa further notes that if we want to understand the high STD rates in Africa, we must look beyond such promiscuity to other causes including poverty and its consequences.[9]

Social and economic development in colonial and post-colonial countries like Ghana generally affects the sexes differentially. The conflation of indigenous and colonial sexism has meant that women have been the last to be educated, to become literate, and to gain access to well-paying positions. Life in the city is expensive, especially as compared to the hometown, where one may live within the bosom of the extended family.

Casual sexual behavior is particularly common in urbanized and commercialized areas with their heterogeneous populations, and it is accentuated by a combination of several factors: the dilution of traditional cultural regulations or controls, the high cost of living, and the traditional financial support that Ghanaian men owe to their women. In the city women may be wives but may also be girlfriends. Polygyny is far less common than in earlier times, but married men commonly have one or two girlfriends. Although it represents a kind of functional polygyny, it is different from polygyny because it is more materially demanding and far less stable, with the result that there is a far greater turnover in partners.

The social and economic reality resulting from culture change is that men have greater earning power than women. "A good deal of female sexual behavior in Africa can best be understood as strategies for economic survival and adaptation to patterns of male dominance in low-income countries."[10] Sexuality is a commodity with a price that can be negotiated, and women bargain to their best advantage.[11] Friendships between men and women or between boys and girls are not necessarily set up with permanency in mind, and neither partner holds power of possession over the other. The courting relationship is marked by much prestation, with a man accommodating his girlfriend's material desires. The actual form and extent of the material support depend upon social and economic expectations. The "sugar daddy phenomenon" in Ghana's cities, as elsewhere in urban Africa,[12] is a natural outgrowth — older, richer men supporting young, attractive, and eligible women.

In the urban area, an uneducated woman's occupational choices have been limited to market trade, domestic service, and prostitution. Market trade requires a substantial capital investment if one is to make any money. Domestic service is pretty much subsistence work. Prostitution can be lucrative and requires no investment. Moreover, there is little traditional concern regarding casual sex; as long as a woman marries (even only briefly) or has a child, she meets the requirements for adult status. Prostitution is an urban phenomenon, and women become prostitutes as a means to survive in the city. This is as true now as it was 70 years ago.

Although sexual freedom has apparently not been perceived as problematic, prostitution has for both local people and government officials, for reasons of morality and health. Prostitution has followed social change. The growing intensity of intercommunication in the colonial period led to greater contacts with strangers. Roads, railroads, and shipping stimulated mobility; people entered unfamiliar disease environments. Rural laborers in towns, mines, and cocoa farms commonly used prostitutes, many of whom were labor migrants themselves. Women from southern Togo went to Accra and other colony towns.

After 1922 prostitution was on the increase.[13] It was also a major problem, because the prostitutes largely hailed from Togo and Nigeria and, thus, were not under the control of either their families or the local Native Authority.[14] In 1925 Central Accra Hausa Chief Kadri English complained to the district commissioner that Hausa women were leaving northern Nigeria for Accra, where "evil influences are somewhat paramount" and were divorcing their husbands "in order to carry on immoral practices."[15] In 1930 the *Gold Coast Independent* wrote that prostitutes and brothels in Accra were swelling in numbers daily and that the prostitutes were foreigners from other African countries.[16]

In fact, it is believed AIDS was brought to Ghana (to Accra) in the mid-1980s by Ghanaian prostitutes working in Abidjan who contracted the disease there. Some were so sick that no driver would bring them back. Because of the extended family system, a dying person could always get care from a family member in the home village and never emerge. Many do not see a doctor, and record keeping in any case has been faulty, thus, it is hard to know who is dying of AIDS.

VENEREAL DISEASES AND THEIR TREATMENT IN PRE-COLONIAL AND COLONIAL GOLD COAST

History of Venereal Disease in the Gold Coast

Venereal diseases (VDs) were well established in Ghana long before the twentieth century, especially along the coast.[17] A European visitor to the Guinea coast in the mid-seventeenth century observed the complications apparently resulting from local sexual activities: "they are . . . much troubled with the Pox [syphilis] . . . Clapdollars, Botches, Worms, Pains in the Head, and Burning Fevers, but these are the favours of their women, to whom they are inexpressibly addicted."[18] In the early eighteenth century, Jean Barbot observed that in the coastal areas of the Gold Coast, fetish priests treated a variety of illnesses, including "the French disease," that is, syphilis.[19]

The Portuguese, Dutch, and other Europeans erected fortifications along the coast of the Gold Coast as they were drawn there for trade as early as the late fifteenth century. The men came alone and were involved with the coastal people on different levels: as hard-nosed entrepreneurs, as interested observers, and as intimates. The arrival of the Europeans in ships and at their forts presented opportunities for the introduction and diffusion of new diseases like smallpox and syphilis.[20]

By the eighteenth century mixed unions in European coastal settlements were a common feature of life. Governor Richard Miles "referred to the African 'wife' by whom he had had seven children."[21] Thus, in contrast to Central and East Africa, most of modern Ghana had experienced centuries of exposure to European diseases by the mid-1800s. The earliest statistics from hospital returns on venereal diseases date to the medical reports entered in the colonial *Blue Book of Statistics* (Table 2.1). In 1867 Colonial Surgeon Thomas Jones wrote that "Syphilis, Gonorrhea, Rheumatism . . . and Remittent fevers are frequent."[22] The Hospital Return

TABLE 2.1

Reported Cases of Sexually Transmitted and Genitourinary Diseases, the Gold Coast, 1872–81

Year	Syphilis	Gonorrhea	Genitourinary	Other Venereal
1872	9	4	—	—
1873	3	1	—	3*
1876	5	7	23	—
1878	—	—	—	6
1879	2	4	—	—
1881	7	—	—	9

Note: These statistics may refer to European, not African, patients because we know that syphilis and gonorrhea were frequent.
*1 herpes, 2 sloughing of the scrotum.

Source: Blue Book of Statistics, Colony of the Gold Coast, National Archives of Ghana, ADM 7/1.

of 1869, written in longhand, was "Disease of Genitourinary Organs" — 6 cases of STDs out of a total of 94 cases of diseases treated.[23]

In 1874 the British established their first West African colony in the Gold Coast and initiated formal public health programs. Until 1881 the hospital statistics are for Cape Coast only, the administrative headquarters of the colonial government until 1874 when they removed to Accra. The first year reporting hospital returns for Accra was 1881, as well. In the 1880s, the Gold Coast Medical Department was established, reporting to the governor through the colonial secretary.

The year 1909 saw the creation of the Sanitary (Health) Branch, responsible for sanitation, vaccinations, and other preventive measures, and in 1919 the Medical Research Institute (Laboratory) Branch for scientific investigations and routine clinical and pathological tests was established.

There is no doubt that venereal diseases spread rapidly from the coast inland during the colonial period, "thanks to social changes and increasing mobility."[24] The Accra Central Hausa chief expressed worry to the British administration that venereal disease was common among his people and resulted from the women fleeing their husbands in Nigeria to come to Accra.[25]

When first studied, gonorrhea, caused by the bacterium *Neisseria gonorrhoeae*, was the most common venereal disease. Syphilis was less common and spread more slowly, perhaps because the agent of syphilis, *Treponema pallidum*, is closely related to the pathogen of yaws, *Treponema pertenue*, commonly prevalent in the area, and victims of yaws acquire partial immunity against syphilis.

Gonorrhea was known to be widespread in Kumase, Accra, and other major towns before World War I. However, until 1907 the annual number of venereal diseases recorded was less than 100 (Table 2.2). European doctors may have seen only small numbers because many African cases went untreated, were self-treated, or were treated by traditional healers.

These figures give the misleading impression of venereal diseases being practically nonexistent in Ghana at this time. This was far from the truth. Between 1880 and 1907 medical officers were anxiously reporting regularly the rifeness of syphilis and gonorrhea and the devastation of their complications in the Keta [Volta] district.[26]

The small numbers listed in Table 2.2 are evidence of a problem in proper reporting, as reinforced by the Medical Department's observation in 1914 that hospital statistics did not adequately represent venereal disease for the colony and Ashanti.[27] The medical officer in Kumase, A.J.R. O'Brien, noted in 1914 that a doctor there believed that almost every male and female over age 20 suffered from gonorrhea. For the Kumase area, O'Brien observed that the alarmingly high prevalence of gonorrhea in villages "induced a native chief to appeal for legislation as a means of dealing with its spread."[28]

The spread of venereal disease was facilitated by the movement of migrant labor and road improvements as cosmopolitan towns like Kumase in Ashanti attracted travellers. Kumase, moreover, was a garrison town, into and out of which soldiers were moving. The 3,000 percent increase in cases of syphilis and gonorrhea between 1906 and 1922 and the previous decade was caused primarily by better reporting and greater use

TABLE 2.2
Reported Cases of Syphilis and Gonorrhea in the Gold Coast, 1898–1907

Year	Syphilis*	Gonorrhea
1898	15	8
1899	17	15
1900	12	5
1905	7	22
1907	272	427

*Many of the venereal ulcers reported as syphilis may have, in fact, been chancroid (Robert Biggar, personal communication).

Source: Stephen Addae, "A History of Medicine in Ghana, 1860–1950," Doctoral dissertation, University of Ghana, 1995, p. 334.

of the health facilities by the Africans, although the diseases also increased in prevalence.

In the early 1920s VD was widespread in southern Ghanaian towns and from them spread to the rest of the country. Carl Reindorf, a native Ghanaian, was appointed medical officer for Akwapim (a region in southern Ghana) in 1919. Although VD did not present a major health problem in the colony,[29] the rates were high enough that he went to England to take a training course, and upon return to Accra in 1921 was given a full-time but temporary appointment as head of the VD clinic in Victoriaborg. The clinic served only Accra and environs. In 1922–23, the Medical Department launched a campaign against VD under the direction of Reindorf. Lectures and pamphlets in English and local languages presented information on signs and symptoms of VD, "the implications of their neglect, the need to report early for treatment and practical preventive measures."[30]

In that same year, according to Reindorf's records,[31] 1.95 percent were treated, but in 1925–26 the proportion increased to 11.79 percent. Reindorf claimed that at that time, "over 75% of the town between ages 18–45 suffer from some form of venereal disease."[32] The reported cases for the country as a whole in 1925 and 1926 were 1,503 syphilis and 3,760 gonorrhea.

During the decade of 1922–32, more than 5,000 cases of venereal disease per year were seen throughout the country, the vast majority at Reindorf's clinic. As the number of syphilis cases reported fell steadily between 1929 and 1944, the Medical Department worried less about that disease, reporting "that syphilis was not a very important disease in Ghana."[33] Gonorrhea was a different story; with the exception of a period of stability between 1927 and 1931, reported cases persistently increased between 1922 and 1946, only then beginning to decline.

The diseases advanced northward, although not arriving in the far North until the late 1920s. According to Addae,[34] syphilis, although common in some southern towns, was brought to the North by migrant laborers returning home in the late 1920s. Gonorrhea, in particular, although it spread slowly in the north, was on the increase; primarily northern men, who as drivers and peddlers had travelled to the south and their contacts, were affected. Eastern Dagomba was unaffected in 1928 but by 1937 had a few reported cases of gonorrhea. The incidence of gonorrhea remained high in the coastal towns.

World War II and the movement of laborers and troops within the country and beyond exacerbated the problem. In 1941 seamen suffering from venereal disease were treated free of charge in accordance with the Brussels Agreement of 1924 to remove any (at least financial) deterrent. Hospitals in seven coastal cities were set up to treat venereal disease and hospital charges were waived. By 1943 the British saw the need for special medical officers in charge of venereal disease. The director of medical services wrote to the colonial secretary on July 23, 1943, that a venereal disease clinic in the major seaport town of Sekondi-Takoradi "would be valuable not only as a means of treating the local population and infected members of ships' crews, but also as a training ground for Medical Officers who will be posted to outstations. Venereal disease is so widespread that the special training of the Medical Staff in its treatment is abundantly justified."[35]

In the mid-1940s the Gold Coast troops (serving with the British) had a 50 percent venereal disease rate.[36] Gonorrhea was by far the most common infection, followed by soft chancre, lymphogranuloma inguinale, and then syphilis. The British administration feared a gonorrhea epidemic in the Northern Territories (NT) with the return of soldiers (about 1,420) to Lawra and Wa Districts. At that time in the NT towns the estimated infection rate for gonorrhea was less than 2 percent, whereas the returnees had been exposed to the disease during their four or more years in Ashanti, the colony, the Gambia, and Sierra Leone. "Should fairly large numbers of infected, or potentially infected, males be returned to their villages it will be a calamity for the peoples of the N.T.s in as much as (1) they have no resistance to the disease, (2) they do not recognise it, and do not know how to control or alleviate it, and (3) even now the maintenance of the population at its present figure is precarious [due to high infant mortality and the burden of sterility due to gonococcal infection driving down the birth rate]."[37]

By 1946–50 in the country at large gonorrhea was nine times as common as syphilis: 82,430 cases of gonorrhea to 9,340 cases of syphilis (Table 2.3). Many more males were seen and treated than females, in part because of care given to soldiers and prisoners (males) and in part because female cases of gonorrhea can be asymptomatic. At the national level venereal diseases apparently had little effect on overall population growth rates in Ghana.

Therapeutic and Control Measures

Therapeutic measures did not begin to catch up with the problem of venereal disease until after 1945 when antibiotics became a powerful weapon.[38] Our seventeenth-century observer noted no local remedies for sexual diseases, but "for the Pox and Clap-dollars, they use much salfa parilla [perhaps parillin, obtained from sarsaparilla root], which the *Hollanders* [Dutch] have furnished them with,"[39] and in the eighteenth century, a "physick" from the fetish priests was used for dysentery and syphilis.[40]

In the early twentieth century a popular treatment was "Potassium Iodide injection and the external application of gray ointment. Although

TABLE 2.3
**Reported Cases of Syphilis and Gonorrhea by Sex in the
Gold Coast, 1913–55**

Year	Syphilis			Gonorrhea		
	Male*	Female*	Total†	Male*	Female*	Total†
1913	281	102	412	714	34	700
1926–27	790	529	1,503	2,333	1,128	3,760
1932–33	439	221	791	2,569	500	3,325
1936	481	263	856	3,562	477	4,416
1940	371	209	695	5,561	1,021	7,336
1946	910	361	1,271	9,111	1,793	10,904
1950	1,368	453	1,821	13,137	4,328	17,465
1955	803	236	1,039	10,454	1,757	12,211

*Cases by sex are for outpatients only until 1942.
†The vast majority of cases were treated as outpatients.

Source: Patterson, *Health in Colonial Ghana*, Table 23.

ineffective, local merchants had taken advantage of importing them, and druggists and others sold them to the public indiscriminately."[41] After establishing his clinic in 1920, Reindorf gave lectures and published pamphlets in Ga and Twi to encourage attendance. He was concerned that infections were increasing and advocated legislation limiting administration of therapy to medically qualified persons; prohibiting patent medicine advertisements; and "establishing the State Serum Institute which has for its main functions the laboratory diagnosis of Syphilis and the maintenance of a Card Index of infected persons."[42]

What really attracted patients to Reindorf's clinic were revolutionary new drugs that unqualified people were forbidden by law to use. To treat syphilis (and yaws), there was Salvarsan (the "magic bullet"), one of the few specific antimicrobial drugs prior to the late 1930s, and Neoarsenobisthmus. Although Salvarsan was effective for its time, Neoarsenobisthmus was regarded as the first wonder drug employed in Ghana. For gonorrhea there was no effective treatment until the advent of sulpha drugs. Penicillin was introduced after World War II.

In the 1940s there were acute staff shortages, and the clinics were expensive to run. Civilian medical authorities were conscious of the venereal disease problem, but it took back seat to other infectious diseases. As far as prophylaxis was concerned, all known methods failed. Throughout West Africa a three month trial of prophylactic centers for soldiers did not reduce venereal disease, because the men would leave camp without permission or bring women into camp. An untreated, heavily infected female population and the failure of male prophylaxis produced a gigantic problem. Because it approached an epidemic, the British administration focussed on educating Ghanaians "to dislike and avoid venereal disease" and on "providing the means by which they could get treated if they became infected."[43]

Among the West African troops, 80–90 percent suffering from gonorrhea responded to sulfonamide. However, if the medical officer did not crush the sulfa tablets and administer them personally, the men would sell them in the town or the village for 1 shilling a tablet. Thus, doctors gave 6 grams in one draught daily for three days, followed by 12 pints of water daily. By 1945 penicillin was available and sulfa-resistant strains could be treated with the new drug. The mass antibiotic therapy against yaws "undoubtedly contributed to a reduced prevalence of both syphilis and gonorrhea after 1953."[44]

In the 1950s, just before independence, there was no department responsible for the treatment of venereal disease as there was for tuberculosis. There was also no agency to follow up contacts.[45] It was suspected that there was much illicit trade in sulfonamides. To prevent this and the consequence of resistant organisms, the pharmacy and poison ordinance provided that "only medical practitioners may treat venereal diseases and the sulfonamides may only be supplied in a doctor's prescription."[46]

SEXUALLY TRANSMITTED DISEASES
IN POST-COLONIAL GHANA

Background

In the 1960s gonorrhea was still the most prevalent venereal disease. The extent of the infection was unknown, because only the most severe cases registered for treatment. The incidence of VD in rural areas appeared to be declining, possibly as a result of the extensive use of penicillin in the treatment of yaws.[47]

According to a small study carried out in November 1992–March 1993, the incidence of STDs in Accra and Kumase was about 1 percent in the adult population.[48] "Genital ulcer diseases (GUD) was found to be uncommon, especially in Accra."[49] A member of the Department of Epidemiology at Korle Bu Hospital projects that there is no statistical significance of syphilis or genital ulcers in the general adult population. The problem lies with gonorrhea, chlamydia (which causes non-specific urethritis), and trichomonas.[50] During 1992 a total of 127 new STD cases were reported at the STD clinic at Adabraka (Accra) Polyclinic. These included urethritis (41), vaginosis (12), gonorrhea (10), trichomonas (2), syphilis (1), and HIV positive (4).[51] The incidence of gonorrhea was declining as compared with the period before 1991. Looking back 40 years we find for Ghana (the Gold Coast) as a whole in 1952 there were 1,985 reported cases of syphilis and 12,948 of gonorrhea. By 1955 they had decreased to 1,039 and 12,211, respectively. This means that there has been a history of increasing and decreasing frequencies. Most recently the decrease in STD numbers is related to the appearance of HIV and a recognition that STDs are dangerous as co-factors in HIV infection.

Among 250 out-of-school youth aged 10–24 surveyed in Accra in 1992,[52] awareness of STDs is high for both sexes (97.6 percent) and knowledge of early symptoms appreciable (67.2 percent for males, 65.6 percent for females). "However, the level of misconceptions is disturbing and females are more likely than males to hold them. For example, the proportion which attributed the transmission of STDs to witches/wizards and act of God/supernatural causes were 50.7% against 36.6%, and 14.7% versus 6.3% respectively."[53]

Treatment and Control

The concern with controlling venereal disease that was stimulated by British concern for British troops went into hibernation with independence in the 1950s. In the 1970s there were no special venereal disease clinics in Ghana to help in prevention of gonorrhea and non-gonococcal urethritis. Clinics had fallen on bad times because of expense and change in priorities for diseases to be treated. Venereal disease treatment was successful with a single dose injection of procaine penicillin, single doses of ampicillin (with or without probenecid), spectinomycin (togamycin) tetracycline, and trimethoprim and sulphamethoxazole (septrim). Unfortunately, 70 percent of the patients with sexually transmitted urethritis were treated by dispensers and non-medical personnel,[54] despite earlier laws to the contrary.

According to Beatrice Mensah, head of the STD clinic at Adabraka (Accra) Polyclinic, a 1985 medical report indicated many Ghanaians expelled from Agege (Nigeria) were suffering from STDs, and they were quarantined in temporary quarters before being sent home. Adabraka Polyclinic was established to care for them under the Communicable Disease Control of Greater Accra Regional Health Administration. Routine examinations were done for trichomonas, candida, and gonorrhea. The clinic was dormant from 1989 until 1991 because there was no resident doctor. Since then the clinic has assumed responsibility for the Regional AIDS Control Program. The Adabraka Polyclinic is a referral clinic. It now also screens all cases for HIV (unless patients refuse) and cares for those diagnosed elsewhere as well as those who present without being referred.

Despite the high incidence of STDs, since 1986 the emphasis in the country was on AIDS. Now the health authorities are trying to bring STD control into the picture. A study of health centers in Accra and Kumase, Ghana's two largest cities, was carried out in spring 1992 with support from the European Economic Community and Family Health International. It was concluded that a basic infrastructure exists for controlling STDs, although there are problems, such as long patient waiting time, scarcity of drugs, and poor service. In addition, doctors did not do physical examinations. There were no vaginal specula. Laboratory tests for STDs were requested in 50 percent of the cases at their first visit. In the rest, tests were requested only when symptoms persisted after treatment. Microscope slides and reagents for Gram staining were not readily available, and none of the laboratories had the means to perform serological tests for syphilis. Some 70 percent of the clinicians started treatment of patients the same day without waiting for the results of laboratory tests. The regimens pursued varied; for example, there are six different regimens for treating gonorrhea, including cefuroxime, spectinomycin, amoxycillin, tetracycline, gentamycin, and cotrimoxazole.

Because facilities for management were inadequate, STDs resulted in a high level of complications, such as urethral stricture, pelvic inflammatory disease, ectopic pregnancy, infertility, cervical cancer, primary hepatocellular cancer, and blindness.[55] Yet the 1992 study revealed that less than 1 percent of consultation time of health care providers in the two cities was spent on STDs.

STD patients were going to private rather than public clinics because of proximity, no queuing, and the shame factor, and the statistics were not passed on to the health authorities.[56] Mary Narday Kotei, head of the Health Education Unit at the Ministry of Health, feared that clients were scared off from rural facilities because of the judgmental attitude of the nurses, doctors, and medical assistants — "you've been to a prostitute, you've been promiscuous, it's your own fault."[57] The Ministry of Health still used an old daily activity report form, which, according to Mensah, includes no syndrome-specific notations like gonorrhea.[58]

AIDS IN GHANA

Extent of the Problem

Facilities for HIV sero-diagnosis were established in Accra in late 1985 at the Noguchi Memorial Institute for Medical Research as well as at Korle Bu Hospital. The first AIDS case was reported from Koforidua (Eastern Region) in March 1986, followed by several more from the same region. "The clinical presentation was similar to the disease described from East and Central Africa."[59] In 1987, the first case of pediatric AIDS was diagnosed, a child born to an HIV-1 positive mother.[60] Until September 1988 reports to the World Health Organization (WHO) did not differentiate between HIV seropositives and AIDS cases and, as a result, there have been discrepancies in reported figures for AIDS.

In Ghana, unlike other areas, there was an initial female predominance. In 1986 90 percent of AIDS victims were women (in contrast to the United States, where most cases have been men, and Central Africa, where the prevalence has been equal). Most were sexually active and 96 percent had recently lived abroad, especially in Côte d'Ivoire. Many had worked as prostitutes.[61] F.I.D. Konotey-Ahulu, a London-based Ghanaian medical researcher, referred to these early AIDS cases in Ghana as "repatriation AIDS."[62] Infection in infants was first detected "because the mothers gave a history of high risk behaviour, that is prostitution."[63] The female-to-male ratio ranged from 11:1 to 7.7:1. By the end of 1986 HIV-1 infections had been documented in 115 Ghanaians; by the end of 1987 276 were known to be infected. The ratio of females to males declined to 6:1 in 1987.[64]

In October 1988 a new AIDS case definition for the country was adopted: "A person is said to have AIDS when he has two of the major signs and one minor sign plus evidence of HIV by the ELISA method, or when he has three major signs with or without a minor sign plus evidence of HIV by the ELISA method. . . . The major and minor signs are the same as in the WHO clinical case definition."[65]

Although it is hard to say how complete AIDS reporting in Ghana is, the total number of reported cases is probably an underestimate (Table 2.4). Many are not seen by qualified medical staff and thus are not reported; sometimes surveillance forms have not been forwarded; in the Northern Region testing facilities are nonexistent in many towns; some patients fear being stigmatized and, therefore, do not attend health institutions.[66]

There are regional differences. For example, in late 1989 and again in mid-1992 the Eastern Region was reported as having the highest incidence. The incidence in the Ashanti Region has also been high, and in January 1991 an average of 50 AIDS cases per month[67] were reported at Kumase's Komfo Anokye Hospital. In 1994 33 percent of the reported AIDS cases were in Ashanti; 70.5 percent were reported from three regions, Ashanti, Eastern, and Greater Accra. Is it that the reporting from those regions is better? The Eastern Region is a base for Krobo women, who go to the Ivory Coast to work. "Although they may intend to work as house servants or waitresses, many end up working as prostitutes in the 'sex industry,' where the earnings are high. They return home for traditional festivals with rich clothes and jewelry. This attracts even more young women. [The returnees] are well groomed, with plucked eyebrows, permed hair and lipstick. Their clothes are smart and modern.

TABLE 2.4
Number of Reported AIDS Cases By Sex in Ghana

Year	Male	Female	Total
1986	7	35	42
1987	18	94	112
1988	114	532	646
1989	499	1,832	2,331
1990	585	1,428	2,013
1991	803	1,638	2,441
1992	926	1,773	2,699
1993	857	1,514	2,371
1994	—	—	2,258

Source: National AIDS Control Program, Disease Control Unit, *The HIV/AIDS Epidemic in Ghana, 1994 Overview* (Accra: Ministry of Health, 1994). The figures for 1994 were provided by Dr. Asamoah-Odei, Epidemiology, AIDS Control Program, Accra, 1995.

They have the confidence of the well-off. What unemployed girl would not envy them and want the same?"[68]

Most AIDS patients of both sexes are aged between 20 and 39, and women continue to constitute 70–75 percent of AIDS sufferers in the country.[69] The female-to-male ratio for 1994 was 1.7:1; "thus the trend is that the female to male ratio is heading toward 1:1 which is consistent with heterosexual transmission of HIV."[70]

According to Mensah, the drug abuse population is not large and thus far no cases have come to light, and because homosexuality does not appear to be widely practiced, homosexual transmission has not been a focus of public health attention.

What may be unique to the Ghanaian context (certainly in comparison with the Western world) is the cosmetic use of razor blades — to cut nails, clean under nails, get rid of dead skin. The chances of cutting oneself are high, people share blades, and although epidemiologists have found little or no empirical evidence that practices involving razors actually spread HIV infection, because sharing razors can spread hepatitis and tetanus, the practice of sharing blades should be discouraged.[71]

In 1986, when the first two cases were seen, none of the 247 blood donors and only 1 percent of the prostitutes in Accra were infected with HIV. However, by 1989 16 percent of the prostitutes tested were seropositive.[72] In July 1993 Tema General Hospital Polyclinic (the port city 15 miles east of Accra) found that 14 percent of 205 blood donations were HIV positive.[73] At Akomfo Anokye Teaching Hospital in Kumase in 1994, out of an STD population of 502 people, 5 percent were confirmed positive for HIV. In Accra in 1995 1–6 percent of pregnant women in Ghana wre HIV positive.[74]

As of the end of 1994 14,913 cases of AIDS were reported to the Ministry of Health.[75] Those working in the AIDS control program believed that these cases represent only the visible part of the epidemic. The actual number was not known because some people did not seek hospital care, some doctors did not record the AIDS diagnosis for fear of stigma, and some rural facilities were not equipped to diagnose AIDS. It was estimated, however, that more than 30,000 cases had actually occurred.[76]

Treatment and Control

Surveillance of AIDS in Ghana began in 1985 following the formation of the National Technical Committee on AIDS (NTCA). This agency was mandated to assess the AIDS situation and advise the government on prevention and control.[77]

In 1987 the U.S. Agency for International Development funded a six-month pilot intervention program with 72 prostitutes and clients. In 1991 a follow-up survey was taken of the pilot group and an additional group of 176 women and their clients. According to the study, condom use among the pilot and expanded group in 1991 was 64 percent, a dramatic increase from 6 percent among the pilot group in June 1987 and 48 percent among the expanded group in January 1988, respectively.[78] Condoms were provided through government-subsidized distribution, although there was a minimal cost.

A medium-term plan for AIDS prevention and control was organized in September 1989 by the NTCA. A five-year program was drawn up by the Ministry of Health and NTCA in collaboration with WHO's Global Program on AIDS to prevent further transmission and spread. Donors included the European Economic Community, France, Britain, and West Germany. The European Economic Community had already agreed to finance STD control as part of the program. The five-year program included laboratory services, screening facilities at blood banks, and development of a zonal banking system. There were also workshops on AIDS. Key groups included progressive organizations (self-help associations), traditional healers, churches, hoteliers, airline workers, and hairdressers. A 24-member National Advisory Council on AIDS has been formed to advise government on policy matters.

Because STDs have been recognized as important co-factors in the transmission of HIV, AIDS provoked an extraordinary interest in and commitment to STD prevention and control, and in 1993 the Ministry of Health combined the STD and AIDS control programs. The general objective of strengthening STD control has been to reduce morbidity of STDs as co-factors in HIV transmission and to reduce complications associated with STDs.[79] Specifically, the program set out to strengthen the capability to do research; to train health workers in prevention, diagnosis, and treatment of STDs; and to promote behavior that will reduce the incidence and impact of STDs in Ghana.

Everyone in the clinical and research establishment agrees that AIDS awareness is high. Even in 1987, when the disease was in its early phase in Ghana, in a survey of 267 men and women living throughout the country, only one person had not heard of AIDS, most knew that it was spread through heterosexual sex, and 97 percent knew that it was fatal. The most common methods for AIDS prevention acknowledged by those surveyed included avoiding indiscriminate sex, staying with one partner, and using condoms.[80] Unfortunately, many did not know of other modes of spread. In 1991–92 211 hospital outpatients in Kumase aged 16 years and older were interviewed randomly. Only one-third to one-half knew that AIDS could be contracted through inoculation or blood transfusion.[81] In the 1992 survey of 250 youth,[82] 97.6 percent knew about AIDS although only about one-fifth had ever seen an AIDS patient. Most knew how AIDS is transmitted, although as with STDs, there were misconceptions, "including kissing, cause by witches/wizards and by act of God/supernatural causes. Again females are more likely than males to hold on to the last two misconceptions (48% versus 34.4%, and 18.7% versus 9.1%)."[83]

People continue to engage in high risk behavior — mainly refusing to use condoms. In Ghanaian culture generally, and among couples particularly, men and women do not talk much about sex or share equally in decisions of a sexual nature. A study of contraceptive attitudes among spouses in Ghana reveals that men dominate the decision-making process in this area. The influence is so pervasive it cuts across all age groups, regions, and ethnicities. "It is so strong that even if a woman's opinion is in line with cultural norms but lacks the husband's support or runs contrary to his own opinion, her opinion is untenable."[84]

When it comes to condom use in general, there are a host of problems. Married couples or regular partners do not want to use condoms, because they believe they are meant for illicit sex. Attitudes toward contraception are dominated by male opinion, and men generally dislike condoms. This is problematic for women engaging in recreational or commercial sex, because they have little leverage over the men's condom usage. Women say that their partners do not like condoms and that they complain of a loss of pleasure. In the Accra intervention on condom use among prostitutes, even those who maintained contact with project staff and knew that HIV can be transmitted by a healthy seeming man or believe that condoms prevent AIDS, "are significantly less likely to use condoms if the client fails to initiate condom use."[85] Yet men are unwilling to use condoms. In one study, 66 percent of the businessmen and professionals who were customers of high-class prostitutes refused to use condoms.[86] AIDS researcher A. R. Neequaye tried to set up a control system, and people started to complain that it would mean legalizing prostitution.

The question is how to translate AIDS awareness into behavior. Ministry of Health public education programs on safe sex focus on the population aged 20–49 years and include women (because they are more vulnerable to HIV and they have little say about condom use),[87] commercial sex workers, the youth, the military, and truck and taxi drivers. The media campaign has been targeted at them, including public service advertisements on television, pamphlets, and posters. Because drinking and sex are linked, public education includes coasters and bottle opener key chains, both proclaiming "AIDS is Real, Use a Condom." Those illiterate in English are contacted through local languages, local workers, community events, and *durbars* (traditional state receptions). There are also seminars and educational programs that involve secondary schools, universities, churches, and mosques. The school curriculum integrates AIDS awareness into family life programs, including human sexuality, reproduction, and issues of peer pressure in coordination with the Ministry of Information. There has been some resistance from the Catholic Church and religious fundamentalists, who do not want elementary school children to hear about sex.

To help prepare the service providers for dealing with the public, the Ministry of Health has commissioned a manual and training seminars. There is more face-to-face educational work at regional and district levels.

An intervention program on condom use among 248 prostitutes in 1987 proved the importance of such personal educational contacts. Four years later, 107 of the women were still engaged in prostitution. "Their level of condom use in 1991 was higher than pre-enrollment but similar to use among prostitutes never enrolled. Sixty-four percent of those followed up reported always using condoms with clients in 1991."[88] Of especial interest is that these users were also more likely to maintain contact with project staff.

Despite high awareness and some fear, the young do not feel at risk. Few people know anyone who has died of AIDS. "Few clinicians have been privileged to see AIDS cases," except in the Eastern and Ashanti Regions.[89] Because people did not express vulnerability in 1993, Minister of Health S. G. Obimpeh made November a month for intensified education on AIDS throughout the country. This included durbars, education talks in schools and churches, leaflets and posters, films in communities, and the distribution of condoms through social marketing programs, the Planned Parenthood Association of Ghana, and Maternal and Child Health programs. Protector Condoms sponsored organized activities, such as dancing evenings where condoms were sold.

Aside from the young, various population groups are at risk. A seminar was held in 1994 with businessmen in Accra, but in fact it is the lower class that has been hit first, along with some white collar workers. Thus, according to Antwi,[90] unlike elsewhere in Africa,[91] Ghana does not yet have the problem of elite men dying of AIDS, but she believes the seeds have been sown. Although elite (professional) men frequent prostitutes and have girlfriends outside of marriage, these men have not been approached directly. Because many of the elite (like all Ghanaians) are religious, they are reached through their churches.[92]

The control program people also went to the clubs where the prostitutes pick up their clients.[93] There is an organization for prostitutes in Accra, the Widows' Association. Some of the leaders have been identified and have been used as a conduit by which to distribute condoms and talk with the women.

Long-distance drivers and taxi drivers are both at high risk. They have been brought together for education sessions by the Adabraka Polyclinic and through the Ghana Public Road and Transport Union. The AIDS Control Program is working with a variety of nongovernmental organizations in the implementation of its programs, including Planned Parenthood, the Young Women's Christian Association, World Vision, the Red Cross, and Catholic hospitals. There is money for the control program, but they need a nongovernmental organization to run it, because the U.S. Agency for International Development (the agency funding the condoms-to-prostitutes project) cannot pay civil servants who are already being paid.[94] For those suffering from AIDS, the Ministry of Health is pushing for home-based care. Home visiting is part of the Public Health system, therefore, the infrastructure is already in place.

Medically, the authorities are just treating opportunistic infection. Zudovudine (AZT) is not available through the control program. In 1994 the control program received from WHO the antifungals Ketoconazone and Niridazole. There are no specific AIDS clinics. At Korle Bu Hospital in Accra, AIDS patients are cared for in the fever-infectious disease unit.

CONCLUSIONS

The issue here is part sociocultural (the traditions that people hold dear, the rituals and relationships they participate in, the status markers they employ) and part economic (how they make a living, how they spread the resources). The highest incidence of AIDS cases has been in the Eastern and Ashanti regions "where definite socio-cultural practices promote young girls to enter prostitution."[95] In Ghana, development has taken place at different rates for different sectors of the population. As a consequence, there are regional, ethnic, socioeconomic, and sexual inequities. They influence the incidence of STDs and AIDS and must be acknowledged by policy makers if these diseases are to be curbed, not to mention eradicated. According to Antwi, head of the AIDS Control

Program in Ghana, it is easier to talk about malaria as a killer than AIDS, and many do, because many children still die of malaria despite the availability of drugs. Moreover, to effectively deal with AIDS means talking about issues of development, a far more complex topic with far more unwieldy solutions: why a girl must become a prostitute. "Why," Antwi asks, "don't we have education for everyone, jobs that are not just financially satisfying but also fulfilling?"[96]

Although far fewer AIDS cases are reported in the north, there are also far fewer economic opportunities in that region; educational institutions are inferior to those in the south. As in the early twentieth century, the north is far less developed and isolated. Also, like 50 years ago when venereal disease was the concern, now there is worry about AIDS sufferers carrying the disease north, where the health care facilities are insufficient.

The southern cities of Accra and Kumase are magnets for those northerners and rural dwellers whose lives are destabilized by poverty. Migrants come to the cities, leaving family or spouse behind, to seek their fortune. Many of the women migrants are uneducated, have few skills, and are dependent upon men to support them. Sex is the bargaining chip. Some migrant men become truck drivers, an occupation that takes them long distances to different towns and people and to the beds of different women. The other end of the social and economic spectrum also has its instability. Many city men who become prosperous as businessmen, members of the military, or professionals are able and willing to support a girlfriend or two. Indeed, just as unmarried women in the city claim that they need a man for financial and social status, many men who are or aspire to be members of the modern elite bask in the reflected glow of having the right girlfriend in tow. This is what Caldwell and colleagues would refer to as a "pragmatic attitude toward sex."[97] In the city the hallowed but old-fashioned tradition of polygyny is translated into having one or more girlfriends in addition to a wife.

Despite this pragmatism, men and women, married or not, do not discuss matters related to sex such as contraception or protection. Men do not like condoms and are willing to make it financially worth the while of prostitutes to dispense with them. Thus, if men stray, their wives or partners may be unknowingly exposed to disease. The silence that attaches to sexual conversations similarly affects attendance at clinics. Many who fall sick are afraid to go to the polyclinics for diagnosis and treatment. Again, like 50 years ago, they fear being recognized and being stigmatized. They have families to whom they can return. Many are accustomed to using traditional doctors and herbalists, who are not part of the AIDS/STDs treatment establishment.[98] Even private doctors do not keep systematic records.

Awareness of AIDS is high and yet people continue to take risks. Because STDs are known to be a predisposing factor to AIDS, awareness of STDs, their causes, and their symptoms must be made greater. The government should enlist the various levels of traditional leadership, those whom the citizenry listen to: chiefs, church leaders, community elders, and traditional healers. Ted Green, for example, has pushed extensively for the involvement of traditional healers in treating STDs, because traditional healers are often consulted before modern medical practitioners. Because the traditional healers "cannot be wished away or legislated out of existence [and] surveys and limited program experience in Africa have shown that traditional healers are highly motivated to learn about medicine," and healers' associations are eager to collaborate with the modern sector, why not develop collaborative health programs and include the traditional healers?[99] Green offers as his most persuasive argument the fact that public health goals are probably not realizable in Africa unless there is collaboration involving traditional healers, because the number and distribution of modern biomedical personnel and facilities are inadequate.[100] As I have written elsewhere, African notions of sex are mystical, carry magical potency, and require observance of social boundaries.[101] According to Green, this helps explain why STDs would fall within the domain of traditional rather than biomedical treatment. He recommends several ways that traditional healers could have an impact on STDs, and, thus, on AIDS risk factors, including referring STD cases or through collaboration treating them, identifying sexual partners of those infected with STDs for treatment, and advocating single partner sexual relationships.[102] They could help people of all ages understand the dangers and the correlations between STDs and AIDS. They could help eradicate inequities that prevent everyone from having access to continuing education and treatment and bridge the gap to behavioral change.

The initial impetus for treating venereal disease was to protect the British soldiers in the service of the colonial administration. With independence and the departure of the British, venereal disease appeared to be less of a priority of the new government. It was not until AIDS hit the country that the newly labeled STDs were taken seriously by the Ghanaian Ministry of Health.

Now there are mechanisms in place to track, diagnose, and treat STDs and AIDS. The Minister of Health has provided strong leadership in the fight. Public education has been put into place. Awareness among the sexually active population is high. Still, there is the political economy of disease. Social and economic change facilitated the movement of people and the spread of venereal disease. Social and economic disappointments have facilitated the spread of AIDS. Hope for alleviation, if not obliteration, of these diseases is possible only if there is transformation of social roles and relationships, especially between men and women, economic rights and opportunities to education and work, and stability of the state and private sector to provide the medical care and social welfare necessary.

NOTES

This chapter incorporates substantially revised material originally published in *Genitourinary Medicine* 70 (1994): 418–23. I am grateful to the publishers of the journal for permission to use this material.

1. Interviewing in Accra was carried out in June 1993 and throughout the spring of 1995. I am grateful to Beatrice Mensah and her colleagues, Comfort Asamoah-Edu and Mike Aryee, at the Adabraka Polyclinic, and at Korle Bu Hospital to Phyllis Entwi, Asamoah-Odei, and Asamoah-Edu in Epidemiology, and Mary Narday Kotei of the Ministry of Health. Stephen Addae very generously printed out a section on the history of venereal disease in Ghana from his doctoral dissertation just prior to his defense. I alone am responsible for any errors.

2. A. R. Neequaye, G. A. Ankrah-Badu, and R. A. Afram, "Clinical Features of Human Immunodeficiency Virus (HIV) Infection in Accra," *Ghana Medical Journal* 21 (1987): 3.

3. Gilbert Herdt, "AIDS and Anthropology," *Anthropology Today* 3 (1987): 2.

4. Charles Geshekter has built his irresponsible and factually vacant essay upon such tales ("Outbreak? AIDS, Africa, and the Medicalization of Poverty" *Transition* 5 [1995]: 9).

5. R. O. Addae, "Guest Editorial: Venereal Disease," *The Medic: Journal of the Ghana Medical Students Association* 1 (1972): 2–3.

6. John K. Anarfi and Phyllis Entwi, "The Study of Factors Affecting AIDS-related Sexual Risk Taking Behaviour Among Out-of-School Youth in Accra," Institute of Statistical, Social and Economic Research, University of Ghana and Ministry of Health, Accra, 1992.

7. Harold J. Monger, Donald W. Dickerson, and Mary T. Mulhern, "Report on Baseline Study of Knowledge and Practices Regarding Family Planning and Health in Ghana," Ghana Family Planning and Health Project, 1993.

8. Ibid., p. 4.

9. Edward C. Green, "The Anthropology of Sexually Transmitted Disease in Liberia," *Social Science and Medicine* 35 (1992): 1458.

10. Edward C. Green, *AIDS and STDs in Africa* (Boulder, Colo: Westview Press, 1994), p. 100.

11. Deborah Pellow, *Women in Accra: Options for Autonomy* (Algonac, Mich.: Reference, 1977), p. 204.

12. For Dakar, see Mariama Ba, *So Long a Letter* (London: Heinemann, 1981).

13. National Archives of Ghana ADM 11/922; 8/20/1925.

14. National Archives of Ghana ADM 11/922; 9/1/1925.

15. National Archives of Ghana ADM 11/922 Prostitution in the Gold Coast (Case No. 25/1925): 5/13/1925.

16. K. David Patterson, *Health in Colonial Ghana: Disease, Medicine, and Socio-Economic Change, 1900–1955* (Waltham Mass.: Crossroads Press, 1981), p. 76.

17. Ibid.

18. Anonymous, *The Golden Coast, or a Description of Guinney* (London, 1665), pp. 10, 76. See also "Michael Hemmersam's Description of the Gold Coast 1639–45" in *German Sources for West African History 1599–1669*, annot. and trans. by Adam Jones (Wiesbaden: Franz Steiner Verlag GMBH, 1983), p. 122.

19. Jones, *German Sources for West African History*, p. 122.

20. Patterson, *Health in Colonial Ghana*, p. 3.

21. Margaret Priestley, *West African Trade and Coast Society: A Family Study. London* (London: Oxford University Press, 1969), p. 7.

22. *Blue Book of Statistics*, Colony of the Gold Coast, ADM 7/1/5.

23. *Blue Book of Statistics*, Colony of the Gold Coast, ADM 7/1/7.

24. Patterson, *Health in Colonial Ghana*, p. 75.

25. National Archives of Ghana ADM 11/922 Prostitution in the Gold Coast (Case No. 25/1925): 5/13/1925.

26. Stephen Addae, *A History of Medicine in Ghana, 1860–1950*, doctoral dissertation, University of Ghana, 1995, p. 334.

27. *Gold Coast Government Report of the Medical and Sanitary Department*, 1914, p. 39.

28. Ibid.

29. "The case incidence between 1906 and 1922 was only some 2% and the cases:population ratio vanishingly [sic] low at less than 0.05%. In 1921 some 2.5% of the population was receiving medical attention for all diseases in Government hospitals and dispensaries. Only 0.05% were due to venereal diseases." Stephen Addae, *The Evolution of Modern Medicine in Ghana, 1880–1960*, doctoral dissertation, University of Ghana, p. 336.

30. *Gold Coast Government Report of the Medical and Sanitary Department*, 1922–23, cited in Addae, *A History of Medicine in Ghana, 1860–1950*.

31. C. E. Reindorf, "The Problem of Venereal Disease on the Gold Coast and the Possibilities of Control," *West African Medical Journal* 1 (1927): 9.

32. Reindorf, "The Problem of Venereal Disease on the Gold Coast," p. 8. The steady decrease may have been because of better information on the disease and its treatment.

33. Addae, *The Evolution of Modern Medicine in Ghana, 1880–1960*, p. 335.

34. Ibid, p. 339.

35. Colonial Service Office 11/1/619, File No. 2001.

36. R. R. Willcox, "Venereal Disease in West Africa," *Nature* 157 (1946): 416–19.

37. Colonial Service Office 11/10/138; File No. 3967; M. P. Brown, Medical Officer, Wa Medical Department, 10/1/43.

38. Patterson, *Health in Colonial Ghana*, p. 77.

39. Anonymous, *The Gold Coast, or a Description of Guinney*, p. 10.

40. Jones, *German Sources for West African History 1599–1669*, p. 122.

41. Addae, *The Evolution of Modern Medicine in Ghana, 1880–1960*, footnote 96.

42. Reindorf, "The Problem of Venereal Disease on the Gold Coast," p. 9.

43. Willcox, "Venereal Disease in West Africa," p. 419.

44. Patterson, *Health in Colonial Ghana*, p. 76.

45. Ghana Government, *Report of the Ministry of Health 1955* (Accra: Government Printer, 1959), p. 9.

46. Gold Coast Government, *Report of the Commission of Enquiry into the Health Needs of the Gold Coast*. [Folio SOE. 148] 1952, p. 52.

47. Irving Kaplan, *Area Handbook for Ghana* (Washington, D.C.: U.S. Government Printing Office, 1971), p. 146.

48. Interview with Beatrice Mensah, STD clinic, Adabraka Polyclinic, June 7, 1993.

49. Ibid.

50. Emil Asamoah-Odei, Epidemiology, Korle Bu Hospital, June 2, 1993.

51. STD clinic, Adabraka Polyclinic, April 1993.

52. Anarfi and Entwi, "The Study of Factors Affecting AIDS-Related Sexual Risk Taking Behaviour," p. 8.

53. Ibid. pp. 9–10. Traditional belief in witchcraft and the powers of *juju* or black magic is found today even among the school-going population. It was told to me some years ago that students from the Volta Region arrived at boarding schools with charms and amulets to protect them against curses.

54. E. D. Yeboah, "Editorial: Modern Treatment of Gonorrhea and Nongonococcal Urethritis," *Ghana Medical Journal* 19 (1980): 131.

55. Executive Summary, *STD Control Programme, 1989–1991* (Accra: Ministry of Health).

56. Interview with Beatrice Mensah, Adabraka Polyclinic, June 6, 1993; Alexander Asamoah-Adu, Korle Bu Hospital, May 8, 1995.

57. Interview with Mary Narday Kotei, April 18, 1995.

58. Interview with Beatrice Mensah, June 6, 1993.

59. Neequaye, Ankrah-Badu, and Afram, "Clinical Features of Human Immunodeficiency Virus," p. 6.

60. J. E. Neequaye, A. R. Neequaye, J.A.A. Mingle, G. A. Ankra-Badu, and A. Asamoah-Adu, "Ghanaian Children of Women Infected with Human Immunodeficiency Virus (HIV)," *Ghana Medical Journal* 22 (1988): 86–89.

61. A. R. Neequaye, J.A.A. Mingle, J. E. Neequaye, V. K. Agadzi, V. Nettey, M. Osei-Kwasi, M. Hayami, K. Ishikawa, G. Ankrah-Badu, C. Bentsi, A. Asamoah-Adu, S. E. Aggrey, W. Ampofo, J. A. Brandful, F. Grant, and R. J. Biggar, "A Report on Human Immunodeficiency Virus (HIV) Infection in Ghana up to December 1986," *Ghana Medical Journal* 21 (1987): 7–11.

62. F.I.D. Konotey-Ahulu, *What is AIDS?* (Worcester: Tetteh-A'Domeno, 1989), pp. 72, 123.

63. Neequaye, Neequaye, Mingle, Ankra-Badu, and Asamoah-Adu, "Ghanaian Children of Women," p. 87.

64. Ibid.

65. E. J. Asamoah-Odei, P. M. Antwi, K. Ahmed, A. Osei, and G. K. Akar, "AIDS in Ghana, 1986–1989: Epidemiological Aspects," *Ghana Medical Journal* 24 (1990): 192.

66. Ibid.

67. Again, these may have been HIV seropositives, not AIDS.

68. Janie Hampton, *Meeting AIDS with Compassion: AIDS Care and Prevention in Agomanya, Ghana* (London: ACTIONAID, 1991), p. 3.

69. Figures are abstracted from short dateline articles in *West Africa*, 1988–93.

70.   Interview with Asamoah-Odei, April 13, 1994.

71.   Personal communication, Ted Green.

72.   A. R. Neequaye, J. E. Neequaye, and Robert J. Biggar, "Factors That Could Influence the Spread of AIDS in Ghana, West Africa: Knowledge of AIDS, Sexual Behavior, Prostitution, and Traditional Medical Practices," *Journal of Acquired Immune Deficiency Syndromes* 4 (1991): 914, 917.

73.   *West Africa*, July 26– August 1, 1993, p. 1312.

74.   Interview with Phyllis Antwi, Head, AIDS Control Programme for Ghana, Accra, April 12, 1995.

75.   National AIDS Control Programme, *The HIV/AIDS Epidemic in Ghana: 1994 Overview* (Accra: Ministry of Health, 1994); interview with Asamoah-Odei, April 13, 1995.

76.   National AIDS Control Programme, *The HIV/AIDS Epidemic in Ghana*, p. 5.

77.   Asamoah-Odei, Antwi, Ahmed, Osei, and Akar, "AIDS in Ghana."

78.   Alexander Asamoah-Adu, Sharon Weir, Matilda Pappoe, Nicholas Kanlisi, Alfred Neequaye, and Peter Lamptey, "Evaluation of a Targeted AIDS Prevention Intervention to Increase Condom Use Among Prostitutes in Ghana," *AIDS* 8 (1994): 242–43.

79.   Policy Statement on Sexually Transmitted Diseases Control, Department of Epidemiology, Ministry of Health, Accra, Ghana, 1993.

80.   Neequaye, Neequaye, and Biggar, "Factors That Could Influence the Spread of AIDS," p. 915.

81.   Emmanuel O. Addo-Yobo and Hermione Lovel, "Hospital Users' Knowledge about Blood Transfusion and Awareness and Attitude towards AIDS/HIV Infection in a Region in Ghana," *Journal of Tropical Pediatrics* 38 (1992): 94–95.

82.   Anarfi and Entwi, "The Study of Factors Affecting AIDS-related Sexual Risk Taking Behaviour," p. 10.

83.   Ibid.

84.   Alex Chika Ezeh, "The Influence of Spouses over Each Other's Contraceptive Attitudes in Ghana," *Studies in Family Planning* 24 (1993): 171.

85.   Asamoah-Adu, Weir, Pappoe, Kanlisi, Neequaye, and Lamptey, "Evaluation of a Targeted AIDS Prevention Intervention," p. 246.

86.   J. E. Neequaye, A. R. Neequaye, J. A. Mingle, D. Ofori-Adjei, M. Osei-Kwasi, F. Grant, M. Hayami, K. Ishikawa, and R. J. Biggar, "Sexual Habits and Social Factors in Local Ghanaian Prostitutes Which Could Affect the Spread of Human Immunodeficiency Virus (HIV)," *Ghana Medical Journal* 21 (1987): 12–15.

87.   *West Africa*, July 12–18, 1993, p. 1215.

88.   Asamoah-Adu, Weir, Pappoe, Kanlisi, Neequaye, and Lamptey, "Evaluation of a Targeted AIDS Prevention Intervention," p. 239.

89.   Interview with Phyllis Antwi, Accra, April 12, 1995.

90.   Ibid.

91.   N. Miller and R. C. Rockwell, "Introduction," in *AIDS in Africa: The Social and Policy Impact*, edited by N. Miller and R. C. Rockwell (Lewiston N.Y.: Edwin Mellon Press, 1988), p. xxv.

92.   Interview wth Mary Narday Kotei, Head of Health Education Unit, Ministry of Health, Accra, April 18, 1995.

93. Interview with Alexander Asamoah-Adu, Korle Bu Hospital, Accra, May 8, 1995.

94. Ibid.

95. Asamoah-Odei, Antwi, Ahmed, Osei, and Akar, "AIDS in Ghana," p. 198.

96. Interview with Phyllis Antwi, April 11, 1995.

97. John C. Caldwell, I. O. Orubuloye, and Pat Caldwell, "Underreaction to AIDS in Sub-Saharan Africa," *Social Science and Medicine* 34 (1992): 1169–82.

98. Green's book, *AIDS and STDs in Africa*, focuses specifically on this issue.

99. Green, *AIDS and STDs in Africa*, p. 36.

100. Ibid., p. 38.

101. Deborah Pellow, "Sexuality in Africa," *Trends in History* 4 (1990): 77.

102. Green, *AIDS and STDs in Africa*, p. 245.

3

Sexually Transmitted Diseases and HIV/AIDS in Côte d'Ivoire

Jeanne-Marie Amat-Roze

Côte d'Ivoire, a state in West Africa bordering the Gulf of Guinea, is a former French colony founded in 1893 and annexed to the French West African Federation in 1899. In 1960 it became independent. For more than 30 years, its president, Félix Houphouët-Boigny, was regularly reelected and remained faithful to a policy of cooperation with France. This young state, an economic leader in francophone West Africa, enjoyed outstanding economic growth for two decades (1960–80) and was an enviable and attractive land, with the capital city of Abidjan as its symbol. However, from 1981 onward, conditions began to decline. Côte d'Ivoire had to cope not just with a serious economic crisis but also with AIDS. Today the country, which had been doing better than others, is faced with the most serious epidemic in West Africa. More cases of AIDS have been recorded there than in the eight other French-speaking West African states combined. A combination of economic and social factors explains the greater vulnerability of Côte d'Ivoire to sexually transmitted diseases (STDs) and to HIV infection.

HISTORICAL EPIDEMIOLOGY

For a very long time it was difficult to obtain reliable information on STDs in Côte d'Ivoire. From the late nineteenth century to the 1920s Europeans did not have exact knowledge about the country's diseases. Interest in one disease or another varied with its local importance, scientific fashion, and the presence or passage of a doctor. The available data on historical conditions could just as easily be a reflection of the level of health care in a region as the extent of a disease. In addition, it was not until the early 1950s that syphilis stopped being confused with yaws, even though Côte d'Ivoire was an area of yaws hyperendemicity. Furthermore, at the beginning of the century, because there was no official registration of the native population, data about ethnic groups were unreliable, and confusion between ethnic and sub-ethnic groups and tribes was common. In contrast, data about the limited European population are well recorded. The doctors present before 1910 reported that syphilis was known in the indigenous population, but they disagreed about its extent. "For some, gonorrhoea was dominant, for others, syphilis."[1] There was also confusion about localization; was the whole colony affected or only a few areas? According to the doctors, the Africans most affected at the time were single infantrymen displaced far from their home regions. As for Europeans, it was impossible to make estimations because of the embarrassed silence that surrounded this topic. It was noted, however, that "syphilis was the oldest known disease in the colony and took severe forms such as premature tertiary complications. In addition to nervous system lesions."[2] For Europeans, Côte d'Ivoire was mainly a male bachelor society; women and children were rather unwelcome in the public services as well as in the private sector. Adults between 25 and 29 years of age accounted for one-third of the French community, and in 1926 men still made up 77 percent of the European community. Despite the popular silence surrounding STDs, "doctors considered venereal diseases to be important and on the increase. According to the health service director such diseases could be contracted either in brothels or by buying or keeping a concubine. In fact there were prostitutes for Europeans who were shared between them." According to the reports of that time, "the employees of commercial companies were the most affected by these diseases, which were made worse by alcohol [use]."[3]

Europeans often came into the dispensary for treatment late in their syphilis infections, after reaching the secondary or tertiary stage. As for Africans, they were very selective about the use of medical care, depending upon whether they believed in the efficacy of European medicine. Malaria and dysentery, for example, rarely led them to consult a doctor. However, they willingly consulted for venereal diseases, yaws, and trauma. Because they considered these latter ailments to be common misfortunes, they only saw a doctor when they felt some discomfort from them. Women consulted European doctors even less often than men. Between 1920 and 1930, venereal diseases accounted for 40–50 percent of the causes of consultation by all indigenous people. Two illnesses dominated: syphilis and gonorrhea.[4] "Syphilis was considered the social plague of big cities . . . and was also well established in towns of some importance situated along the busiest roads." For instance, Dr. Francois, during a medical visit to Agnéby circle in March 1921, noticed that all the villages located near Abengourea Road were affected.[5]

According to the annual medical report of 1929, "gonorrhoea, less often mentioned, was considered rather as the 'high wage' disease because all the employees of large urban areas were affected."[6] A 1932 report emphasized the importance of STDs among indigenous people in Africa; Côte d'Ivoire, along with Senegal, were the colonies said to be most stricken.[7] Among Europeans, at least according to health service records in 1931, venereal diseases were the main reason for seeking a medical consultation among men (30 percent of visits); for women, the leading causes were fractures and wounds.[8] However, for many years STDs produced a litany of disillusioned comments from the medical profession and, because they did so in a self-selecting manner, the increasing number of Africans who sought treatment did not yield more precise information about their extent within the population. After World War II, syphilis was considered the most common of the colony's social diseases, but doctors usually remained tight lipped about the figures. It was said to be as widespread among Africans as among Europeans, and even more so after 1946 because of the return of many infantrymen from France.[9] From the early 1950s syphilis could be reliably distinguished from yaws, but the necessary serodiagnostic screening could be done only at a hospital. Thus, in practical terms, risks of confusion could not be completely ruled out. Among Europeans gonorrhea and related infections seemed more frequent than syphilis, but this was perhaps only because screening was easier. Between 1946 and 1951 the number of cases of gonococcus infection doubled in the colony. Was this due to better screening? "Soft chancre and lymphogranuloma did not seem very frequent and were not the object of a regular census."[10] In 1946 among the main causes of exemption of Africans from military service were physical underdevelopment (due to malnutrition in most cases), locomotor system problems, hernia, and syphilis.[11] Given all the unknowns and uncertainties concerning venereal diseases, the fact that syphilis came first among social diseases revealed how important the disease was. Venereal diseases were a major public health problem in the colony. The years following independence brought no further development of knowledge about the state of STDs in the colony. Syphilis, chlamydia, and other STDs remained under a taboo of silence.

In fact, it was not until a new plague (AIDS) arrived and was recognized by the state authorities that the silence surrounding all these diseases was broken. The recognition of the role of STDs as co-factors in infection and requests for studies by international organizations speeded up this process. Since the mid-1980s epidemiologists have increased their investigations of the prevalence of STDs in various groups of society. According to a national survey carried out in 1989 and reported by Dédy and Tapé, 18 percent of the inhabitants of Côte d'Ivoire between the ages of 15 and 24 interviewed reported they had contracted an STD in the past 12 months, compared with 10 percent of those over 40. Among young people, females seemed the most exposed. Some 23 percent of women between 15 and 19 stated that they had an STD in the preceding 12 months, compared with 13 percent of men the same age.[12] Regular epidemiological testing of prostitutes who came to an Abidjan STD clinic provided information about the number of infections involved: 29 percent gonococcal, 25 percent trichomoniasis, 25 percent syphilis, 21 percent genital ulcerations, and 5 percent chlamydia. These figures are considered to have been relatively steady over recent years.[13] Thus, STDs remained a threat to Côte d'Ivoire's youth, but in a decade of HIV infection they became an even more serious threat.

AIDS was first recognized in Côte d'Ivoire in 1985, and the country quickly became the epicenter of the epidemic in West Africa. In 1994 1 million people were estimated to be infected with HIV.[14] By May 31, 1995, Côte d'Ivoire had officially reported a cumulative total of 25,236 cases of AIDS to the World Health Organization (WHO);[15] that is 43 percent of all cases reported to the WHO by West African states. This was much higher than Ghana, Togo, and Burkina Faso, which followed with 25 percent, 8.4 percent, and 6.1 percent, respectively, of the cases reported. (The latest cases reported in Burkina Faso go back to December 31, 1993.) The number for Côte d'Ivoire was probably an underestimate despite the high quality of the epidemiological surveillance, particularly in Abidjan, where Retro-CI, an international collaborative research center, has studied HIV/AIDS since 1987. The notification of AIDS cases and the collection of the results of seroepidemiological surveys provide a means of assessing the sociospatial evolution of infection and AIDS.

In 1987 seroepidemiological surveys carried out in Abidjan on samples of pregnant women gave very variable results. Denis and colleagues found that 3.3 percent of the pregnant women in Abidjan were infected with HIV, although Odehouri and colleagues came up with a figure of 10 percent.[16] In 1988 a survey confirmed the rapid emergence of AIDS in Abidjan; out of 1,501 patients, the overall prevalence of infection was 43 percent in men and 28 percent in women, and AIDS "accounted for 19% and 9% respectively of medical admissions to the two hospitals and for 33% of medical deaths in hospital."[17] In 1989 a survey in the total adult population (15–65 years old) living in the five urban and rural regions showed the rapid spread of HIV in the country (Table 3.1), revealing a situation of considerable concern.[18]

The crude prevalence rates ranged from 2.2 percent in the north to 8.3 percent in the south. The highest seroprevalence rates were observed in urban areas, as had been previously described in other countries. Another survey confirmed these results in urban areas other than Abidjan. The

TABLE 3.1
Distribution of HIV Infection in the Adult Population of Côte d'Ivoire in 1989

Region	Number Tested	Percent HIV-Positive
North	252	2.2
West	617	4.2
Center	607	6.0
East	366	7.3
South	470	8.3

Source: Guy-Michel Gershy-Damet, Konan Koffi, N. Soro Benoît, Adama Coulibaly, David Koffi, and Koudou Odehouri, "Seroepidemiological Survey of HIV-1 and HIV-2 Infections in the Five Regions of Ivory Coast," *AIDS* 5 (1991): 462-3.

overall seroprevalence rate was 7.3 percent in urban areas and 4.9 percent in rural areas;[19] in 1989 levels of HIV infection among Abidjan blood donors and pregnant women were approximately 10 percent.[20] In 1990 it was observed that "AIDS has become the leading cause of death in terms of potential years of life lost in adult men, followed by unintentional injuries and tuberculosis. In women, AIDS is the second leading cause of death and premature mortality, after deaths related to pregnancy and abortion,"[21] and "AIDS accounted for 15% of adult male deaths and 13% of adult female deaths."[22] The most recent data have confirmed this high seroprevalence. With a rate of 14.8 percent detected in 1992 in a sample of pregnant women, Abidjan was by far the most affected town in West Africa.[23] However, considering that the infection rate among pregnant women in Abidjan was about 10 percent in 1987, it should be noted that the epidemic in the total population had not spread at the same rate as that observed in the big cities of the Great Lakes region.

The AIDS epidemic in Côte d'Ivoire shows some unique features related to the presence of two HIV infections: HIV-1 and HIV-2. Both immunodeficiency viruses have been isolated in patients and mixed infections with HIV-1 and HIV-2 in the same individual are common. In 1988 in the two largest hospitals of Abidjan, "50% of AIDS patients were positive for HIV-1 only, 4% for HIV-2 only, and 46% reacted serologically to both viruses."[24] However, "The increases in infection rates have been largely due to transmission of HIV-1, whereas rates of HIV-2 have remained stable or have declined."[25] Among pregnant women, the increase in prevalence was particularly related to HIV-1, and to the HIV-1–HIV-2 combination as well. HIV-2 infection has largely declined in men with STDs; female prostitutes had the highest rate of dual reactivity (34 percent).[26]

As observed in the other sub-Saharan countries, AIDS has affected mostly young adults; women have also been more susceptible than men to infection. In 1993 Dédy and Tapé reported that "Despite the awareness campaign, HIV infection and AIDS continue to spread among the inhabitants of the Côte d'Ivoire in general and in the youth in particular (15–24 years old) essentially through sexual transmission (80%)."[27] AIDS cases in men and women reported by Project Retro-CI (from 1987 to 1993) show "the majority of cases occurred in people between 20 and 49; the most heavily affected age ranges were 30–39 years old for men and 20–29 for women."[28] In 1989 among 1,501 HIV-positive patients admitted to Abidjan hospitals, the median age of male patients was 36 (with a range of 15–88) and of female patients 30 (with a range of 15–83).[29] Among pregnant women, in Abidjan again (from 1990 to 1992), maximal seroprevalence occurred in the 15–30-year-old range, but differences were observed according to the virus involved. "HIV-1 infection was concentrated in women younger than 30 years of age, whereas the highest prevalence of HIV-2 infection was in women aged 30–39 years."[30] At first the epidemic in Côte d'Ivoire showed a very unbalanced male-to-female sex ratio: 4:8 in 1988. Since then the gap steadily narrowed, and in 1993 the sex ratio was 1:9.[31] Both HIV-1 and HIV-2 gradually spread among young adult women, who increasingly became the primary victims of the epidemic.

However, male patients with an STD and female sex workers have been most at risk, as clearly shown by the results of several seroepidemiological surveys in Côte d'Ivoire and other countries of sub-Saharan Africa. In both groups prevalence reached alarming levels. "The overall prevalence of HIV infection in male STD clinic attenders increased from 9% in 1987 to 27% in 1992."[32] On average 28–30 percent of the men consulting anti-venereal dispensaries were estimated to be seropositive. Prostitutes, however, had among the highest rates. The most recent surveys showed infection rates at or above 80 percent. In 1992–93[33] as in 1994[34] studies showed that in confidential clinics for female sex workers of the city, 80 percent of the women were HIV positive and "Female sex workers in Abidjan had the highest absolute (30%) and proportional rate (38%) of dual sero-reactivity yet described in any population."[35] Overall rates of HIV infection were among the highest observed on the continent.

HIV infection appears to have become an important cause of morbidity in children from birth to the age of five in Abidjan, but rates remained fairly constant from the late 1980s into the 1990s. Studies conducted in 1989, 1991, and 1992 among children in Abidjan's hospitals showed that overall HIV seroreactivity was respectively 10 percent, 8 percent, and 8.5 percent.[36] According to the 1989 survey, 92 percent of seroreactive children of all ages had an HIV positive mother. The remaining seropositive children had a history of receiving blood transfusions, and infection in this group was entirely with HIV-1.[37]

POLITICAL, CONTROL, AND
THERAPEUTIC MEASURES

The economic boom of colonial times made Côte d'Ivoire the most prosperous colony of the French West African Federation. Already considered a leading country in development circles, French health policy contributed greatly to its expansion. As early as 1893 a health service was set up. It stagnated, however, for lack of staff, resources, adequate medical knowledge about tropical diseases, and because of the absence of any clearly determined purpose other than that of keeping the European population in good health. Two diseases were given priority: yellow fever, which periodically decimated the European population, and smallpox.[38] From 1905 attention to the health of the native population led to the creation of a special service called Indigenous Medical Aid. This body was of no help for venereal diseases, which were ignored.

In 1924 a new health policy arose in response to new goals. Developing the country required a large work force — which did not exist at the time — and increased population mobility. The minister of colonies, E. Daladier, assigned the health services a new mission: "the preservation and spread of races."[39] To achieve this, emphasis had to be placed on social and preventive mass medicine, along with the development of hygiene and health education. Doctors had to go out and visit the population to practice the provision of medical assistance on a mass scale. The obligation of providing general social welfare required the control of social diseases, an increase in the number of dispensaries for their detection and treatment, the regulation of prostitution, and the development of public education. Curative and individual medicine were relegated to secondary and tertiary positions. This policy, maintained until independence, involved a reorganization of health services. The system was organized hierarchically. Every district had to include a local hospital. The main towns had to have a social medicine dispensary for disease detection, consultation, and treatment with clinic days planned to coincide with important meetings, markets, or celebrations. In addition, Mobile Hygiene Units (part of the General Service for Mobile Hygiene and Prophylaxis) were charged with reaching the most isolated villages and made regular rounds among the population. Finally, there was a need for better knowledge of the population's health situation through centralization of all information in the hygiene and demography departments of the Health Service.[40] This was an ambitious policy. However, because of the inertia of the Health Services, the size of the job, inadequate resources (the funds were absorbed by salaries), and too few staff (a situation that was not specific to this colony but concerned the whole of French West Africa), these directives did not have any effect.[41]

In 1934 the Economic Conference of Metropolitan and Overseas France in Paris reasserted and relaunched the policy it had established in 1924, but did so at a time when the state had very limited means to pay for it.[42] Nevertheless, the number of health services increased on average by 17.3 percent a year between 1933 and 1936, and in 1936 the health budget accounted for 10 percent of the budget of the colony.[43] All the same, this progress was still quite insufficient to meet the requirements of the policy of mass preventive medicine. During World War II "the difficulties arising from the war might have led us to expect a limitation of the health services resources, but this was not the case."[44] The health budget showed growth higher than that of the colony itself (an average of 24.3 percent a year between 1937 and 1945, compared with 17.8 percent for the colony's budget overall). Infrastructure and hospital accommodation capacity grew. Between the end of the war and independence the policy defined in 1924 was not questioned. During this time the colony experienced the highest economic growth of its history and of the whole of French West Africa (which was dissolved in 1958). Parallel to this growth, health and social services had an unprecedented rise. In 1950 the Social Affairs Service was set up and was, among other things, in charge of health education. Despite the silence surrounding them, venereal diseases were a cause for alarm, and it fell to this service to improve their detection. This was in line with the continuing policy of developing mass medicine focused on hygiene and prophylaxis. However, most of what was achieved concerned medical treatment rather than preventive medicine.

Before 1920 the governor had tried without success to control prostitution in the biggest cities, Bassam and Abidjan. In 1930 in Bassam (the first colonial capital), weekly examinations of prostitutes with obligatory hospitalization of infected women were established. Because the equivalent did not exist in Abidjan, all the prostitutes moved to this city. In 1932 a decree regulating prostitution remained in place to no effect. In 1940 a health department was created in every health center for surveillance of female prostitutes, providing for jail sentences and fines.[45] In 1942 another decree was promulgated: Every woman diagnosed with a venereal disease was to be isolated and treated. Subjected to control by the constituted authorities, she was not to be allowed to resume work until complete recovery was certified. Neither of these measures had any effect. A woman needed only to be married (or perhaps merely to claim to be in a formal union) to escape any medical examination.[46] In 1945 the General Service for Mobile Hygiene and Prophylaxis and its Mobile Hygiene Units were given a treponematosis department, but this arm of the health service started operating only in 1949 in Senegal and Niger. In 1953 11 units made the rounds throughout French West Africa (4,425,000 km²), including to Dalou in Côte d'Ivoire, a location considered to be hyperendemic.[47] In 1946 Houphouët-Boigny, then a deputy, had a law passed that was to have appreciable consequences for health supervision. The law, which abolished forced labor, gave the work force greater freedom but also increased its mobility. It was accompanied by measures relaxing administrative regulations, which, as far as health was concerned, consisted of suppressing the medical consultations that had accompanied labor recruitment and departure. This medical supervision network was abolished just when populations began to travel more, a situation favoring the circulation of pathogens. The measures taken in 1953 also did not reinforce prophylaxis. The roadblocks and surprise visits in markets and villages instituted primarily to fight trypanosomiasis were so unpopular that they were abandoned in 1955.[48]

As for traditional medicine, at the turn of the century the people of West Africa used tamarind seeds to treat gonorrhea and peanut leaves against syphilis. Western physicians at the time used mercury salts or potassium iodide. In 1925 specialized units within dispensaries treated syphilis patients with arsenobenzol injections. However, the treatment was usually not completed, because once the first signs of skin bleaching occurred (a side effect of these injections), the patients disappeared. Until 1942 arsenic-based treatments were still the most commonly used, although administered sparingly to avoid creating drug resistance. From 1942 sulphonamides were introduced; one of them, Dagenan, raised the same concerns about resistance as the previous arsenic-based treatments, particularly in view of its wide availability. As a rule, the patient population could not be relied upon to finish any treatment. Penicillin, although very effective, was scarce and, hence, reserved for the European population.[49] After the war sulphonamides and penicillin were used. However, doctors continued using the far more dangerous bismuth and mercury-based arsenic preparations. The hopes raised by the introduction of sulphanomides and antibiotics were dashed. The usual unreliability of patients to come to the clinic and the free availability on the black market of certain of these drugs led to inappropriate use by patients and abandonment of the dispensary. More ominously, it led to microbial resistance to sulphanomides and penicillin. This led doctors to prescribe fewer antibiotics and to use other drugs more, which, although less effective, would not have the same consequences of developing resistance.[50]

In spite of these disappointing early results in the treatment of venereal diseases using antibiotics, health care became increasingly effective. The first to benefit were city dwellers, and modern medicine became routine for the better-off urban population. However, in the hinterlands and among the poor, traditional medicine still came first. It was through the action of the Mobile Prophylaxis Group that modern medicine was slowly introduced to the most remote areas. In this final decade of the twentieth century both types of medicine often still coexist, with modern medicine often being sought as a last resort. However, since the onset of AIDS in the early 1980s modern medicine has been unable to respond to this hope. HIV infection threatens it with failure after a triumphant century of success in the fight against infectious disease. The war against AIDS is, thus, multifaceted, and never before has a disease been the focus of so many different specialties. Research into HIV has in fact led to progress both in medical science and in the social sciences, working together in a joint effort to cure and protect. As long as medicine is unable to cure, prevention is the only way to sever the links in the epidemiological chain that spreads the HIV epidemic. To achieve this taboos have had to be broken and habits changed. As with many other African countries, Côte d'Ivoire has been slow in implementing a policy of prevention. However, there is now a general desire to make up for lost time.

The national Anti-AIDS Program was set up in 1987 with the help of the WHO. Since then numerous agencies have sprung up, which in sheer numbers put Côte d'Ivoire ahead of other French-speaking countries. Most of these organizations are urban based, and they are mainly located in Abidjan. The AIDS Information and Prevention Campaign was started in 1988, targeting the general public and using a variety of technical channels and networks: the media (with the international cooperation of Italy and France), groups of musicians and actors, and public lectures. At the beginning of 1989–90 the National Anti-AIDS Committee organized the free distribution of condoms. Since 1991 their sale has been subsidized under the trademark Prudence (a box of four costs 100 CFA francs, about $0.20). In 1992 the government organized the first National Anti-AIDS Day. Later that year an Anti-AIDS Information and Prevention Center, financed by the United States Agency for International Development, was opened in Abidjan, the first in West Africa. It targeted the sexually active population by offering four different types of services: information, counselling (pre- and post-testing), confidential testing, and promotion of community awareness. City dwellers have been the main beneficiaries of those policies, and there has been little regular follow-up. It remains to be seen what has been or will be the effect of these activities on HIV infection rates.

Since 1987 numerous anti-AIDS initiatives were implemented through international cooperation, which brought in staff and resources. In that year the Ministry of Health and Social Security signed an agreement with the United States Centers for Disease Control for a project to study HIV epidemiology, based in Abidjan: Retro-CI. In 1990 this agreement was extended for another five years. Since 1991 Retro-CI has been the most important Centers for Disease Control research facility in Africa, with a staff of 60, including 13 doctors. It has multiple objectives, and its studies aim to accomplish at least one of the following goals: to prevent the spread of the infection in the population at large, to delay the onset of AIDS in HIV-infected patients, to support the Health Services in their fight to control the epidemic, and to study the relationship between HIV and associated opportunistic diseases. In October 1992 Retro-CI opened a clinic in Abidjan (named *Confiance*, or Trust) to offer free STD treatment to local prostitutes and study the interaction between AIDS and STDs. In 1991 the European Community financed a complete renovation of the National Center for Blood Transfusion.

Numerous nongovernmental organizations were also recruited to disseminate knowledge of anti-AIDS practices among the sexually active population. They have experimented constantly in their attempts to raise awareness through techniques, such as AIDS Days, parties, organized activities, theatrical performances, wall posters and slogans, and leafleting. Since 1994 AIDS information stalls have been set up at local markets and other popular meeting points. To reach the most people most efficiently, the channels for action were greatly diversified. Many workplaces became springboards of anti-AIDS campaigning. The spreading of information at worksites has been a valuable addition to national efforts and has helped to offset some of the deficiencies in public health initiatives. This policy of raising awareness started first in anglophone Africa. Since 1994 Côte d'Ivoire has been at the forefront of such activities in francophone Africa. The Federation of Employers wrote a charter to establish guidelines, and the workplace became a public health resource. Companies took on a dual role of training medical and paramedical staff in the proper management of patients and of spreading information, education, and communication programs to raise the awareness of AIDS among employees. In 1995 there were about 20 such innovative business enterprises in Côte d'Ivoire. Those with a leading role included Filitisac, based in Abidjan with 1,500 employees, and the Côte d'Ivoire Electricity Board. With 3,000 employees spread throughout the country, the board has been able to disseminate information to all regions.[51] At the same time that prevention has been improving, so has care of the HIV-positive and AIDS-affected populations. From 1990 on, hospitals have tried to coordinate the medical and psychological handling of both the HIV-positive and the ill. At the same time, health care workers have received specialized training. The first centers for care and counselling were opened in hospitals in Abidjan and the larger provincial cities. The will to organize and develop these centers exists, but the resources available are laughably small compared to the needs. To remedy this at a local level, in 1994 the French Ministry of Cooperation financed the creation of a mobile unit for the HIV-positive population of Abidjan. Also in Abidjan, three STD clinics began offering specialized treatment. In 1994, however, the clinics were sorely underfunded. There was a lack of political interest and lack of coordination with the anti-AIDS program even though, in principle, the fight against STDs is part of the larger struggle against HIV.[52]

SOCIAL, CULTURAL, AND ECONOMIC DIMENSIONS

As elsewhere in sub-Saharan Africa, colonization caused a weakening of traditional societies. Formerly self-sufficient, they became dependent on trade. The population, which had been comparatively stable and rural, became much more mobile and urbanized. In Côte d'Ivoire, the showcase of the colonial empire, these changes were particularly notable. Those who were first in answering the challenge were mainly young adult males, whether from France or Africa. Colonial development of Côte d'Ivoire was very patchy. The coastal areas saw large projects in agriculture, forestry, road building, urban development, and the improvement of port facilities. Originally sparsely populated, the coast became a magnet for labor migration to the detriment of neighboring regions.[53] Before 1946 migration and settlement were regulated by a system of forced labor, with recruits confined in camps. After 1946 abolition of this system increased the instability of the work force at just the time the economic boom of the coastal areas was calling for more workers. New migratory movements led to the mixing of populations, providing ideal conditions for the spread of pathogens. Camps, worksites, and travel routes became centers of casual, multi-partnered sexuality, and, thereby, served as nodes in initial chains of infection and zones of high transmission in full-blown epidemics. Reliable observations have confirmed this in the case of non-sexually transmitted diseases, such as smallpox and trypanosomiasis. For venereal diseases much less is known. As early as 1921, François observed the process at work in the Agnéby Social Club.[54]

West Africa has been a region of intense migration since at least colonial times. Historically, internal migratory paths were mostly north-south. All roads and railways run perpendicular to the coast — the only exception being the Bamako-Dakar line. The coastal states of Côte d'Ivoire, Ghana, Senegal, and Nigeria (with its oil miracle of the 1970s) have been lands of immigration, but the landlocked Sahel states are lands of emigration. These patterns, however, have proven to be very sensitive to economic and political circumstances. Difficult economic conditions during the 1980s in Senegal, Ghana, and Nigeria shifted the flow of migration toward the more prosperous Côte d'Ivoire, which became the West African country with the highest immigration ratio. Of 13 million inhabitants in 1988, almost 4 million were foreigners. Thirty years of peace and 20 years of prosperity (exceptional in much of Africa) made Côte d'Ivoire a powerful economic magnet. Immigrants came from all over Western Africa, but the most established sources were Burkina Faso, Mali, and Nigeria. The latest census (1988) gives a breakdown of the origin of those immigrants. By far the largest contingent came from Burkina Faso (42 percent of annual migration between 1987 and 1988), far ahead of Mali (21 percent). To traditional migratory patterns have been added movements because of political instability; the conflicts of the mid-1990s in neighboring Liberia and Sierra Leone caused thousands to seek refuge in Côte d'Ivoire.

The migrants, whatever their origin, prefer the southern half of the country, where labor demands are concentrated; 79 percent of them settle there.[55] This includes a large group of seasonal workers from Burkina Faso and Mali who leave their villages during the dry season (when no agriculture is possible) to seek work on plantations, forest lumbering operations, or in the port of Abidjan. This historic tradition was accentuated during the 1970s when climatic crises of the Sudan and Sahel regions and the economic crisis of the neighboring coastal nations led to an increase in east-west migration.[56]

The growth of Abidjan indicates the attraction exercised by Côte d'Ivoire: A small fishing village in 1890, in 1900 it still had fewer than 1,000 inhabitants. In 1930 the population was estimated at 6,000. In 1975 it reached the 1-million mark, and this doubled by 1990, giving it 45 percent of the country's urban population. Its growth rate was greater than 10 percent over a 30-year period. Such growth is among the highest ever recorded. The city was the nation's capital until 1983 and is still its economic capital, having retained most of the benefits of the country's economic growth. The urban region is the foremost employment region not only of the nation but of all French-speaking West Africa, with a continuous influx of population from the rest of Côte d'Ivoire as well as its neighbors.

This positive migratory balance has been matched by a high birth rate. Between 1960 and 1992 the annual growth rate of the Côte d'Ivoire population was 3.9 percent. At this rate the population will double by 2010. The total fertility rate was 7.4 in 1992, one of the highest in the world. This has given Côte d'Ivoire a young population, with 48 percent of all inhabitants under 15 years of age. The sex ratio in Abidjan reflects this situation: In 1957 it was 1.39:1[57] and in 1988 1.5:1 for the population between 20 and 49. Traditionally, the majority of the migrants have been young male adults, although there has been strong female involvement along certain routes, particularly from parts of Ghana. The cultural uprooting of men and imbalanced urban sex ratios created a situation favorable to the spread of STDs. These consequences were analyzed and formulated by De Cock and colleagues in 1989 in an epidemiological study of AIDS carried out in the two largest hospitals of Abidjan.[58]

The high proportion of males in the 20–49 year age group come from elsewhere in the country and from neighbouring countries to seek employment. About 40% of Abidjan residents were not born in the Côte d'Ivoire. (For the purpose of the study a resident of Abidjan was defined as a person who had been living in Abidjan for at least 3 months before admission). Twenty-one countries of origin were represented with the study population. 33% of the 1421 patients whose country of birth was known were born outside the Côte d'Ivoire. The observations on sex ratios, the rapid development of the epidemic in Abidjan, and the apparently high risk of AIDS among foreign-born people (many of whom are in Abidjan without family), raise the possibility that female prostitution may have had an important role here in the spread of AIDS.[59]

Observing the evolution of the sex ratio is instructive; men exposed to the risk of infection by prostitutes have gradually transmitted the virus to the general female population within Abidjan, in surrounding areas, and also in neighboring countries when men returned home. Such a demographic and epidemiologic explosion became dramatically worse when economic development declined from 1980 onward. From 1960 to 1980 economic growth was remarkable. The increase in national wealth, on the order of 6–7 percent per year (more than double the population growth rate), was accompanied by a policy of development of infrastructure, industrialization, and job-creating social investment. After these two decades of prosperity, economic difficulties hit the country, which has the highest per capita debt in the world. The economic development of Côte d'Ivoire was mainly financed from abroad, and the slowdown of economic activity made it impossible to honor debts. The debt burden and the drop in coffee and cocoa prices since 1981 (Côte d'Ivoire is the world's biggest cocoa producer and the fifth biggest producer of coffee) forced the country to declare itself insolvent on May 28, 1987. In response, international organizations imposed a reduction of the public deficit with the consequences of accentuating social imbalances and reducing public health spending. These reductions came even though health care was the weakest point of the social system (one doctor for 16,670 inhabitants in 1990, a life expectancy of 51.6 in 1992) and needs were increasing.[60] For example, the number of tuberculosis patients handled in the tuberculosis clinics of Abidjan rose continuously, from 3,004 in 1989 to 3,600 in 1991, while the budget of these clinics decreased an average of 17 percent per year for that period.[61]

Against a background of increasing economic difficulties, Côte d'Ivoire had to face the fastest population growth in its history. City populations grew without the economic development that would justify such growth, so that in 1990 almost one-third of urban dwellers were living below the poverty level.[62] Abidjan, where one inhabitant in two had no regular job, was a focus for all these problems, forming a fertile breeding ground for infections such as AIDS: new living conditions linked to social and cultural upheaval; deteriorating sanitary and social conditions marked by the precariousness of employment, health, and housing; and an increase in the number of cases of distress, especially among women.

Despite the progressive actions of the Ivorian government regarding AIDS, and given the context of rapid social change and increasing poverty, young Ivorian males can also, by their behavior, further circulate HIV. Studies of social behavior since 1989 to determine the state of knowledge about AIDS and sexual behavior have shown that young people have a high degree of knowledge about the way AIDS is transmitted, but may be failing or unable to put this knowledge into practice. According to a 1989 national study reported by Dédy and Tapé, 91 percent of those aged 5–19, and 89 percent of those in the 20–24 age group knew how HIV is transmitted.[63] However, there was much less knowledge about condoms and how to use them. The authors write: "Those in the 'always' group, ie. those who always use protection, barely surpass 10%" and the study revealed that "43% of Côte d'Ivoire inhabitants of both sexes and all ages believe that condoms reduce sexual pleasure. Young people state this even more affirmatively . . . they prefer 'natural' sexual relations." On average first sexual relations were at age 15, an age at which, as the authors stress, "there is great [emotional] instability, which can lead to a high-risk situation if there are both precocity and multiple partners." Given the low rates of condom usage, young men are at more risk; according to this study, for each woman with multiple partners there are four men. In addition, almost 10 percent of young people between 15 and 24 years of age have had sexual intercourse involving payment to professional prostitutes or informal sex workers; in 85 percent of the cases condoms were not used. The risk is, thus, quite high, even more so because young people today are more precocious sexually than were those who are now in the 45–49 age group. This change is more marked with men than with women. In 1993 Côte d'Ivoire inhabitants using condoms were still a minority.[64] Dédy and Tapé cite three reasons that explain this "irresponsible sexuality":

the sexual exploration and freedom that often accompanies adolescence — despite the fact that young people state that STD prevents them from "living it up" or "enjoying life" (using two terms by which they mean living one's sexuality to the full);

the inadequacy of family education or censorship boards to counteract more modern models spread by the media (television, cinema, and popular romances); and

the attraction of money and an uncontrollable or illegal lifestyle to which the young resort in pursuit of it.

DEMOGRAPHIC AND ECONOMIC OUTLOOK

As with most African nations, poorly functioning systems of vital registration mean that official Côte d'Ivoire statistics are less than reliable. It is, thus, quite difficult to measure the demographic consequences of AIDS at the national level.[65] Nevertheless, whereas a long decline in the mortality rate had been observed, from 1986 onward this trend changed, except for the birth to four-year-old age group. A recent study in Abidjan indicates this. Garenne and colleagues analyzed both the mortality rate and causes of death in the city's hospitals.[66] They estimated that "almost 25,000 people died of AIDS here between 1986 and 1992, more than doubling the mortality rate, and this impressive increase is said to have already diminished the life expectancy of 15-year-old men by 4.3 years, and that of 15-year-old women by 1.1 years."[67] All levels of society have been affected, but it has been primarily young adult males who have paid the heaviest toll during this first phase of the epidemic (70 percent of all AIDS deaths). It should be noted, however, that although figures for men are probably reliable, the mortality rates of women and young children are underestimates. The authors further estimated that "we can expect an average of about 7,000 cases of AIDS per year in the city up to the year 2000." These figures confirm the worries expressed in 1989 based upon the results of a study carried out between 1983 and 1988 in two major hospitals of the city.[68] "Review of records showed that fatality rates (deaths per 1,000 admissions) in adult medical patients increased by 54% between 1983 and 1988, with increases of 106% and 98% in men 20–29 and 30–39 years of age, respectively, and 199% and 42% in women of the same age ranges. Over the same period, official mortality statistics for the city showed reduced mortality rates in children and women 20–29 years of age, but an increase in mortality rates of 54% in men 20 years of age and older, and of 28% in women ages 30 years and older."[69]

AIDS was already the major cause of the increase in the number of deaths observed in the city and had reversed the steady trend of reduced mortality observed since the end of World War II. At the national level, "we can now state with certainty that AIDS is the leading cause of mortality in men, and the second cause in women, after maternal mortality, but it is swiftly becoming clear that it will be the first cause of death in women too. . . . Almost half of the deaths in coming years will be entirely due to the AIDS pandemic."[70] Two hypotheses have been put forth by Abbas Senoussi as estimates of the demographic impact of the epidemic up to the year 2003. One predicts an evolution of the epidemic to a peak rate of 15 percent in 2000, the other to a rate of 20 percent. According to the first hypothesis, 1.5 million people have been or will be infected with HIV between 1993 and 2003. According to the second, more than 2 million people will be infected. Furthermore, in ten years 1.5 million people will die according to the first hypothesis, and almost 1.7 million according to the second.[71] The most recent demographic projections estimate that in the absence of AIDS the population of Côte d'Ivoire would have reached 19 million by 2003. AIDS will, thus, eliminate about 8 percent of the country's expected population.

The economic and social impact of AIDS on affected families and companies in Côte d'Ivoire are still mainly unknown. The same is true for health care services. The first study of the impact of AIDS on the health care system of Côte d'Ivoire is underway as of this writing. Nevertheless, the reports of the tuberculosis treatment centers give some indication of likely effects. Studies carried out in Abidjan and reported by Djomand and colleagues[72] show the high rate of HIV infection in adults with tuberculosis. In 1989, "overall rates of HIV infection were 40% in patients with tuberculosis, and 'only' 10% in blood donors."[73] Since 1991, this rate has been more than 45 percent,[74] and 32 percent of deaths among people with AIDS are due to tuberculosis.[75] The incidence of tuberculosis (as a percentage of the general population) is below that of the 1960s. This results from the quality of care in the country's eight anti-tuberculosis centers (two of them in Abidjan). However, because of the joint impact of economic difficulties and AIDS, the rate is no longer falling. AIDS is, thus, imposing an increasingly heavy burden on health care structures and exacerbating other infections that pose serious health problems in their own right. "In infectious disease and pulmonary medicine wards, more than two-thirds of beds are now occupied by HIV-infected persons."[76]

What has been the cost of AIDS to business? Here again there is little, and only partial, information. A pioneering sectoral study was carried out in May–June 1994 involving four private firms in the food and agriculture sector in Abidjan. One of its goals was to measure the cost of care for sick workers.[77] E. Gnaore, National Plan to Combat AIDS coordinator for Côte d'Ivoire, reported preliminary results in an interview: "thus, the total cumulative cost for 1993–1998, assuming an infection rate for these workers of 10%, would be in the neighborhood of 500 million francs CFA. For a rate of 15%, it would be a thousand million francs CFA."[78]

Given that the main group affected by AIDS is young, economically active adults, in May 1992 Côte d'Ivoire launched a study aimed at analyzing the economic and social consequences of the illness for families and the coping strategies they might employ. Preliminary results indicate a weakening of social support networks, disrupted by "the fear inspired by the epidemic, and the over-burdening of some forms of social solidarity."[79] AIDS appears, not surprisingly, to have very serious consequences for the professional activities of its victims. "Among those who have a profession, more than half (52%) report changes in their professional activity since the start of their illness: more than 40% had to leave their jobs, 3.4% were dismissed, and 16% suffered other changes."[80] It is easy to imagine the added distress caused by this situation, but it is still too early to discuss the exact patterns of family response to illness of members.

We must also take into account the effects of one more factor: the increasing instability of migratory networks. Population movements have acquired increasingly complex spatial dynamics. Shifts in the patterns of movement have accelerated in response to the economic differences between countries and their immigration policies. More and more, migration has taken place outside of traditional support networks. Mobility has become individual, informal, precarious, and opportunistic, relying on highly temporary networks. All these factors, besides favoring the spread of the virus, make control of the pandemic a more complicated matter. Plans to counter the disease and prevent it must be conceived and applied at a transnational level, here more than elsewhere, and now more than ever, in Côte d'Ivoire.

CONCLUSION

The economic and social conditions of the colonization of Côte d'Ivoire a century ago led to the disappearance of an old equilibrium and the emergence of complex new forces in population health. On one hand, the continuous drop in mortality rates and the successful eradication of smallpox have been successfully launched within this disequilibrating context. On the other hand, the rampant spread of STDs, including AIDS, points to more negative health consequences of these changes. In this final quarter of the twentieth century, HIV infection has found a particularly favorable terrain in Côte d'Ivoire, mainly because of the antagonism between development and underdevelopment internal to the country. Its major impact is still to come, but the inhabitants of Côte d'Ivoire, with those of Abidjan on the front line, have been mobilized, encouraged, and helped by a considerable international effort. Nevertheless, at a time when an enormous infrastructure must still be developed, especially in the provinces, the exceptional and exemplary effort seen in Abidjan is itself a fragile one, dependent as it is on foreign aid. Uncertainty about whether certain forms of external aid will be maintained puts the future of many important anti-AIDS commitments, such as Retro-CI, at risk. Economic difficulties and Côte d'Ivoire's continued dependence on international aid maintain levels of poverty that nourish the system of infection.

NOTES

1.   Danielle Domergue-Cloarec, *La santé en Côte d'Ivoire 1905–1958* (Paris: Association des publications de l'Université Toulouse-Le Mirail, Académie des Sciences d'Outre-Mer, 1986), p. 163.
   2.   Ibid., p. 195.
   3.   Ibid., p. 194.

4. Ibid., p. 444.

5. Ibid.

6. *Rapport médical annuel* (Abidjan: Service de santé de Côte d'Ivoire, 1929) cited in Domergue-Cloarec, *La santé en Côte d'Ivoire*, p. 444.

7. Jean Grosfillez, "Les principales maladies observées dans les colonies et les territoires sous mandat en 1932," *Annales de Médecine et de Pharmacie Coloniale* 32 (1934): 219.

8. *Rapport médical annuel* (Abidjan: Service de santé de Côte d'Ivoire, 1931), p. 32.

9. Domergue-Cloarec, *La santé en Côte d'Ivoire*, p. 1037.

10. Ibid., p. 1038.

11. Ibid., p. 1176.

12. Séry Dédy and Gozé Tapé, "Comportements sexuels et sida en Côte d'Ivoire Rapport préliminaire, PNLS, 1991, Abidjan," in *Jeunes et préservatifs en Abidjan, une recherche d'ethno-prévention du sida et des NST*, edited by François Deniau (Bingerville: Actes de l'atelier du CRES, 1993), p. 107.

13. Mathieu Verboud, "Que font les centres de recherche occidentaux à Abidjan?"*Le journal du SIDA*, Nos. 67–68 (1994): p. 14.

14. Ibid.

15. *Weekly Epidemiological Record* 70 (1995): 193.

16. François Denis, Françoise Barin, and Guy-Michel Damet-Gershy, "Prevalence of Human T-lymphotropic Retrovirus Type III (HIV) and Type IV in Ivory Coast" *Lancet* 1 (1987): 408; Koudou Odehouri, Kevin M. De Cock, John W. Krebs, Jacques Moreau, Mark Rayfield, Joseph B. McCormick, Gerald Schochetman, Raymond Bretton, Genviè Bretton, Daniel Ouattara, Paul Herouin, Jean-Marie Kanga, Bernard Beda, Ezany Niamkey, Auguste Kadio, Elisabeth Gariepe, and William L. Heyward, "HIV-1 and HIV-2 Infections Associated with AIDS in Abidjan, Côte d'Ivoire," *AIDS* 3 (1989): 509.

17. Kevin M. De Cock, Koudou Odehouri, Jacques Moreau, Justin C. Kouadio, Anne Porter, Bernard Barrere, Lacina Dialy, and William L. Heyward, "Rapid Emergence of AIDS in Abidjan, Ivory Coast," *Lancet* 2 (1989): 408.

18. Guy-Michel Gershy-Damet, Konan Koffi, Benoît N. Soro, Adama Coulibaly, David Koffi, and Koudou Odehouri, "Seroepidemiological Survey of HIV-1 and HIV-2 Infections in the Five Regions of Ivory Coast," *AIDS* 5 (1991): 463.

19. Benoît N. Soro, Guy-Michel Gershy-Damet, Adama Coulibaly, Konan Koffi, Victor S. Sangare, David Koffi, Roger Houdier, Roger Josseran, Jérôme Guelain, Eba Aoussi, Koudou Odehouri, Armand Ehouman, and Nangbele Coulibaly, "Seroprevalence of HIV Infection in the General Population of the Côte d'Ivoire, West Africa," *Journal of AIDS* 3 (1990): 1195.

20. Kevin M. De Cock, Bernard Barrere, Marie-France Lafontaine, Lacina Dialy, Emmanuel Gnaore, Daniel Pantohe, and Koudou Odehouri, "Mortality Trends in Abidjan, Côte d'Ivoire, 1983–1988," *AIDS* 5 (1991): 393.

21. Kevin M. De Cock, Bernard Barrere, Lacina Dialy, Marie-France Lafontaine, Emmanuel Gnaore, Anne Porter, Daniel Pantobe, Geoarges C. Lafontant, Augustin Dago-Akribi, Marcel Ette, Koudou Odehouri, and William L. Heyward, "AIDS, the Leading Cause of Adult Death in the West African City of Abidjan, Ivory Coast," *Science* 249 (1990): 793.

22. Ibid.

23. Mamadou O. Diallo, Virginie Traore, M. Maran, J. Kouadio, K. Brattegaard, A. Makke, E. Van Dycke, M. Laga, and Kevin M. De Cock, "Sexually Transmitted Diseases and HIV- 1/HIV-2 Infections among Pregnant Women Attending an Antenatal Clinic in Abidjan, Ivory Coast," Seventh International Conference of AIDS in Africa, Yaounde, Cameroon, December 8–11, 1992, poster T.P.041.

24. De Cock, Odehouri, Moreau, Kouadio, Porter, Barrere, Dialy, and Heyward, "Rapid Emergence of AIDS," p. 408.

25. Gaston Djomand, Alan E. Greenberg, Madeleine Sassan-Morokro, Odette Tossou, Mamadou O. Diallo, Ehounou Ekpini, Peter Ghys, Benoît Soro, Kari Brattegaard, Achy Yapi, Koudou Odehouri, Doulhourou Coulibaly, Issa-Malick Coulibaly, Auguste Kadio, Emmanuel Gnaore, and Kevin M. De Cock, "The Epidemic of HIV/AIDS in Abidjan, Côte d'Ivoire: A Review of Data Collected by Project Retro-CI from 1987 to 1993," *Journal of AIDS* 10 (1995): 363.

26. Ibid., p. 360.

27. Séry Dédy and Gozé Tapé, "Jeunesse, Sexualité et sida en Côte d'Ivoire," in *Jeunes et préservatifs en Abidjan, une recherche d'ethno-prévention du sida et des NST*, edited by François Deniau (Bingerville: Actes de l'atelier du CRES, 1993), p. 83. The figure of 80 percent sexual transmission seems low for this age group; the remaining 20 percent of infections may have been caused by transfusions or nosocomial infection.

28. Djomand, Greenberg, Sassan-Morokro, Tossou, Diallo, Ekpini, Ghys, Soro, Brattegaard, Yapi, Odehouri, Coulibaly, Coulibaly, Kadio, Gnaore, and De Cock, "The Epidemic of HIV/AIDS," p. 362.

29. De Cock, Odehouri, Moreau, Kouadio, Porter, Barrere, Dialy, and Heyward, "Rapid Emergence of AIDS," p. 409.

30. Djomand, Greenberg, Sassan-Morokro, Tossou, Diallo, Ekpini, Ghys, Soro, Brattegaard, Yapi, Odehouri, Coulibaly, Coulibaly, Kadio, Gnaore, and De Cock, "The Epidemic of HIV/AIDS," p. 360.

31. Ibid., p. 363.

32. Verboud, "Que font les centres," p. 14.

33. Virginie Ettiègne-Traoré, Peter D. Ghys, Mamadou O. Diallo, Marie Laga, Félix Lorougnon, and Kevin M. De Cock, "Dual HIV-1 and HIV-2 Reactivity in Female Commercial Sex Workers in Abidjan, Côte d'Ivoire," Eighth International Conference of AIDS in Africa, Marrakech, Morocco, December 12–16, 1993, Session T.R.T.023.

34. Peter D. Ghys, Mamadou O. Diallo, Virginie Ettiègne-Traoré, Kouadio M. Yeboué, Emmanuel Gnaore, Félix Lorougnon, Marie-Jeanne Teurquetil, Marie-Laure Adom, Alan E. Greenberg, Marie Laga, and Kevin M. De Cock, "Dual Seroreactivity to HIV-1 and HIV-2 in Female Sex Workers in Abidjan, Côte d'Ivoire," *AIDS* 9 (1995): 955.

35. Ibid.

36. Djomand, Greenberg, Sassan-Morokro, Tossou, Diallo, Ekpini, Ghys, Soro, Brattegaard, Yapi, Odehouri, Coulibaly, Coulibaly, Kadio, Gnaore, and De Cock, "The Epidemic of HIV/AIDS," p. 361.

37. Hélène D. Gayle, Emmanuel Gnaore, Georgette Adjorlolo, Ehounou Ekpini, Ramata Coulibaly, Anne Porter, Miles M. Braun, Marie Louise Klein

Zabban, Joseph Andou, Adjoua Timite, Jèrôme Assi-Adou, and Kevin M. De Cock, "HIV-1 and HIV-2 Infection in Children in Abidjan, Côte d'Ivoire," *Journal of Acquired Immune Deficiency Syndromes* 5 (1992): 513.

38. Domergue-Cloarec, *La santé en Côte d'Ivoire*, p. 69.

39. Ibid., p. 204.

40. Anonymous, "Instructions relatives au développement des services de médecine préventive, hygiène et assistance dans les colonies," Paris, December 30, 1924, *Journal Officiel de la Côte d'Ivoire*, 1925, p. 72.

41. Domergue-Cloarec, *La santé en Côte d'Ivoire*, p. 245.

42. *Conférence économique de la France métropolitaine et d'Outre-mer, Rapports généraux et conclusion d'ensemble* (Paris: Larose, 1935), p. 22.

43. Domergue-Cloarec, *La santé en Côte d'Ivoire*, p. 364.

44. Ibid., p. 586.

45. Ibid., p. 655.

46. *Rapport médical annuel 1942* (Abidjan: Service de santé de Côte d'Ivoire, 1942), p. 27.

47. Domergue-Cloarec, *La santé en Côte d'Ivoire*, p. 1107.

48. Ibid., p. 1154.

49. Ibid., p. 655.

50. Ibid., p. 1038.

51. Evelyne Chevalier, "La lutte contre le sida, des initiatives du côté des grandes entreprises privées du secteur industriel à Abidjan," *Sidalerte* No. 40 (1995): 32.

52. Domergue-Cloarec, *La santé en Côte d'Ivoire*, p. 14.

53. Jeanne-Marie Amat-Roze, "Les inégalités géographiques de l'infection à VIH et du sida en Afrique sub-saharienne," *Social Science and Medicine* 36 (1993): 1252.

54. Domergue-Cloarec, *La santé en Côte d'Ivoire*, p. 444.

55. Anonymous, "Recensement Général de la Population et de l'Habitat, Répartition spatiale de la population et migrations, Tome 2," (Abidjan: République de Côte d'Ivoire, 1992), p. 54.

56. Jean-Claude Arnaud, "Les migrations africaines vers la Côte d'Ivoire," *Cahiers de Géographiques de Rouen*, No. 30 (1988): 53.

57. Domergue-Cloarec, *La santé en Côte d'Ivoire*, p. 1171.

58. De Cock, Odehouri, Moreau, Kouadio, Porter, Barrere, Dialy, and Heyward, "Rapid Emergence of AIDS," p. 408.

59. Ibid., pp. 408, 410.

60. *Rapport mondial sur le développement humain, publié pour le Programme des Nations Unies pour le Développement (PNUD)* (Paris: par Economica, 1994), p. 164.

61. Bi Tah Nguessan, "Aspects économiques de la prise en charge du sida, exemple de centres antituberculeux d'Abidjan." in *Jeunes et préservatifs en Abidjan, une recherche d'ethno-prévention du sida et des NST*, edited by François Deniau (Bingerville: Actes de l'atelier du CRES, 1993), p. 197.

62. *Rapport mondial, 1994*, p. 177.

63. Dédy and Tapé, "Jeunesse, sexualité et sida," p. 85.

64. *Rapport médical annuel, 1931*, p. 46.

65. Jeanne-Marie Amat-Roze and Gèrard-François Dumont, "Le sida et l'avenir de l'Afrique," *Ethique* 2 (1994): 38.

66.   Michel Garenne, "Population africaine et sida," *La chronique du Ceped* 16 (January–March 1995): 2. The quality and reliability of statistics derived from health services have improved considerably since the colonial era. Furthermore, since the mid-1980s epidemiologists have increased the number of investigations into the prevalence of STDs among various population subgroups. The major sources of bias in these statistics at present are thought to stem from underestimates in mortality among women and children.

67.   Ibid., p. 4.

68.   De Cock, Barrere, Lafontaine, Dialy, Gnaore, Pantobe, and Odehourri, "Mortality Trends in Abidjan, Côte d'Ivoire, 1983–1988," p. 395.

69.   Ibid., p. 393.

70.   Abbas Senoussi, "Le sida en Côte d'Ivoire: projections démographiques et épidémiologiques, 1988–2003," in *Jeunes et préservatifs en Abidjan, une recherche d'ethno-prévention du sida et des NST*, edited by François Deniau (Bingerville: Actes de l'atelier du CRES, 19931995), 282.

71.   Ibid., p. 283.

72.   Djomand, Greenberg, Sassan-Morokro, Tossou, Diallo, Ekpini, Ghys, Soro, Brattegaard, Yapi, Odehouri, Coulibaly, Coulibaly, Kadio, Gnaore, and De Cock, "The Epidemic of HIV/AIDS," p. 361.

73.   Kevin M. De Cock, Emmanuel Gnaore, Georgette Adjorlolo, Miles M. Braun, Marie-France Lafontaine, Gilberte Yesso, Geneviève Bretton, Issa M. Coulibaly, Guy-Michel Gershy-Damet, Raymond Bretton, and William L. Heyward, "Risk of Tuberculosis in Patients with HIV-I and HIV-II Infections in Abidjan, Ivory Coast," *British Medical Journal* 302 (1991): 496.

74.   Djomand, Greenberg, Sassan-Morokro, Tossou, Diallo, Ekpini, Ghys, Soro, Brattegaard, Yapi, Odehouri, Coulibaly, Coulibaly, Kadio, Gnaore, and De Cock, "The Epidemic of HIV/AIDS," p. 362.

75.   Verboud, "Que font les centres," p. 14.

76.   Djomand, Greenberg, Sassan-Morokro, Tossou, Diallo, Ekpini, Ghys, Soro, Brattegaard, Yapi, Odehouri, Coulibaly, Coulibaly, Kadio, Gnaore, and De Cock, "The Epidemic of HIV/AIDS," p. 363.

77.   Evelyne Chevalier, *Sida et entreprises, enquête en Côte d'Ivoire* (Lyon: Impact Sida et entreprise, 1995).

78.   Emmanuel Gnaore, "RCI: 40% de cas de sida en Afrique de l'uest," *Sidalerte* No. 38 (1994): 17, 31.

79.   Nathalie Béchu, Eric Chevallier, Agnès Guillaume, and Bi Tah Nguessan, "Les conséquences socio-économiques du sida dans les familles africaines (Burundi et Côte d'Ivoire), premiers jalons, premières réflexions," in *Jeunes et préservatifs en Abidjan, une recherche d'ethno-prévention du sida et des NST*, edited by François Deniau (Bingerville: Actes de l'atelier du CRES, 1993), pp. 219–33.

80.   Béchu, Chevallier, Guillaume, and Nguessan, "Les conséquences socio-économiques," p. 229.

4

A History of Sexually Transmitted Diseases and AIDS in Senegal: Difficulties in Accounting for Social Logics in Health Policy

Charles Becker and René Collignon

Historians still recall the fear aroused in Europe late in the fifteenth century by a certain cataclysmic new disease that broke out near the Kingdom of Naples. It emerged suddenly amid the armies of France and Spain during Charles VIII's expedition to Italy in a troubled context of war and loosening moral standards. It was so new then that there was no name to identify it. The French called it the Neapolitan disease and Italians the French disease. Upon returning to their homes after demobilization, Charles VIII's mercenaries — who were natives of many countries — spread the disease widely throughout Europe. The prestige of the Italian Renaissance contributed largely to popularizing the name *morbus gallicus* for this new scourge and its alleged American origin (which, although controversial, has found advocates throughout the centuries in an ongoing and open-ended debate).[1] French medical practitioners suggested other nomenclature: venereal disease or great pox. Girolamo Fracastoro was the first to propose the name syphilis,[2] which gained wide acceptance only at the end of the eighteenth century; the term most commonly used by doctors and lay people until then was "great pox."

However that may be, it is interesting to note how much syphilis has been, from the very beginning, branded the other's disease or the foreigner's disease. How, then, was this peculiar, devilish, contagious, venereal disease represented a few centuries later within the special context of colonial confrontation between Europeans and Africans? In 1897 the libertarian press, playing with words, ironically referred to the so-called civilizing mission of French soldiers in Madagascar as promoting "syphilization in Madagascar."[3] This philippic echoed the famous saying attributed to Krafft-Ebing, "civilization is syphilization." The eminent German professor[4] was an illustrious representative of a *fin de siècle* Europe marked by an obsessive fear of the taints of civilization. These taints included alcoholism and syphilis, which were regarded as "social scourges."[5] It was precisely during this time that the Old World was launching its colonial conquests. This enterprise was perceived by some propagandists as presenting opportunities for the regeneration of a failing nation still in the throes of the trauma of defeat in the 1870 war with Germany.[6]

European wayfarers had been travelling along the West African coast for many years, at first (and for quite a long time) trading human beings and later for legitimate trade that paved the way for colonization. It was not until the nineteenth century that long-term settlement prospects materialized with the establishment in Senegal of permanent administrative structures. An order dated November 5, 1830, made the French common law enforceable in that colony. Through a specific so-called assimilation policy, the French institutional and administrative model was applied in the parts of Senegal under direct administration. Hence, four communes with full rights were created in this way: Saint Louis and Goree (1872),[7] Rufisque (1880), and Dakar (1887). All of these communes were founded before the establishment in 1895 of a federation of West African territories named *Afrique Occidentale Française* (AOF). Natives of the AOF were French colonial subjects and ruled by so-called indigenous laws. The European residents of the communes, in contrast, were *orginaires* and were granted French citizenship. Although our purpose in this chapter is to focus on Senegal, we shall also consider other territories under French colonial rule in West Africa. This is appropriate because, after the far-reaching reorganization of the AOF from 1902 to 1905, medical and sanitary policy was elaborated at the federal level for the whole group of West African colonies until independence in 1960.

AWARENESS OF VENEREAL DISEASES

Awareness of venereal diseases and proof of their existence in AOF started fairly early in urban areas with initial reference to two specific groups: prostitutes and the military. In September 1882, the internal affairs officer, acting as head officer, informed the civil physician in Saint-Louis (capital of Senegal), "In view of the considerable number of venereal disease cases in town, serious measures should be taken and loose girls sent regularly to the hospital for check up."[8] The doctor was requested to examine those "girls" carefully and to keep in hospital those who presented with questionable signs until they were totally recovered. Full cooperation with the administrator was expected from the physician, who was also to prepare a status report on prostitution in Saint-Louis.[9] In his reply, dated September 28, Duchoud indicated that:

Authorized prostitution in Saint-Louis did not include brothels. Girls were not subjected to weekly consultations. Prostitutes registered directly with the police. On my arrival there were ten to twelve of such girls registered. Three of them have died, one is in prison, and another one is in hospital suffering from typhus. The police list has been given to the hospital staff so that they will report any absences from regular consultations. As for underground prostitution, the most dangerous form — which exists according to rumors — the police are in a better position to provide the most accurate information. Certainly, common and hereditary syphilis are very prevalent and considered to be normal by people who declare they have it without any shame and often without basis. Out of an average of 600 newborns per year, about 60 die. This figure is twice that in France and it is unfortunate that general treatment that needs to be of a long duration is unaffordable due to exaggeratedly high drug prices.[10]

On the preceding day, September 27, the police superintendent of Saint-Louis informed the internal affairs officer that he had "ordered women whose behavior is notably unhealthy to be taken to the hospital for a detailed examination."[11] In a letter dated June 8, 1897, the AOF governor general informed the internal affairs director of a high prevalence of venereal diseases among military troops based in Saint-Louis and Dakar and requested all municipalities to undertake surveillance in this regard.[12] A few days later, the governor of Senegal stated:

The conditions under which prostitution was occurring in Senegal made preventive measures such as those implemented in European cities impracticable. For it is not in the streets that such actions take place that would have facilitated surveillance by vice squads who could then keep records on those indulging in such an activity. As for controlling prostitution in brothels, it is easier to imagine than to actually establish because those ready to undertake such commerce are yet to be located, and no such request has been reported so far. The attempt made [to establish a brothel] some years ago at Ndar Toute[13] was not successful but some local entrepreneurs are likely to take it over. The Public Administration can not achieve efficient surveillance unless cases of infected women, and brothels where infection is detected are reported. If military officials could provide such information — which should be easy since a number of their soldiers have had hazardous contacts — police could then track down women thus reported and necessary steps could be taken to cure them.[14]

During the same month, Colonel Pujol, the Senegal troops' commander-in-chief, informed the AOF governor general of the sanitary measures taken against venereal diseases and wrote to the internal affairs director on July 1, 1897, about an African soldier in the Saint-Louis garrison suffering from a venereal disease.[15]

The first overall picture of the venereal disease problem in the colonial territories was given at the beginning of the twentieth century by an inspector general in charge of health in the colonies. After he reviewed various medical reports received at the Ministry for Colonies from 1890 onward, Inspector Kermorgant noted that the colonies had acquired a bad reputation and had been considered high prevalence areas for venereal diseases for quite some time.[16] He reinstated the 1888 measures taken by the *Ministère de la Marine et des Colonies* to prevent importation of such diseases into France.[17] Those measures focused on the military and prostitutes; any contaminated person was detained for treatment in hospital until the complete disappearance of the first visible symptoms. After that he or she was still regularly controlled and received drugs; a constant control was imposed on prostitutes. Kermorgant further noted that doctors in the colonies put a greater emphasis on diseases specific to tropical countries. Yet medical reports from the colonies convinced him of the need to protect the African colonies and elsewhere against diseases from abroad. This decision was made despite the difficulties in implementing preventive steps (caused, for example, by the governors' fears of alienating the populations they governed or confronting elected assemblies in the four Senegalese communes).

Kermorgant observed that in Senegal — where prostitution was neither regulated nor controlled — venereal diseases were quite common. Blennorrhagia (gonorrhea) was prevalent among the military. It was also found in its acute form among newly arrived Europeans and in its chronic form among black soldiers. In 1898 venereal diseases accounted for 177 out of 1,000 days of treatment for Europeans and 270.2 out of 1,000 days of treatment for Africans according to hospital statistics. Kermorgant concluded that venereal disease infections were highly prevalent, especially considering that 90 percent of Africans admitted to the hospital for other infections also had chronic urethritis and almost all of them had syphilis.[18] According to the same author's data, however, some years later (1905 and 1906) AOF ranked last among French colonies along with New Caledonia in prevalence of venereal infections among the European military. In these colonial territories there were 11.4 cases of syphilis per 1,000 population, 17.5 blennorrhagia cases per 1,000, and 53.6 cases per 1,000 for all venereal diseases combined. Yet, morbidity among African troops appeared to be about one-third of that among European soldiers. This may be explained by the fact that African soldiers were authorized to live with their spouses. Presumably they had less opportunity of becoming infected than Europeans. In addition, African troops were often assigned to geographically remote positions without doctors, and so often were missed in medical examinations and reports.[19]

In addition to an interest in assessing the scope of public health problems arising from sexually transmitted diseases (STDs), there were new concerns about sanitation. After the establishment of administrative authority over the whole country (Senegal and other territories of AOF) there was a pressing need for more physicians to respond to the needs of the increasing population under colonial rule. Physicians were also need-ed to treat colonial personnel and to confront the diverse disease ecologies of an expanding colonial domain. In a report to the AOF governor gener-al, Rangé, inspector of civil health services, proposed training young physicians who would be posted to pacified areas and provide medical assistance to African populations. An order dated February 8, 1905, insti-tuted Medical Assistance to Natives after poor health conditions and dreadful mortality were revealed among populations of West Africa.[20] In a circular dated April 12, 1905, Governor General Ernest Roume ordered that surveys be conducted in each colony of AOF in order to determine the causes of mortality and how they might be prevented, particularly among children.[21] The resulting civil health service inspection report[22] indicated excessively high mortality because of two major types of dis-eases: ordinary diseases caused by poverty, poor hygiene, and "dirt" (tuberculosis ranked first, followed by syphilis and alcoholism) and dis-eases that were presented to be specific to those countries at that time (endemic beriberi, leprosy, trypanosomiasis, malaria, and epidemic cere-brospinal meningitis, typhoid fever, and smallpox).

Venereal diseases were dealt with in the context of an interest in these so-called diseases of misery — an interest that was new in the colonies. Such an approach may sound like a sociological perspective. More pre-cisely, the general point of view of the report reflects the deep influence of the new perspective introduced in France by the hygienists on health matters at the end of the nineteenth century. The promotion of the trio of tuberculosis, syphilis, and alcoholism to the rank of "social scourges"[23] by European hygienists was based on a convergence of social fears and sta-tistical observations. These theories came about in the context of urban-ization and industrialization characterized by unhealthy living conditions and promiscuity — conditions denounced in the first studies in medical geography and sociology. This era was also characterized by the influence of Social Darwinism. Among the elite, Social Darwinism comforted the fear of human degeneration, which was thought to be the inevitable result of the abuses in the popular classes, such as venereal disease and alcohol abuse. Hygienists of this period were also fascinated by the use of statis-tics, despite their doubtful and deceptive nature at the time. During this period the French government became haunted by the fear of depopula-tion and passed two major modern laws on gratuitous medical assistance (1893) and on public health preservation (1902).[24] High-level health authorities in both the metropolitan ministry offices and in the West African colonies adopted a similar perspective.

In his report Gallay indicated that it was impossible to state definitely the number of syphilis cases in AOF.[25] He did, however, give some general (and sometimes contradictory) information about forms of the disease, its geographic distribution, and its sequelae. For example, he observed that secondary and tertiary attacks accounted for half of the consultations in county clinics, especially in Podor (on the bank of Senegal River), at the trade points along the river, and along the railway running from Saint-Louis to Dakar. Demand for potassium iodide in these locations often overwhelmed the scanty budgets and supplies. The Animist populations in the Southern colonies of Ivory Coast and Dahomey seemed less affected by syphilis than the Islamic peoples of the North,[26] but were more affected by the consequences of increasing alcoholism. The greatest concerns raised by syphilis among these populations in the minds of colonial sanitation authorities related to its effects on child mortality, abortion, premature childbirth, and child mental deficiency. To prevent the depopulation of the colonies, Gallay recommended the creation of an autonomous smallpox vaccine service to be staffed by a corps of native medical assistants. This was accomplished in the order dated January 7, 1906.[27]

WORLD WAR I AND THE DEMOGRAPHIC OBSESSION

World War I heightened this demographic obsession because of such factors as the poor health of young Africans, which became more apparent during the massive process of recruiting black troops at the beginning of the war. Furthermore, the high demographic cost of the conflict exacerbated the urgent need for manpower to develop the colonies and prompted the colonial party to launch an active campaign for the development or promotion of so-called "colonial reservoirs."[28] This strong trend in metropolitan public opinion turned into a large development program of which Albert Sarraut was one of the keenest defenders.[29] Sarraut emphasized the role that the colonies could play in increasing the greatness of France after World War I. He argued that the colonies had a threefold purpose of serving France: to increase its population and give it greater manpower, to make a financial contribution to the nation, and to supply France with the raw materials it needed.[30]

The Inter-War Years

In the aftermath of the war, the native health issue in AOF was clearly connected to concerns about labor shortage and, thus, was expressed in terms of (re)production, "the native race had to be developed qualitatively and quantitatively." Governor Carde's slogan, *"faire du noir"* ("produce 'Blackies'"), was relayed over the years by the administrators. In his journal of the Dakar-Djibouti ethnography mission, Michel Leiris noted the following on July 14, 1931, at the French National Feast in Tonkoto (a gloomy subprefecture of French Sudan): "After the distribution of small presents, the administrator closing the ceremony, had the following statement translated, after he read it very loudly in French: 'Now, you will go to bed and work to get babies! Because when there are a lot of babies, there is a lot of income tax!' ... The interpreter repeated faithfully the formula and everybody went away light-hearted."[31]

This attitude brought a radical change in the doctrine of action regarding STDs; a ministerial circular dated December 10, 1924, ordered that "curative medical assistance had to give way to social preventive medicine." This change was supported by a considerable increase in medical staff. The circular of Governor General Merlin dated April 12, 1921, confirmed by a circular of Governor General Carde dated March 12, 1924, emphasized the social role to be played by African auxiliaries. The circulars spoke of the need to increase the numbers of auxiliaries and to encourage midwives to visit African families in a sustained effort to improve child health and to advocate hygiene. Carde's circular of February 15, 1926, gave specific instructions about these objectives and the means by which to implement them.[32] A circular of March 5, 1927, relates the first results recorded from these activities and provides some supplementary guidelines to their implementation. The circular of August 1, 1930, focuses on infant protection and worker health.

The inter-war years were marked by a substantial fear of syphilis by French medical administrative authorities in both France[33] and AOF. During this time the picture of the threat of venereal disease became denser and more complex in colonial medical reporting. The ever-present demographic concern led to a close retrospective look at data on stillbirth rates and infant mortality recorded in health facilities in Dakar between 1890 and the early 1920s.[34] In 1923 Thiroux compared these figures from Senegal to more recent data on the ravages of congenital syphilis (such as abortions and infant mortality) given by Hata[35] for Japanese women with a positive Wassermann reaction (but without clinical signs of syphilis). Several childhood afflictions among native populations in West Africa and more specifically athrepsia (marasmus) were sequelae of congenital syphilis as evidenced by blood tests, and "the superiority of sulfasenol treatment over vegetable soups [that is, a nutritious diet]"[36] was confirmed. The relative immunity of Africans to venereal syphilis as suggested by Jeanselme in 1904 and possible diagnosis errors were major issues.[37] The assumed immunity of Africans seemed to be based on the mildness of symptoms or on the fact that the African adult was relatively resilient to malaria as compared to the white population, for whom malaria-associated syphilis was seen to be extremely virulent.[38] Fournier referred to this combination of diseases as "exotic syphilis."[39] The extreme malignancy of exotic syphilis in Europeans was thought to be due to co-infection with malaria, as demonstrated by thorough etiological analysis of blood slides. Thiroux[40] noted on the contrary that if African adults were not very sensitive, their children were hardly affected by malaria,[41] which, he stressed, had a major effect on the virulence of syphilis.

New Specialized Facilities and Medicines

With more appropriate specialized institutions and facilities gradually put in place — *Institut Prophylactique*,[42] *Institut d'Hygiène Sociale*,[43] community clinics, and specialist consultants[44] — Africans were followed more closely and their diseases detected through new scientific methods. Hence the deceitful and sly nature of the epidemic among them[45] was better understood. A new conviction that "Certain ethnic groups like the Fulani and Tukulor, were almost all infected with syphilis" appeared in the medical reports, and some doctors stated that "eighty percent of the population of Dakar were infected."[46] The scope of the problem did not dwindle with the passing years, although results of treatment were generally positive; reporters delighted in underscoring the quick curative action of arsenical medications. These drugs were replacing the other inter-war anti-syphilis medications because of their easy administration and ready acceptance by local populations.[47]

Therapeutic options had, of course, evolved greatly since the medical instructions of 1876 issued for posts without doctors.[48] These old recommendations included the use of a mixture of copaiba and cubeb (local emollient baths), zinc sulfate injections, lead acetate, and calomel. However, at the beginning of the twentieth century the soda salt from arsenic acid (atoxyl) that Thomas and Breinl in Liverpool proved effective for treating trypanosomiasis[49] in 1905 was used by French practitioners to treat syphilis in West Africa. In 1908 Bargy at Gaoua, Sudan, reported 32 cases of syphilis (6 primary, 17 secondary, and 9 tertiary) that were rapidly and successfully treated using this method, apparently to the patients' great satisfaction.[50] Injections of Van Swieten liquor and mercury were used alternatively in the cure of a same person. Bargy reported the constant, rapid, and successful results of this new specific treatment for the great pox and the absence of medical complications (common with mercury injections). It was also painless. However, he recommended not giving more than 4 grams because this drug was a poison. Because of its toxicity, its usage was abandoned and some other products proposed.

In Frankfurt, Ehrlich had developed in 1910 an organic arsenical preparation injected intravenously called 606 (or Salvarsan, an arsphenamine), which was later modified into the more easily used 914 (Neo-Salvarsan or novarsphenamine).[51] In 1921 Sazerac and Lavaditi discovered the treponemocide properties of bismuth. With arsenical medications and bismuth doctors claimed they could defeat the disease.[52] A Health Service inspection report made to the governor general of AOF dated August 1, 1922, recommended preventive measures.[53] In particular, it suggested that abortive or curative treatment of primary syphilis at community clinics, maternity wards, examination rooms for prostitutes, or hospitals be provided through the use of mercury salts, arsenic, or bismuth. These were drugs preferred in the absence of arsphenamines, which, although having a more powerful bleaching effect (easing of the symptoms), were quite expensive. For tertiary lesions, the report suggested the use of iodide in association with mercurial medications. Iodide was very expensive and required high doses in a prolonged course of treatment. Thus, its use in a mixed iodide treatment was prioritized for pregnant women and young children with hereditary syphilis.[54] On the contrary mercury salts were to be distributed generously to patients. Budgetary constraints were still bitterly felt as demand increased for arsenical products within a population that was appreciative of the successful results of injections.[55] In the context of global economic crisis during the 1930s, bismuth- and mercury-based medications were to be given priority once again.[56]

Difficulties and Blaming Africans' Attitudes

However, the hopeful prospects introduced by the new therapeutic possibilities[57] were thwarted by constant difficulties in implementation in the field among African populations. The medical community constantly implicated African attitudes as the root of the problem. It was as if the physicians wanted to exculpate themselves from their helplessness by blaming their patients. They denounced the "natives' unbelievable lack of privacy," "excessive copulation,"[58] and their patients' indifference to blennorrhagia and the symptoms of primary syphilis.[59] When physicians were not busy excoriating Africans for their sexual behavior, they were complacently pointing to popular local beliefs and prejudices according to which blennorrhagia was held to give males special procreative abilities. This was thought to be because of the special erethism of the penis caused by urethral irritation. Virtually all authors stressed the "natives' incredible carelessness" about the disease and its treatment.[60] The infection was also believed to make the semen "thicker."[61] According to another prejudice, sexual intercourse with a virgin was supposed to cure chronic blennorrhagia.[62]

Colonial confidence in the civilizing mission of promoting and improving the health conditions of Africans was often shattered by the harsh realities in the field where diagnosis was difficult. For instance, after the era of symptom-based diagnosis, the Wassermann reaction (discovered in the first decade of the twentieth century) revealed that the scope of syphilis infection was larger than ever suspected.[63] It seemed to be even more so with the advent of large scale big yards in Senegal and West African colonies and the significant labor migrations they produced. Railways and the new road networks also indirectly contributed to the expansion of STDs in AOF.[64] Furthermore, prevention was complicated by the frequently overlooked sequelae of blennorrhagia and by late or incomplete treatment.[65] Arsenical medications were also attacked.[66] Although their quick action, easy administration, and acceptance by patients prompted intensive use, they were often not used long enough to do more than merely mask symptoms. It gradually became apparent that neither clinical observation nor laboratory tests could definitely establish whether recovery was complete. Hence, the health service's strategy was to emphasize a reorientation to pathogen-focussed control efforts, for syphilis at least, that stressed identification and treatment.[67]

The limited reach of the institutes of hygiene or anti-venereal clinics situated in urban areas was to be supplemented in rural practice by the administration of polyvalent medications at sufficiently high dosages to ensure long-lasting cure of the infection. This practice accommodated the common impatience with long-term treatment among African populations. The context of global economic crisis in the 1930s coupled with repeated warnings — from Marcel Léger[68] in particular — about the risks of relapsed infection from inadequate treatment with arsenical prescriptions prompted a renewed preference for bismuth- and mercury-based drugs. Treatment with sublimate pills was to be left to patients only under exceptional conditions. Treatment at dermato-venereology clinics in towns was improved through regular blood testing and prevention-oriented home visits conducted by nurses.[69] In 1932 a special place for STD consultation was opened in Sor, a suburb of Saint-Louis. External treatment of blennorrhagia by repeatedly applying washing conducted in sanitary facilities had a chance of succeeding only in a restricted category of disciplined and well-informed patients (referred to as evolved in colonial ideological discourse). For other more restive patients, gonacrine injections were successfully used. The African population was favorably impressed by injections and its yearning was to be cured in one single consultation. However, over the entire range of therapy, there was no product that was genuinely effective for the masses.

THE NEW ERA OF ANTIBIOTICS

The advent of antibiotics, starting with the introduction of penicillin in 1943, began a new era in the biomedical treatment of STDs. In the early 1950s extencillin allowed mass treatment with one single low-cost injection. It was a true revolution. Meanwhile, major changes were made to the doctrine instituted by Jamot when he was head of the Permanent Mission for the Prevention of Trypanosomiasis. Jamot had initiated mobile medicine in 1926 in Cameroon and in 1932 in AOF. The Independent General Service for Sleeping Sickness was created in 1939 with biochemistry and entomology laboratories. A nursing school was also set up in Bobo-Dioulasso to organize control activities throughout AOF (which was divided into sectors). Mobile preventive medicine employed trained African staff who took laboratories to rural areas. Following the Brazzaville Conference in June 1944, the Independent General Service for Sleeping Sickness became the General Mobile Hygiene and Preventive Service and was concerned with several major endemic diseases including syphilis (bejel, a variant of endemic, non-venereal syphilis). The importance of such a service was to be fully realized only after 1949, with the creation of a mobile group conducting investigations in the Sahelian areas of Niger (in Djerma-Songhai lands) and Senegal River Valley (in Podor). The General Mobile Hygiene and Preventive Service thus included treponematoses. In 1955 mass campaigns were extended to other treponematoses (pian, or yaws)[70] in forest areas. In 1957 intensive control activities were conducted under international guidance and using international means, such as the intensive use of slow-release penicillin.[71]

Problems of Differential Diagnosis among Treponematoses in the 1950s

Research on various aspects of the treponematoses problem increased, with special attention paid to the diagnosis of congenital syphilis.[72] The importance of pian became a clear indicator of social changes and progress in health education and hygiene and was more of a social issue than a medical one.[73] Gradually, a focus endemic syphilis[74] was clearly identified in Senegal, mostly affecting the Fulani nomad people's grazing lands.[75] Treponematoses prevalence rates among various sedentary populations that were previously overlooked were being assessed among the Bedik people in East Senegal[76] and the Serer around the groundnut growing area.[77] Epidemiological data based on patient records at the Institut d'Hygiéne Sociale provided information about syphilis for both urban dwellers[78] and some rural ones[79] (Figure 4.1).

The disturbingly high frequency of positive blood tests that remained positive after treatment was a major concern. This raised the difficult issue of differential diagnosis between endemic syphilis, congenital syphilis, and the latent forms[80] and emphasized the limited reliability of serological reactions. It also may have had direct administrative consequences for some African workers and constituted a social injustice if used in rejecting for international labor migration African candidates coming from regions with (sometimes unknown) focus of endemic syphilis.[81] Western medicine has enormous difficulties in establishing scientific criteria for differential diagnosis between venereal syphilis and

FIGURE 4.1
Focuses of Endemic Syphilis in Senegal, Circa 1965

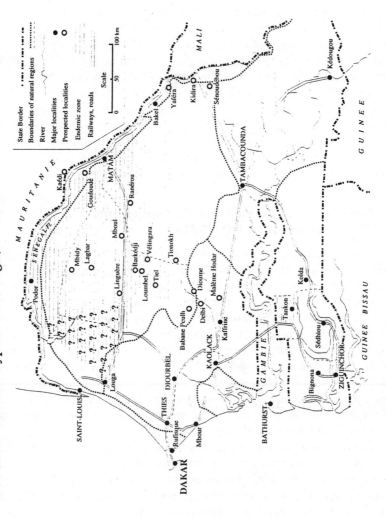

Sources: Adapted from Basset et al. (1963, p. 176) and Boiron et al. (1965, p. 410).

other remaining human treponematoses.[82] An increasing number of elements tend to substantiate the unity of the parasite (*Treponema pallidum*) in the on-going and open-ended debate between the partisans of a unitarian concept of treponematoses and the defenders of a plurality of germs.[83]

Although we do see similarities between the AOF case — at least on its main principles — and the analysis by Megan Vaughan[84] of British colonial views of the syphilis epidemic in Baganda-land (Uganda) at the beginning of the century and of the colonial efforts to overcome it, British and French colonial views on certain issues were not identical. In francophone West Africa, for instance, the Christian missionary lobby had a lesser impact on sexual matters in countries that were heavily involved in Islamic culture. The church-state separation that occurred in French political life at the beginning of the twentieth century (1904) soon applied in the colonial administration's context with deeply anti-clerical components. This is highlighted in the slight socio-moralizing tone of colonial papers dealing with STDs. Prejudices in colonial medical circles as reflected in medical reports stigmatized — in lay terms — the African population's indifference or carelessness in the face of STDs rather than viewing the issue as one of African immorality. The oldest texts did, however, stigmatize Africans for "excessively copulating." This obsessive fear of morbid copulation[85] was common in that period of the twentieth century marked by the fears of degeneration of humankind. These fears derived from popularized ideas of Social Darwinism. The French historian Alain Corbin[86] stresses how in the continuous dialogue between medicine and society, medical staff and their discourse (the hereditary syphilis theory, for instance) merely translated the collective fantasies of their times into scientific language. In this respect, the prejudices and attitudes of colonial doctors toward African populations were not so different from those of their counterparts in Europe at the time who held a mixture of contempt and fear toward the European lower classes, another category of people who were regarded as immature.

Prostitution

The history of prostitution in Senegal is still to be constructed. Archival materials on the issue are rather scarce, thus showing how the regularizing system, or French system,[87] found it more difficult to operate in this domain than anywhere else. The regularist project — first designed by Parent-Duchâtelet[88] — considered the management of prostitution as a "matter of refuse collection," of maintaining order and decency along public ways and in public places. Prostitution was not an offense per se, because criminal law only condemned public indecent exposure as an offense against public decency (*Code pénal*, Article 334). Prostitutes were, therefore, not subject to police or magistrates' courts, but only to local municipal regulations and administrative authority (which tended to be arbitrary in terms of enforcement).

There are many examples of the difficulties faced by the public authorities in the AOF trying to regulate prostitution and in finding managers for identified brothels that were supposed to be easily controllable under regulation. Some hygienists, however, suggested the establishment of a vice squad that would collaborate with the preventive medical service.[89] Whereas European prostitution seemed to be under control[90] its native counterpart escaped virtually all control. Lhuerre deplored the fact that the vice squad did not apply to African and mulatto prostitutes in the provisions of the order of January 13, 1926. The colonial practice of *"prendre mousso"*("to take a native woman," in the colonial jargon of French Sudan) also contributed to restricting prostitutes from being referred to health facilities. Military doctors tacitly encouraged this practice among male colonial staff, believing that it would guarantee sanitary safety. African companions were supposed to "entertain, care, dispel boredom and thus prevent Europeans from indulging in alcoholism and sexual depravity that were unfortunately so frequent in hot climates."[91] However, because the transformations of the African social and economic order called almost exclusively for male labor, large-scale migrations ensued and indigenous prostitution developed. Another characteristic of modern prostitution in much of Africa is that organized procuring seldom exists.[92]

THE AIDS ERA IN SENEGAL

In Senegal, as in many other African countries, AIDS occurred with the emergence, resurgence, or persistence of other major health problems: the resistance of malaria to conventional drugs, the reappearance of cholera after some 80 years of silence, and the persistence of cerebrospinal meningitis, tuberculosis, malnutrition, and diarrhoeal diseases. There is often a discrepancy between degree of medical awareness of a problem's existence and scope and the layman's social awareness. Initial lay reactions to AIDS include denial or the use of a discourse minimizing the existence and seriousness of the disease. An analysis of such reactions highlights the opposite rationales invoked by the various actors and their differing and competing discourses about the epidemic.[93] Before 1986 the Senegalese media were giving information on the epidemic's development elsewhere in the world and in other African countries at the same time that local scientists were actively involved in research on human and simian retroviruses. In 1985–86 these scientists played an active part in the discovery of HIV-II.[94] Yet the presence of the infection in the country had still not been announced. By mid-1986, though, the first cases were reported and were considered to be of foreign origin.

The National AIDS Prevention Program

Structures for confronting the epidemic were rapidly established, however. The Senegalese scientists who were participating in research and who kept abreast of the epidemic's spread in Africa and elsewhere around the world were convinced of the need to promote prevention. Yet the media and those engaged in common discourse persisted in overlooking the presence of the disease and its impact. The policy for managing the epidemic remains deeply marked by previous STD control models; HIV infection and AIDS are viewed as social diseases similar to other STDs. A National Multidisciplinary Committee for AIDS Prevention (*Comité National Pluridisciplinaire de Prévention du Sida* [CNPS]) was created in 1988. Located at the Institut d'Hygiène Sociale, the committee has a more or less conscious perception of AIDS as a social disease inspired by the pattern of STDs that makes it focus on preventive specific human measures more difficult to implement than those regarding other transmitted infections. However, two medical units are playing a key role: the Bacteriology/Virology Laboratory, which conducts blood testing of STDs and AIDS and epidemiological follow-up of these diseases, and the Infectious Diseases Ward of Fan's University Teaching Hospital, which conducts clinical studies and carries out patient treatment.

The CNPS encourages control and research and leaves a large action-oriented share of prevention work to nongovernmental organizations and other associations. Epidemiological surveillance, testing in blood collection units, and medical care are combined under the CNPS's authority. Both prevention and control have their advocates within the CNPS, which has been expanded while keeping its autonomy from the Ministry for Health. The leading members of CNPS have held their posts since its inception, despite frequent reshuffling within the ministry. Its guidelines and actions have been praised in international conferences by such foreign organizations as the World Health Organization and the United Nations AIDS Organization, which support national AIDS control programs.

Assessments of awareness of HIV/AIDS have been attempted since the first cases were reported. In 1989 a study was conducted on the population of Dakar and its suburbs, as well as a standardized knowledge, attitudes, beliefs, and practices survey initiated at the request of the World Health Organization. However, findings concerning Senegal have not been published; the reasons for this are unknown. Studies using more sophisticated methodologies and implemented in selected rural areas revealed that the regions of Kaolack,[95] Ziguinchor,[96] Fatick,[97] and Kolda[98] were very little affected by HIV. These studies provided a better picture of rural perceptions of STDs and indicated that rural populations were not well aware of AIDS. There has heretofore been no in-depth study on the most affected regions (Saint-Louis, Louga, Diourbel, Thiès, and

Tambacounda), which would have allowed the evolution of awareness to be followed, and the impact of past and recent initiatives for prevention and education to be assessed. In 1992–93 a demographic and health survey largely confirmed the relative scarcity at the national level of knowledge about AIDS, its modes of transmission, and methods of prevention.[99]

Yet, academic work on HIV/AIDS is developing, especially in the medical field. There have been some 200 doctoral theses on HIV, AIDS, and STDs at the Faculty of Medicine and Pharmacy of the University of Dakar (90 percent of which have been submitted since 1986);[100] presentations on AIDS at international meetings; publications in journals;[101] sustained participation in international research on HIV (particularly on HIV-II); and facilitation of regional and continent-wide training courses organized regularly in Dakar since 1993.

Epidemiological Data

One of the CNPS's main tasks has been to follow the evolution of the pandemic in Senegal through data collected by the sero-epidemiological surveillance group. Sentinel surveillance for AIDS only, on six target groups (blood donors, pregnant women, prostitutes, men with STDs, hospital patients, and tuberculosis patients) was initially restricted to four towns but was extended to six in 1992. It also now includes surveillance on other STDs, notably syphilis. In addition, forecasts have been made[102] that give grounds for optimism on the part of public health authorities, with an estimated prevalence rate lower than 1 percent among the adult population. Case reporting is still limited. As Figure 4.2 indicates, there were 1,846 cumulative cases between 1986 and January 1996. For 1993 the estimated figures were 54,042 HIV positive people and 3,468 AIDS patients.[103] In 1994 the estimated adjusted seroprevalence rate for the general population over 15 years of age was 0.95 percent or 36,485 people with HIV infection (including 23,969 men). The cumulative number of deaths was thought to be 8,188.[104]

The information available on HIV/AIDS in Senegal generally relates to epidemiological, virological, clinical, and treatment issues. Few data are available on the social issues, with the exception of sexual behavior,[105] migration,[106] and prevention efforts among Dimba and Lawbe women.[107] There has been more research in urban than rural areas. Data on rural locations are scattered and primarily concern Casamance, the Kedougou area,[108] Sine,[109] and the Senegal River area where migration to countries both within and outside of Africa has been correlated to the presence of HIV-I.[110]

A review of media reports shows a slow evolution in the social perception of AIDS and reveals the reluctance to confront the epidemic long shared by the general public and newsmen. Newspapers started reporting on

FIGURE 4.2

Cumulative AIDS Cases Reported from Senegal, 1986 to January 1996

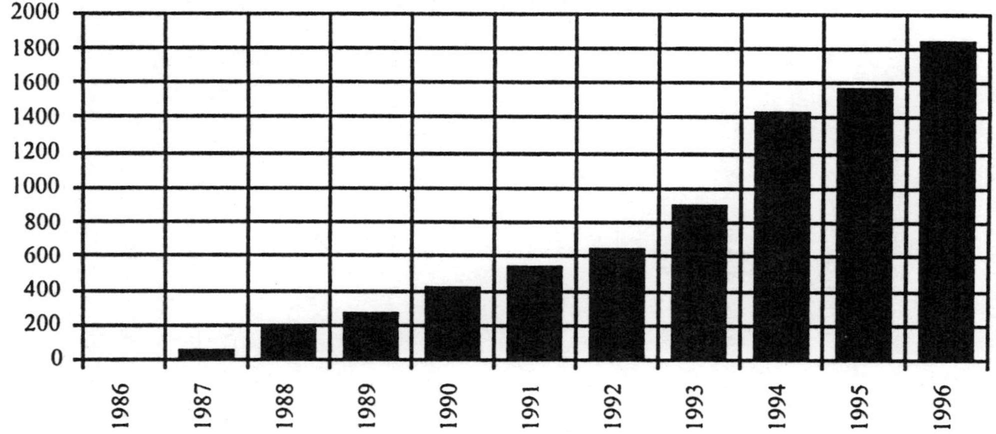

Source: Compiled by authors from data provided by the Senegal National AIDS Control Program.

AIDS as a problem in Senegal only in 1986. Earlier, brief articles located the disease elsewhere and conveyed very negative views on the disease and those afflicted with it. These reports rejected the idea of an African origin for HIV by emphasizing that the virus was first identified and reached high prevalence in the United States and Europe. Following official reports of the first cases in Senegal in 1986, newspaper coverage included both new and recurring topics, often reporting reactions of denial similar to those recorded elsewhere in Africa. Because the epidemiological situation was regarded as less alarming than in other African countries, the journalists made reference to specific concerns. They stressed the need for more scientific studies and more preventive action, but they did not refer to the therapeutic activities and other counseling and support activities by biomedical staff and nongovernmental organizations.

Since the very first cases — considered as imported — there are regular accounts of the role played by migrants and other high risk groups (prostitutes, drug addicts, homosexuals) in spreading the epidemic. Reference to risky behaviors is often just euphemistic talk that does not conceal the assumed relationship of AIDS to certain social groups. Designating migrants from a given region or an ethnic group as the vectors of epidemics constitutes an obstacle to prevention. Furthermore, AIDS has often been compared by politicians and newsmen to other fatal diseases like malaria with an intent to highlight that there were other health priorities aside from HIV.

There has been a large gap between the active involvement of Senegalese scientists in international research work[111] and the common understanding of this complex epidemic and its scope, which even the Senegalese intellectuals find difficult to comprehend. This is particularly reflected in the abundance of accounts of scientific meetings and the emphasis on the role played by Senegalese scientists, as compared to the scarcity of data on the spread of the epidemic in Africa and the problems it raises for health care systems and African societies. Nevertheless, in 1986 research authorities who were actively involved in CNPS activities focused more on education and prevention, but the results were less important than the expected achievements. Using epidemiological statistics, health authorities have often vehemently claimed an illusory control over epidemics — not only AIDS but also cholera and yellow fever. At the same time their claims are met with reluctance from non-medical circles to talk about health-related social issues (especially those raised by AIDS) and shyness about offering reflections on the pandemic.

Social Actors Facing AIDS

The possible role of traditional healers and their pharmacopoeia in STDs and AIDS prevention and management is seldom dealt with in Senegal and has so far given rise only to brief debate. This debate has highlighted old conflicts. Journalists have shown little interest in the possible contribution of traditional medicine, and certain doctors have firmly rejected it. Yet in order to have a significant impact on the spread of STDs and AIDS in Africa, an active cooperation between the modern and traditional health care systems has been underscored as desirable, normal, and inevitable.[112] Reflection on this issue is still insufficient in Senegal and has not yet led to the development of collaborative approaches.[113]

The publicity given to events organized by associations or in outlying regions is part of the strategies devised by various groups suggesting varying solutions and cautiously advising the use of condoms. Events organized and publicized by local associations in outlying regions are part of a diverse set of strategies devised by local actors. These strategies suggest varying solutions to the problem of AIDS founded on traditional and religious values, which are very reluctant to advise the use of condoms. Moral and religious leaders who long stood back from debate and action have recently become involved. The causes and modalities of that new commitment, which has been promoted by the AIDS Control and Prevention project,[114] require further analysis.

Because of the atmosphere of denial surrounding the epidemic, prevention has not been easy to implement. Prevention has too exclusively been targeted at risk groups, such as prostitutes, and neglected other groups. Furthermore, there are difficulties in devising specific messages for other groups. Despite some experiments conducted over the past years in three towns (Dakar, Kaolack, and Ziguinchor) and in the most heavily AIDS-affected regions, very few programs have been directed to youth — to apprentices, workers of varying status, pupils, and students.

Furthermore, reflections on the ethical and legal aspects of AIDS are not well developed in Senegal, even though the CNPS includes a subcommittee dedicated to such issues that was established fairly early. This may be related to the low prevalence rate recorded and published in the country and the epidemic's virtual invisibility suggested by the official discourse. Current debates in more severely stricken countries (in Eastern, Central, and Southern Africa)[115] about drug trials, testing, confidentiality, rights of people with HIV, and related issues are not yet well developed in Senegal. However, a national team has been formed, and it has participated in the Dakar Consultation of June 1994 that formalized the establishment of the African network on ethics, law, and HIV. The Dakar Consultation adopted a declaration stating ten basic principles to safeguard the rights of infected people.[116] The development of associations of people with HIV seems to be partly hindered by a desire to keep secret the identity of infected individuals in a context of low prevalence and fear of stigmatization.

The Senegalese community has been unequally confronted with the HIV epidemic from region to region, and the infection has spread less rapidly than in other African countries.[117] The model by which the epidemic has been managed is considered by CNPS and UNAIDS authorities[118] to explain this slower rate of spread; but other factors including religious, moral, and social factors are also thought to contribute. As everywhere else, the community's perception of AIDS was initially limited before the disease became visible and a directly noticeable reality. For a large majority it remains so, and denial is still frequent. In areas that seem least affected most people are not aware of AIDS and even deny its very existence.[119] In the absence of a genuine knowledge of the infection based on experience, popular discourses about AIDS, such as traditional African representations associated with evil, disease, and misfortune, may just express a personal denial to believe in this very special disease that is a serious and frequent occurrence for others. Such public discourses may disseminate and reactivate a lot of traditional representations associated with evil, its origins, and modes of transmission. These profoundly grounded representations, largely shared, do not facilitate the acceptance of a modern medical message in the absence of genuinely effective medicine and appropriate counseling and support.

PROVISIONAL CONCLUSION

The history of STDs, health policies, and conceptions implemented by colonial rulers highlights an often ambiguous relationship between the demographic themes of concern over population growth and health for the development of colonies and the theme of sanitation that has been recurring in venereal disease control programs. Some practices are constant, particularly those pertaining to the status of the diseases long considered as social scourges and stigmatized as such. Because they jeopardized the population growth desired by the colonial administration and were more difficult to control than other diseases, they were classified as separate from other kinds of afflictions and were dealt with very much as AIDS is today.

Recent historical research on West African demographic evolution during the last century underlines the interactions between the four parameters constituting the demographic regime: fertility, nuptiality, migrations, and mortality. This approach put forward the study of mortality (subsequently study of attached morbidity), because this parameter lies at the confluence of demography and health. Mortality often reflects sanitary crises or progress, as it appears through demographic and health statistics. This approach focuses on the inception of the demographic transition in Africa and encompasses concerns of ill health and death among the African population. Despite the limits and the distortions of colonial statistics[120] as well as of postcolonial ones, these data can be taken into account. Nevertheless, the too few available studies need to be expanded and widened for a better understanding of the positive and negative factors affecting past mortality, especially "the social context of health and illness in contemporary Africa, the inequalities in terms of access to good health."[121] The first historical studies on demography and health in Senegal pointed out that sanitary measures, especially vaccination programs, may have had a real impact on the course of demographic development in reducing mortality since the 1930s.[122] However, the precise consequences of the measures against STDs in the decrease of mortality cannot be defined with any certainty, but were probably limited insofar as the concerned diseases — contrary to what colonial doctors thought and wrote — seemed not so widespread in Senegal in the past. Priority was broadly given to epidemics and endemics, which were targeted first by the sanitary measures. A wide field of investigations remains open on themes and questions scantily raised in this contribution about social, economic, and political factors related to health, reproductive health, and mortality.

Nevertheless, it may be recognized that, as in the cases of other compulsorily reportable diseases, the struggle against STDs has been marked, since the end of the past century, by its internationalization and the desire for control and eradication under the supervision of doctors. Recent campaigns for controlling rapid population growth are also conducted at international levels with similar methods. In both cases, contradictions appear within communities where authorities want to implement voluntary actions — and where health programs are imposed — without taking into account the various social actors' point of view, rationales, and initiatives.

NOTES

The authors are indebted to Gary Engleberg, Robert Franklin, Michel Garenne, Milton Lewis, and Philip Setel for their critical comments and kind suggestions. This chapter was written in May 1996.

1. Claude Quétel, *Le mal de Naples. Histoire de la syphilis*, (Paris: Séghers, 1986); Jon Arrizabalaga, "Syphilis," in *The Cambridge World History of Human Disease*, edited by Kenneth F. Kiple (Cambridge: Cambridge University Press, 1993), pp. 1025–33; Olivier Dutour, György Palfi, Jacques Bareto, and Jean-Pierre Brun, eds., L'origine de la syphilis en Europe avant ou après 1493? (The origin of syphilis in Europe before or after 1493?) (Toulon: Centre archéologique du Var, 1994).

2.   Quétel, *Le mal de Naples*, p. 68). This disciple of Copernicus at Padua University entitled his book — published in 1530 — *Syphilis sive morbus gallicus*. The volume was translated into French in 1753 under the title *Syphilis ou le mal vénérien. Poème latin de Jérôme Fracastor* (Syphilis or the venereal disease. Latin poem by Jerome Fracastor).

3.   *Le Père Peinard*, November 28–December 5, 1897, quoted by Alain Corbin, *Les filles de noce. Misère et prostitution (19e siècle)*, (Paris: Aubier Montaigne, 1978), p. 401. It should be noted that some experimental syphilization was attempted in the mid-nineteenth century by Auzias Turenne (1844), who issued several publications on the matter over some 30 years. The experimentation consisted in repeatedly inoculating the same individual with soft chancre until a negative reaction or the expected curative effect was obtained. This syphilis "immunization" has been dropped and is now just one of many vain attempts at preventing the disease (see J. Rollet, "Syphilisation,"in *Dictionnaire encyclopédique des sciences médicales*, vol. 14, edited by Dechambre [Paris: Asselin and Cie, Masson, 1884], pp. 678–91).

4.   His book *Psychopathia sexualis* published in 1886 was translated into French in 1892.

5.   See, in particular, Olivier Faure, *Histoire sociale de la médecine (XVIIIe-XXe siècles)*, (Paris: Anthropos, 1994), pp. 199–220, and the analyses by Claudine Herzlich and Janine Pierret, *Malades d'hier, malades d'aujourd'hui. De la mort collective au devoir de guérison* (Paris: Payot, 1991); Quétel, *Le mal de Naples*, p. 348; Alain Corbin, "Le péril vénérien au début du siècle: prophylaxie sanitaire et prophylaxie morale," *Recherches* No. 29 (December 1977): 245–83; A. Corbin, *Les filles de noce*.

6.   See Raoul Girardet, *L'idée coloniale en France de 1871 à 1962* (Paris: La Table Ronde, 1972).

7.   The order dated August 10, 1872, promulgated in Senegal on September 20, 1872, established in the colony municipal institutions similar to those in France (with counsellors elected by universal suffrage). Gorée and Saint-Louis, however, had had municipal status since 1848, each with a mayor appointed by the governor.

8.   *Archives Nationales du Sénégal* [hereafter *ANS*] series H (Santé) H42, letter no. 621.

9.   *ANS*, H42.

10.   Ibid.

11.   *ANS*, H42, letter no. 35.

12.   *ANS*, H46.

13.   Ndar Toute is a fishermen's district in the city of Saint-Louis located on a sandy littoral band at the mouth of Senegal River called "Langue de Barbarie"and separate from the city center, which is on an island.

14.   *ANS*, H42, letter no. 149, June 19, 1897, to the AOF governor general.

15.   *ANS*, H46, letter no. 995.

16.   A. Kermorgant, "Aperçu sur les maladies vénériennes dans les colonies françaises,"*Annales d'Hygiène et de Médecine coloniales* 6 (1903): 428–60.

17.   These measures were taken in answer to a wish expressed by the *Académie de Médecine*.

18.   Kermorgant, "Aperçu sur les maladies vénériennes," p. 435.

19.   A. Kermorgant, "Maladies endémiques, épidémiques et contagieuses

dans les colonies françaises en 1906," *Annales d'Hygiène et de Médecine coloniales* 11 (1908): 379–80.

20.   Henry Gallay, *Trois années d'Assistance médicale aux indigènes et de lutte contre la variole. 1905, 1906, 1907* (Paris: Emile Larose, 1909), p. 13.

21.   Circular letter drafted by Civil Health Service Inspector Rangé.

22.   Report prepared by Gallay, Rangé's successor (reproduced in Gallay, *Trois années d'Assistance médicale*, pp. 14–45).

23.   See Faure, *Histoire sociale de la médecine*, pp. 199–220; Herzlich and Pierret, *Malades d'hier, malades d'aujourd'hui*, pp. 193–211.

24.   July 15, 1893, Loi sur l'assistance médicale et gratuite (République française, *Bulletin des Lois*, 1893; no. 1583, p. 841); February 15, 1902, Loi relative à la protection de la santé publique (République française, *Journal Officiel*, February 19, 1902, p. 1173).

25.   Gallay, *Trois années d'Assistance médicale*, p. 20.

26.   There was a commonly held view that Africa was infected through the double influence of Europe and Islam (see Henri Baudet, *Extension actuelle de la syphilis dans les pays de nouvelle colonisation* [Paris, Legrand, 1936], MD thesis).

27.   *Bulletin Administratif du Sénégal*, 1 (1906): 54, 59. The Independent Service of the Vaccine represented a major and even a prioritizing investment in the colonial health policy for many years and reached a very large part of the population in the countryside as well as in the cities. Important data on its activities, its forceful methods, the various reactions from the populations, and its effects are available in the archives and in medical journals from the colonial period. (cf. René Collignon and Charles Becker, *Santé et population en Sénégambie des origines à 1960. Bibliographie annotée*, [Paris: INED, 1989], pp. 85–109, 305–7).

28.   Christophe Bonneuil, *Des savants pour l'Empire. La structuration des recherches scientifiques coloniales au temps de la "mise en valeur des colonies françaises" 1917–1945* (Paris: Orstom, 1991).

29.   Albert Sarraut, *La mise en valeur des colonies* (Paris: Payot, 1923). Appointed at the Ministry of Colonies in January 1920, Sarraut stayed for more than four years.

30.   Michael Crowder, *Senegal: A Study of French Assimilation Policy* (London: Methuen, 1967), pp. 31–32.

31.   Michel Leiris, *L'Afrique fantôme* (Paris: Gallimard, Quarto, 1996), p. 148.

32.   *Journal Officiel du Sénégal*, 1926, no. 1318, p. 193.

33.   Quétel, *Le mal de Naples*, p. 238.

34.   See Maurice Nogué, "Note sur le fonctionnement de la polyclinique de l'Hôpital indigène de décembre 1918 à juillet 1919," *Bulletin de la Société médico-chirurgicale française de l'Ouest africain* 1 (1919): 28–33; Ferdinand Heckenroth, "Quelques renseignements démographiques sur Dakar," *Bulletin de la Société médico-chirurgicale française de l'Ouest africain* 2 (1920): 132–41.

35.   Hata, *Revue Internationale d'Hygiène Publique* 1921, p. 368, quoted by André Thiroux, "Les maladies vénériennes dans les colonies françaises," *Bulletin de l'Office international d'Hygiène publique*, 1923, p. 194.

36.   Thiroux, "Les maladies vénériennes," p. 195.

37.   Ibid., p. 196; Hermant, "Les maladies transmissibles observées dans les colonies françaises et territoires sous mandat pendant l'année 1928," *Annales de Médecine et de Pharmacie coloniales* 29 (1931): 5–139.

38. Kermorgant, "Aperçu sur les maladies vénériennes."

39. Alfred Fournier, *Traité de la syphilis* (Paris, Rueff, 1906), p. 841. Fournier was one of the leading figures in syphilography in France and was hailed by Léon Daudet as "the first syphilographer of his time and probably of all times." Herald of the crusade against this venereal disease, his numerous works since 1857 are authoritative on the subject. In 1901 he founded the French Association for Sanitary and Moral Prevention. He was also the father of dispensaries (community clinics), elaborated the idea that the disease was not threatening just those who passed it on, and stressed the number of underserved contaminations among women and children (see Quétel, "L'ère de Fournier," in *Le mal de Naples*, pp. 165–9).

40. Thiroux, "Les maladies vénériennes," p. 195.

41. The ratio of malaria patients (determined using Koch's method based on the percentage of infected children) was 60–70 percent in Senegal early in the century (André Thiroux and L. d'Anfreville, *Le paludisme au Sénégal pendant les années 1905, 1906* [Paris: Baillière et fils, 1908], p. 59).

42. An advisory committee on venereal diseases in the colonies was set up in 1929 at the *Institut Prophylactique* (established in 1916) where Marcel Léger was appointed after spending several years as head of the *Institut Pasteur* in Dakar. Cazanove presented to this committee his report on syphilis control at the Port of Dakar (Frank Cazanove, "Les enseignements de deux années de lutte anti-vénérienne au Port de Dakar," *Archives de l'Institut prophylactique* 5 (1933): 32–42).

43. Opened in 1921, the Institute of Social Hygiene comprises six departments including an anti-venereal one. In 1927 some 87,723 consultations were made (H. Lhuerre, "Notes sur le fonctionnement de l'institut d'hygiène sociale de Dakar," *Bulletin de la Société de Pathologie Exotique* 21 [1928]: 329–34).

44. After 1919 in Dakar an anti-venereal clinic and consultation service annexed to the native maternity ward operated in the mornings (J. Kerneis, "Fonctionnement de la maternité indigène de Dakar," *Bulletin de la Société médico-chirurgicale française de l'Ouest africain* 2 [1921]: 107–18). In 1926, in compliance with the Brussels International Arrangements of December 1, 1924, a health station was created with a syphilis laboratory at Dakar Port. It was charged with providing care to merchant navy men suffering from STDs. Its testing and care services were gradually extended to the fluctuating population of the port vicinity and to natives in Dakar city center and Medina, a separate ward that was set up exclusively for women. Mercurial pills recommended by Dr. Vernes were manufactured locally from a formula provided by Marcel Léger. The pills were easy to take, were without side effects, and were very popular among Africans (Cazanove, "Les enseignements"). Blood testing was being developed at the syphilis laboratory at Hôpital Principal. The Institut Pasteur in Dakar used Bordet-Wassermann's reaction to test blood serum and cerebrospinal fluid (Marqué, "Les maladies transmissibles dans les colonies françaises et territoires sous mandat pendant l'années 1931," *Annales de Médecine et de Pharmacie coloniales* 31 [1933]: 123–323).

45. Marcel Léger, *Conférence de la défense sociale contre la syphilis* (Nancy: Procès-Verbaux de la conférence, 1928), pp. 53–56.

46. Ibid.

47. Hermant, "Les maladies transmissibles"; Grosfillez, "Les principales

maladies observées dans les colonies françaises et territoires sous mandat pendant l'année 1932," *Annales de Médecine et de Pharmacie coloniales* 32 (1934): 153–268.

48. *ANS*, H38, "Instructions médicales pour les postes n'ayant pas de médecin," manuscript, p. 24ff.

49. The pathogenic agent in human trypanosomiasis has similarities with the *Treponema pallidum* — syphilis treponema — that had been also discovered in 1905. Trypanosomiasis was a major public health concern in British East Africa and in some AOF territories. This led to the establishment of a specific control device that made Jamot famous (see Jean-Pierre Dozon, "Quand les Pastoriens traquaient la maladie du sommeil," *Sciences sociales et Santé* 3 (1985): 27–56; Jean-Pierre Dozon, "D'un tombeau l'autre," *Cahiers d'Etudes africaines* 31 (1991): 135–57.

50. "Wonderful, your injections!" as an infantryman from Sudan exclaimed in December 1907 in response to the rapid and spectacular results of Bargy's injection treatment (Bargy, "L'Atoxyl dans le traitement de la syphilis en Afrique occidentale," *Annales d'Hygiène et de Médecine coloniales* 11 (1908): 617–29.

51. 914 has apparently been very popular in the Senegal River basin, according to Abdoul Sow, a Halpulaar investigator of the Tukulor ethnic group, personal communication, February 1996.

52. Quétel, *Le mal de Naples*, p. 179.

53. *ANS*, H130.

54. In the mid-1920s stovarsol tablets were introduced as a specific treatment of pian in Ivory Coast where the infection was widespread. This treatment soon appeared as the most advisable treatment technique for heavily infected communities. Its success was evidenced by the local population's increasing demand. It thus became a policy instrument: From 25 kg in 1926, its intake went up to 150 kg in 1929 (Anonymous, *Les Services de l'Assistance Médicale Indigène en Afrique Occidentale Française* [Paris: Agence économique de l'AOF, 1931]).

55. *ANS*, H186, letter to the governor of Senegal, from the files of the Medical Assistance Department.

56. G. Ledentu, "Les maladies transmissibles observées dans les colonies françaises et territoires sous mandat pendant l'année 1933," *Annales de Médecine et de Pharmacie coloniales* 33 (1935): 765.

57. The malaria therapy suggested by Wagner von Jauregg in 1917 (for which he won the Nobel Prize in 1927) does not seem to be have been applied in the African context where, as we have seen, there were few cases of general paresis, tabes, and neuro-syphilis. There were, however, records in Dakar of several strains of malaria sent to Sainte-Anne Hospital in Paris for malaria therapy of French mental patients.

58. Gallay, *Trois années d'Assistance médicale*.

59. Ledentu, "Les maladies transmissibles observées," pp. 552–816; G. Ledentu and M. Peltier, "Les maladies transmissibles observées dans les colonies françaises et territoires sous mandat pendant l'année 1935," *Annales de Médecine et de Pharmacie coloniales* 35 (1937): 748–1335.

60. Thiroux, "Les maladies vénériennes," p. 206.

61. Ledentu, "Les maladies transmissibles observées," p. 781.

62. Ibid.

63. Thiroux, "Les maladies vénériennes."

64. Hermant, "Les maladies transmissibles."

65. G. Ledentu, "Les maladies transmissibles observées dans les colonies françaises et territoires sous mandat pendant l'année 1929," *Annales de Médecine et de Pharmacie coloniales*, 29 (1931): 661–851.

66. Grosfillez, "Les principales maladies observées." Authors at the time insisted on the importance of early and prolonged treatment. Some of them were also aware of the limitations of treatment capacities of medical facilities in the face of increasing demands for care (Marqué, "Les maladies transmissibles").

67. Ledentu, "Les maladies transmissibles," p. 764.

68. Marcel Léger was correspondent of Académie des Sciences Coloniales. Medical officer of the Corps de Santé Colonial, he created the Institut de Biologie de l'AOF in Dakar (1920) that became Institut Pasteur de l'AOF in 1924. He pursued scientific investigations on syphilis diagnosis and he initiated many colonial physicians to the new techniques of diagnosis and treatments they applied in the African colonies.

69. In 1933 25,734 syphilis patients were under treatment in health care delivery units, as opposed to 19,042 in 1932. An average of 17 injections per patient was delivered in 1933, as opposed to 9 per patient in 1932 (Ledentu, "Les maladies transmissibles," p. 765).

70. This recommendation came from several international conferences, the most important being the one held at Enugu, Nigeria in November 1955. International pressure on colonial powers to show a greater concern about improving the welfare of populations under their rule was growing during that period. The Hot Springs conference (May–June 1943) committed them to take care of malnutrition. A large scale survey for an anthropological study of AOF native populations was conducted over a period of 30 months under the leadership of Colonel Dr. Palès. See Léon Palès, *Rapport No. 1, Sénégal* (Dakar: Direction générale de la santé publique, 1946); Léon Palès, *Le bilan de la mission anthropologique de l'AOF (janvier 1946–août 1948)* (Dakar: Gouvernement de l'AOF, 1948); Michael Worboys, "The Discovery of Colonial Malnutrition between the Wars," in *Imperial Medicine and Indigenous Societies*, edited by David Arnold (Manchester: Manchester University Press, 1988): pp. 208–25.

71. Financially autonomous, the General Mobile Hygiene and Preventive Service was funded from the general AOF budget (about 1 billion F CFA in 1958). (US$1 - 600 F CFA.) A 258 million F CFA fund provided for programs to be implemented in 1956–57 and 250 million in 1957–58 prompted international organizations, such as UNICEF, to grant important assistance for mass campaigns (268 million F CFA in 1957). Such campaigns were undertaken simultaneously with massive anti-yaws campaigns launched with international assistance, in The Gambia, Liberia, Ghana, and Nigeria (see Pierre Richet, *Le Service Commun de lutte contre les Grandes Endémies de l'Afrique occidentale française. Rapport d'activité depuis sa création* [Dakar: ANS, 1958], 111 pp. mimeo.; Makhone Douta Seck, *Le Service de Lutte des Grandes Endémies du Sénégal*, MD Thesis, (Dakar, 1968).

72. Jean Sénécal and René Souvestre, "A propos du diagnostic de la syphilis congénitale chez le nourisson africain," *Bulletin et Mémoire de l'Ecole de Médecine de Dakar* 1 (1952–53): 113–17; Jean Sénécal, G. Trapet, and René Souvestre, "Etude de la sérologie dans la syphilis congénitale en Afrique," *Semaine des hôpitaux* 29 (1952): 3263–70; Jean Sénécal, H. Dupin, and René Souvestre, "Le diagnostic précoce de la syphilis congénitale," *Bulletin médical* 10 (1954): 251–57; René Souvestre,

A propos du diagnostic de la syphilis congénitale chez le nourrisson dakarois (Bordeaux: Imprimerie moderne de Guyenne, 1953); Monique Castets, *Sérologie de la syphilis et protidémie chez les Africains de Dakar* (Paris: Librairie Arnette, 1958).

73. Marcel Augustin Vaucel, "Le pian dans les territoires africains français," *Bulletin of the World Health Organization* 8 (1953): 183–204. The annual prevalence rate of pian in AOF was 4 percent, with a downward trend reported from Ivory Coast (an area of hyperendemicity) up to the Sahelian territories (0.1 percent in Senegal) in areas of hypoendemicity.

74. This was only suspected until the early 1960s; its existence had not yet been confirmed in Senegal. It does not appear on WHO maps by T. Guthe and R. R. Willcox, *Chronique de l'Organisation Mondiale de la Santé* 8 (1954): 42.

75. A. Basset, P. Boiron, P. Brès, M. Castets, M. Basset, and E. N. Moyne, "A propos du foyer sénégalais de syphilis endémique," *Bulletin de la Société de Pathologie Exotique* 56 (1963): 173–81; A. Basset, J. Malleville, and I. Faye, "Nouvelle enquête sur la syphilis endémique au Sénégal. Etude clinique et épidémiologique. Etude sérologique, isolement d'une souche de tréponème," *Bulletin de la Société de Pathologie Exotique* 62 (1969): 1017–34; A. Basset, J. Malleville, J. Malgras, Y. Privat, I. Faye, M. Basset, E. Heid, H. Rusher, and S. Ermolieff, "Nouvelle enquête sur un foyer de tréponématose en Casamance (Sénégal)," *Bulletin de la Société de Pathologie Exotique* 65 (1972): 66–78; H. Boiron, A. Basset, I. Faye, A. Debroise, and M. Mallet, "Etude des limites du foyer sénégalais de syphilis endémique," *Bulletin de la Société médicale d'Afrique Noire de Langue française* 10 (1965): 408–11.

76. P. Cicera, C. Bouloux, and J. Gomila, "La fréquence des tréponématoses chez les Bedik du Sénégal," *Bulletin de la Société de Pathologie Exotique* 63 (1970): 666–75.

77. J. Linhard, R. Baylet, G. Diebolt, and S. Diop, "Prévalence sérologique des tréponématoses dans deux populations sérèr," *Bulletin de la Société de Pathologie Exotique* 66 (1973): 701–6.

78. H. Bah, E. Maffre, R. Baylet, I. Wone, and Ch. Gueye, "Maladies vénériennes suivies à l'Institut d'Hygiène Sociale de Dakar. Aspects épidémiologiques 1956–1964," *Bulletin de la Société médicale d'Afrique Noire de Langue française* 10 (1965): 230–36.

79. In a report on hygiene and health prepared for the First Development Plan of the Senegalese government, Anne Laurentin highlighted all the shortcomings related to the actual awareness of the epidemiological impact of the various treponematoses in several rural areas. She became famous for her work on the effects of incident venereal diseases on the decrease in birth rates in Black African countries (Upper Volta, now Burkina Faso, and Central African Republic). Anne Laurentin, ed., *Rapport Hygiène-Santé*, 2 vol. (Rapport enquête CINAM-ORANA 1959–60, ANS bi I 4° 160); Anne Retel-Laurentin, *Causes de l'infécondité dans la Volta noire* (Paris: PUF, 1979); Anne Retel-Laurentin, *Un pays à la dérive. Une société en régression démographique. Les Nzakara de l'est africain* (Paris: J.-P. Delarge, 1979); P. Peretti and R. Michel, "Bilan de dix ans de dépistage sérologique et de traitements des tréponématoses au Secteur des Grandes Endémies de M'Bour (Sénégal)," *Bulletin de la Société médicale d'Afrique Noire de Langue française* 16 (1971): 201–6.

80. As acknowledged by A. Basset, it is only in 1958, further to Anglo-Saxon works in Uganda and in Bechuanaland reserves, that the French great endemics' department (Service des Grandes Endémies) with Richet started research on

endemic syphilis in West Africa (A. Basset, "Tréponématoses en Afrique de l'ouest," *Afrique médicale* 5 [1966]: 37–40). This affliction had thus far apparently been confused with congenital syphilis. H. Boiron, A. Boisset, M. Basset, and M. Castets, "Contribution à l'étude de la syphilis au Sénégal," *Bulletin de la Société de Pathologie Exotique* 55 (1962): 98–116; Basset, "Tréponématoses en Afrique de l'ouest"; S. Dauchy and R. Baylet, "Réflexion sur les problèmes posés par la positivité de la sérologie tréponémique en Afrique de l'Ouest," *Médecine d'Afrique Noire* 19 (1972): 843–48.

81.   G. Niel and M. Gentilini, "Sérologie tréponémique des travailleurs de l'Ouest africain transplantés (A propos de 1,000 examens en immunofluorescence et en floculation de Kline)," *Bulletin de la Société de Pathologie Exotique* 63 (1970): 180–94; S. Dauchy and R. Baylet, "La syphilis: évaluation de l'importance accordée à cette maladie dans les dispensaires au Sénégal," *Médecine d'Afrique Noire* 19 (1972): 655–58.

82.   A. Basset, H. Boiron, P. Brès, M. Castets, M. Basset, and E. N. Moyne, "A propos du foyer sénégalais de syphilis endémique," *Bulletin de la Société de Pathologie Exotique* 56 (1963): 173–81; A. Basset, J. Maleville, J. Malgras, Y. Privat, I. Faye, M. Basset, E. Heid, H. Rusher, and S. Ermolieff, "Nouvelle enquête sur un foyer de tréponématose en Casamance (Sénégal)," *Bulletin de la Société de Pathologie Exotique* 65 (1972): 66–70; Arrizabalaga, "Syphilis," p. 1032.

83.   Kenneth F. Kiple, "Syphilis, Nonvenerial," in *The Cambridge World History of Human Disease*, edited by Kenneth F. Kiple (Cambridge: Cambridge University Press), pp. 1033–35; Kenneth F. Kiple, "The Treponematoses," in *The Cambridge World History of Human Disease*, edited by Kenneth F. Kiple (Cambridge: Cambridge University Press), pp. 1053–55; Arrizabalaga, "Syphilis," p. 1032.

84.   Megan Vaughan, *Curing Their Ills: Colonial Power and African Illness* (Stanford: Stanford University Press, 1991), pp. 129–54; Megan Vaughan, "Syphilis and Colonial East and Central Africa: The Social Construction of an Epidemic," in *Epidemics and Ideas: Essays on Historical Perception of Pestilence*, edited by Terence Ranger and Paul Slack (Cambridge: Cambridge University Press, 1992), pp. 269–302.

85.   The role of sexuality and venereal overindulgence in disease transmission was thought to be relevant not only to syphilis but also to tuberculosis, another of the so-called social diseases, and was also associated with alcohol use in European hygienists' literature.

86.   Alain Corbin, "L'hérédosyphilis ou l'impossible rédemption," *Romantisme* 31 (1981): 131–49.

87.   Corbin, *Les filles de noce*, pp. 24–34.

88.   Parent-Duchâtelet, *De la prostitution dans la ville de Paris, considérée sous le rapport de l'hygiène publique, de la morale et de l'administration* (Paris: publisher unknown, 1836).

89.   Lhuerre, "Notes sur le fonctionnement"; H. Lhuerre "Sur la prostitution à Dakar," *Bulletin de la Société de Pathologie Exotique* 21 (1928): 703–7.

90.   Five brothels were registered in Dakar in 1942. They received regular medical visits, and the women working there were given periodic blood tests and long lasting treatments. Seventy native prostitutes were reportedly admitted in hospital that same year (*ANS* 1, H29, subdossier 1 — Venereal Diseases in AOF between 1938 and 1943).

91. Francis Simonis, "Splendeur et misère des moussos. Les compagnes africaines des Européens du cercle de Ségou au Mali (1890–1962)," in *Histoire africaine au XXe siècle. Sociétés - Villes - Cultures*, edited by Catherine Coquery-Vidrovitch (Paris: L'Harmattan/UA Tiers-Monde-Afrique Paris VII/CNRS, 1993), p. 209.

92. Catherine Coquery-Vidrovitch, ed., *Les Africaines. Histoire des femmes d'Afrique noire du XIXe au XXe siècle* (Paris: Desjonquères, 1994), pp. 189–206.

93. Didier Fassin and Jean-Pierre Dozon, "Les Etats africains à l'épreuve du SIDA," *Politique Africaine* 32 (1989): 79–85; Jean-Pierre Dozon and Didier Fassin, "Raison épidémiologique et raison d'Etat. Les enjeux socio-politiques du SIDA en Afrique," *Sciences Sociales et Santé* 7 (1989): 21–36; Gilles Bibeau, "L'Afrique, terre imaginaire du sida. La subversion du discours scientifique par le jeu des fantasmes," *Anthropologie et Sociétés* 15 (1991): 125–47; Gill Seidel, "The Competing Discourses of HIV/AIDS in Sub-Saharan Africa: Discourses of Rights and Empowerment vs Discourses of Control and Exclusion," *Social Science and Medicine* 36 (1993): 175–94.

94. Francis Barin, Souleymane M'Boup, and François Denis, "Serological Evidence for Virus Related to Simian T-lymphotropic Retrovirus III in Residents of West Africa," *Lancet* No. 2 (1985): 1387–89; Phyllis J. Kanki, Francis Barin, Souleymane M'Boup, J. S. Allan, J. L. Romet-Lemorre, R. Marlink, M. F. McLane, T. H. Lee, B. Arbeille, and F. Denis, "New Human T-lymphotropic Retrovirus (HTLV-IV) Related to Simian T-lymphotropic Virus Type III (STLV-IIIagm)," *Science* No. 232 (1986): 238–43. According to the media, the first doctoral dissertation by Fatou Dieng Samb related the identification of a "non-pathogenic AIDS virus" in Senegal (Fatou Dieng Samb, "Enquête sur le Sida au Sénégal: perspectives de vaccination," doctoral dissertation, Dakar, 1986, p. 120).

95. Myriam de Loenzien, Alpha Wade, Yves Charbit, and Souleymane M'Boup, "Attitudes de la population rurale face à la maladie et au sida," in *La population du Sénégal*, edited by Yves Charbit and Salif Ndiaye (Dakar: DPS, 1995), pp. 435–66.

96. Gilles Pison, Bernard Le Guenno, Emmanuel Lagarde, Catherine Enel, and Cheikh Seck, "Seasonal Migration: A Risk Factor for HIV Infection in Rural Senegal," *Journal of the Acquired Immune Deficiency Syndromes* 6 (1993): 196–200.

97. Charles Becker, *Etude anthropologique sur les migrations, la nuptialité et les comportements sexuels chez les Sereer du Sénégal* (Report ANRS 1990, 4 volumes, 1991); Charles Becker, "Facteurs de risque du SIDA liés aux migrations et aux comportements sexuels: une étude en milieu rural sénégalais," paper presented at the sixth International Conference on AIDS in Africa, Dakar, December 16–19, 1991.

98. Mame Birane Ibrahima Camara, *Etude socio-culturelle des MST dans la région de Kolda (Casamance)*, Dakar, MD Thesis, 1991, p. 123.

99. Salif Ndiaye and Mohamed Ayad, "Maladies sexuellement transmissibles et sida," in *Enquête démographique et de santé au Sénégal (EDS-II) 1992/93*, edited by Salif Ndiaye, Papa Demba Diouf, and Mohamed Ndiaye (Dakar: DPS, 1994), pp. 161–70.

100. Charles Becker, *Thèses de Médecine et de Pharmacie sur les maladies sexuellement transmises et les virus l'immuno-déficience humaine. Répertoire analytique des thèses soutenues a Dàkar* (Dakar: Comité National de Prévention du Sida, 1997), p. 82.

101. Since 1985, when HIV-II was identified in Senegal, implementation of research and epidemiological investigation showed that the West African region — especially southern Senegal, Bissau-Guinea and Gambia — seems to be a focus of the HIV-II endemicity. Several publications on the characteristics of HIV-II (epidemiology, pathogenicity, natural history, clinical aspects, relations with tuberculosis, and so forth) have been issued over the past 12 years by Senegalese research teams, working closely with U.S. and French institutions (Harvard University, University of Tours-Limoges, Agence nationale de Recherche sur le sida, ORSTOM/Institut français de recherche scientifique pour le développement en coopération). One of the most significant contributions is that of Souleymane M'boup in the most recent synthesis on AIDS in Africa: Max Essex, Souleymane M'boup, Phyllis J. Kanki, and Mbowa R. Kalengayi, *Aids in Africa* (New York: Raven Press, 1994), p. 728; Souleymane M'boup and Guy-Michel Gershy-Damet, "HIV's and AIDS in West Africa," in *Aids in Africa*, edited by Max Essex, Souleymane M'boup, Phyllis J. Kanki, and Mbowa R. Kalengayi (New York: Raven Press, 1994), pp. 613–49. A large overview on the publications about AIDS in Senegal is given by Michel Etchepare and Christine Etchepare, *Sida en Afrique. Bilan d'une décennie. Analyse par pays* (Dakar: Enda, 1993), pp. 210–19, 293–94, 301.
102. *Bulletin épidemiologique, HIV* 5 (1994): pp. 31–34.
103. *Bulletin épidemiologique, HIV* 4 (1993): 31.
104. *Bulletin épidemiologique, HIV* 5, (1994): 34.
105. Michel Garenne, Charles Becker, and Rosario Cardenas, "Heterogeneity, Life Cycle and the Potential Demographic Impact of AIDS in a Rural Area of Africa," in *Sexual Behaviour and Networking: Anthropological and Socio-Cultural Studies on the Transmission of HIV*, edited by Tim Dyson (Liège: Derouaux-Ordina, 1992), pp. 269–82; Catherine Enel and Gilles Pison, "Sexual Relations in the Rural Area of Mlomp (Casamance, Senegal)," in *Sexual Behaviour and Networking: Anthropological and Socio-Cultural Studies on the Transmission of HIV*, edited by Tim Dyson (Liège: Derouaux-Ordina, 1992), pp. 249–67.
106. Emmanuel Lagarde, Gilles Pison, Bernard Le Guenno, Catherine Enel, and Cheikh Seck, *Les facteurs de risque de l'infection à VIH2 dans une région rurale au Sénégal* (Paris: INED — Museum d'Histoire Naturelle, 1992), p. 29.
107. Cheikh Ibrahima Niang, "The Dimba of Senegal: A Support for Women," *Reproductive Health Matters* 4 (1994): 39–45; Cheikh Ibrahima Niang, "Sociocultural Factors Favoring HIV Infection and the Integration of Traditional Women's Association in AIDS Prevention Strategies in Kolda, Senegal" (Washington D.C.: International Center for Research on Women, 1994), p. 5. Studies conducted in the Kolda region among a group of women therapists (*dimba*) and in Kaolack among *lawbe* women who have special knowledge on sexuality, tended to involve prevention activities among people reputed to have extensive traditional knowledge.
108. Bernard Le Guenno, Gilles Pison, Catherine Enel, Emmanuel Lagarde, and Cheikh Seck, "HIV-2 Seroprevalence in Three Rural Regions of Senegal: Low Levels and Heterogeneous Distribution," *Transactions of the Royal Society of Tropical Medicine and Hygiene* 86 (1992): 301–2.
109. Pierre Lemardeley, A. Diallo, A. Gueye, E. Sarr, Charles Becker, Souleymane M'boup, and Jean-Loup Rey, "Evaluation des risques de MST et d'infection par VIH en zone rurale sénégalaise (1991)," *Cahiers Santé* 5 (1995): 43–48.
110. Fadel Kane, Michel Alary, Ibra Ndoye, Awa M. Coll, Souleymane

M'boup, Aïssatou Guèye, Phyllis J. Kanki, and Jean R. Joly, "Temporary Expatriation Is Related to HIV-1 Infection in Rural Senegal," *AIDS* 7 (1993): 1261–65.

111. Supra note 101.

112. Edward Green, *AIDS and STDs in Africa: Bridging the Gap Between Traditional Healing and Modern Medicine* (Boulder, Colo.: Westview Press, 1994), pp. xi–276.

113. The issue of the ambivalent relationship of the two care delivery systems in Senegal deserves a specific historical study. Although the interest in traditional medicine seemed rather timid at first, there were early publications by colonial doctors and pharmacists on the topic — even in the *Journal Officiel du Sénégal* (the official gazette) which at the turn of the century welcomed this type of information. In his outstanding book on Senegalese traditional pharmacopeia, Joseph Kerharo (*La pharmacopée sénégalaise traditionnelle. Plantes médicales et toxiques* [Paris: Vigot, 1974]) makes an inventory of and describes about 100plants commonly used in STD treatment. He further proposes a historical approach to research work on medicinal plants and flora and their therapeutic uses in indigenous medicine. Colonial doctors, however, had a negative attitude toward traditional healers, whom they considered quacks. Variolization (vaccination) as practiced by native populations was put down and stigmatized by the colonial health authorities. In the 1950s, the deliberate inoculation of children of certain groups (nomadic Fulha in Niger region) with *Treponema pallidum* was mentioned with reference to the high syphilis prevalence rates among those populations (Basset, "Tréponématoses en Afrique de l'ouest," p. 38). This has nevertheless not been confirmed in Senegal.

114. AIDS Control and Prevention Project was founded by the United States Agency for International Development and implemented by Family Health International since August 1991. AIDS Control and Prevention Senegal is based in CNPS, and its interventions in Senegal (as in other countries) were built on three strategies: communicating, improving treatment and prevention of other STDs, and increasing access to and correct use of condoms.

115. Seidel, "The Competing Discourses of HIV/AIDS in Sub-Saharan Africa"; Green, *AIDS and STDs in Africa*.

116. These ten basic principles, stated in the Dakar Declaration, are those of: responsibility, engagement, partnership and consensus-building, empowerment, non-discrimination, confidentiality and privacy, adaptation, sensitivity in language, ethics in research, and prohibition of mandatory HIV testing (UNDP, *African Network on Ethics Law and HIV*. Proceedings of the Intercountry Consultation, Dakar, Senegal, June 17—July 1, 1994, pp. 1–2. The Senegalese country team contributed "Senegal Country Paper," ibid., pp. 49–55.

117. Jeanne-Marie Amat-Roze, "Dynamique de l'infection à VIH et du sida en Afrique noire" in *Maladies, médecines et sociétés. Approches historiques pour le présent. Actes du VIe colloque Histoire au Présent*, vol. I, edited by François Olivier Touati (Paris: L'Harmattan/Histoire au présent, 1993), pp. 86–103; Jeanne-Marie Amat-Roze, "Les inégalités géographiques de l'infection à VIH et du sida en Afrique sud-saharienne," *Social Science and Medicine* 36 (1993): 1247–56; Gérard Rémy, "L'espace épidémiologique de l'infection par le virus de l'immunodéficience humaine VIH-2 en Afrique sud-saharienne," *Médecine tropicale* 53 (1993): 511–16; Gérard Rémy, "Image géographique des infections à VIH en Afrique de l'Ouest.

Faits et interrogations," *Médecine d'Afrique Noire* 40 (1993): 15–21; Gérard Rémy, "Image géographique des infections à VIH en Afrique de l'Ouest. Faits et interrogations. II. Epidémiologie géographique des infections dans la population générale," *Médecine d'Afrique Noire* 40 (1993): 81–86; Gérard Rémy, "Image géographique des infections à VIH en Afrique de l'Ouest. Faits et interrogations. III. Dynamique socio-spatiale des infections à VIH," *Médecine d'Afrique Noire* 40 (1993): 161–64.

118.   The provisional report on *The Status and Trends of the HIV/AIDS/STD Epidemics in Sub-Saharan Africa* (Arlington, Va.: MAP), p. 6, presented at an Official Satellite Symposium of the Tenth International Conference on STD and AIDS in Africa, Abidjan, December 3–4, 1997, stated that there are several factors that may explain the control of HIV epidemic in Dakar (and in Senegal). Some of them are linked with the situation before the emergence of the HIV epidemic (regulation of sex work, a long tradition of associations and movements, solid system of blood transfusion banks, and strong social control of women's sexuality); other factors are linked with the early response of the society, including: integration of STD and HIV prevention and care activities since 1989, high response of the civil society, large media coverage, and production of IEC material. "These efforts would have been impossible without political stability, *including a particularly strong national AIDS program*" (pp. 30–31, emphasis added).

119.   Supra notes 96–100, 106.

120.   Raymond Gervais, "État colonial et savoir démographique en AOF, 1904–1960," in *AOF: réalités et héritages. Sociétés ouest africaines et ordre colonial, 1895–1960*, vol. 2, edited by Charles Becker, Saliou Mbaye, and Ibrahima Thioub (Dakar: Direction des Archives du Sénégal, 1997), pp. 961–80.

121.   Dennis D. Cordell, Joel W. Gregory, and Victor Piché, "African Historical Demography: The Search for a Theoretical Framework," in *African Population and Capitalism: Historical Perspectives*, edited by Dennis D. Cordell and Joel W. Gregory (Boulder, Colo.: Westview Press, 1987), p. 31.

122.   Charles Becker, "Past Social Responses to Epidemics and the Present Outbreak of HIV-AIDS in Senegal: Community Responses of the Past and Current Ethical Issues" in *African Network on Ethics Law and HIV. Proceedings of the Intercountry Consultation*, Dakar, Senegal, June 27–July 1, 1994, pp. xiv–220. Charles Becker and Mohamed Mbodj, "Dynamiques régionales au XXéme siècle," in *La population du Sénégal*, edited by Yves Charbit and Salif Ndiaye (Dakar: DPS, 1994), pp. 467–86; Charles Becker and Mohamed Mbodj, "Perspectives historiques," in *La population du Sénégal*, edited by Yves Charbit and Salif Ndiaye (Dakar: DPS, 1994), pp. 31–58; Charles Becker, Mamadou Diouf, and Mohamed Mbodj, "L'évolution démographique régionale du Sénégal et du Bassin Arachidier (Sine-Saloum) au vingtième siècle, 1904–1976," in *African Population and Capitalism: Historical Perspectives*, edited by Dennis D. Cordell and Joel W. Gregory (Boulder, Colo.: Westview Press, 1987), pp. 76–94.

5

Medicine and Morality: A Review of Responses to Sexually Transmitted Diseases in Uganda in the Twentieth Century

Maryinez Lyons

The history of sexually transmitted diseases (STDs) in Uganda exemplifies the complexities of human health and the tensions between two schools of thought in the history of medicine itself — prevention versus cure. The most recent disease in this history, HIV/AIDS has evoked many familiar responses and provides a window on the dissension existing between the often acrimonious proponents of these two views. STDs, by their very nature related to a most private, even ritually important aspect of human life and reproduction, arouse powerful emotional and irrational responses. Such responses complicate the very different approaches of the curative versus the preventive in public health programs for STDs.

The history of STDs in Africa is further complicated by a racism that echoes deeply entrenched European attitudes and fantasies of black sexuality. Early in the dramatic epidemic of HIV in Africa, the scientific and medical community constructed a definition for African AIDS distinct from that of the epidemic in the West.[1] In the West, clearly defined risk groups, albeit most often marginalized and socially disapproved, were identified as the foci of information and education campaigns. The problem in sub-Saharan Africa was how to explain the widespread and heterosexual nature of the epidemic. As one clinician expressed it, "In Uganda there is not a clearly defined risk group . . . the whole population should be considered at high risk."[2] The stereotype, so widespread in the European subconscious, of the promiscuous, highly sexed African contributed greatly to the perception, shared by many African observers, that the real cause of the AIDS epidemic in Africa was immorality and promiscuity.

This was a view shared by the earliest European medical experts and colonial administrators in Africa.[3] The cause of the AIDS epidemic in Africa was HIV, the transmission of which is now known to be greatly enhanced by a number of co-factors including the presence of other STDs, especially those leading to lesions. Other co-factors in the transmission of the virus include inequality of gender relations, economic status and opportunity, mobility, and interaction of populations. A significant co-factor in the epidemiology of STDs is the level of health care provision and the health care seeking behaviors of clients.

In this chapter, I will sketch the history of STDs in Uganda bearing in mind the broader historical context in which they occur. Seemingly intractable for generations of Ugandans, STDs are now known to be important co-factors in the transmission of HIV. In order to understand more fully the extensive nature of the epidemic of HIV/AIDS in Uganda, it is essential to examine the broader history of all STDs.

UGANDA

STDs have been an integral part of the history of Uganda from the time of its inception as a British Protectorate in 1894. Within a decade of its establishment STDs were being cited as a major cause of infertility, morbidity, and mortality,[4] and they were perceived as a major threat to colonial notions of development. The historical record of much of the twentieth century contains many references to the ravages of these diseases, which, it was feared, would exterminate whole populations of potential laborers and taxpayers. Epidemiological projections in the early 1990s of HIV prevalence and AIDS mortality echo the decades-long fear of a dying population in Uganda. The accompanying medical discourse, like its antecedent, often minimized the broader context of disease.

Emerging from decades of disintegration and decay, Uganda by the 1990s was well on the road to recovery with the assistance of a host of international aid agencies. It was a cruel irony that at the same time the country appeared to be one of the most seriously affected by the terrible virus. The president of Uganda, Yoweri Museveni, was the first political leader in sub-Saharan Africa to acknowledge frankly the epidemic and set a precedent that opened his country to assistance. In 1989 Uganda was one of the first countries to establish a national AIDS control program. Aware of its wider implications for the entire political economy of the country, by 1991 Museveni was describing AIDS as a developmentally linked disease that resonated with the history of STDs. Although AIDS is the preeminent public health threat of our time, socioeconomic factors, crucial in the transmission of AIDS and other STDs, have deep historical roots. In Africa STDs, such as gonorrhea and syphilis, were a big health hazard before the advent of modern Western medicine.[5]

SEXUALLY TRANSMITTED DISEASES IN UGANDA

STDs were first noted by foreigners in 1863 when the explorer John Speke "hinted at seeing syphilitic lesions" on individuals in Buganda. By 1879 syphilis was said to be widespread in the two dominant kingdoms, Buganda and Bunyoro.[6] STDs continued to be regularly cited throughout the colonial period (1894–1962) as widespread, and the authorities repeatedly noted that they constituted a grave threat to the population and development of the colony. Albert Cook of the Church Missionary Society began keeping statistics on these diseases in 1897, and he soon concluded that about 80 percent of the Baganda[7] had at one time or other had syphilis. According to Cook, the "drive against venereal diseases" was the second great medical campaign against diseases threatening the population of Uganda, the first having been against sleeping sickness.[8]

The Venereal Diseases Campaign

By 1906 the situation was so worrying that Governor Hesketh Bell appealed to the secretary of state for the colonies, and in 1907 Colonel F. J. Lambkin, venereologist of the Royal Army Medical Corps, was commissioned to study the situation. His report, "An Outbreak of Syphilis on Virgin Soil," substantiated Cook's claims and greatly alarmed the authorities.[9] He concluded that "venereal" diseases were widespread and included syphilis, gonorrhea, and soft chancre. Gonorrhea was said to "exist to a fearful extent" and was thought to be the cause of very high miscarriage and infant mortality rates.[10] Lambkin warned that unless steps were taken the "population stands a good chance of being entirely exterminated in a very few years, or left a degenerate race fit for nothing."[11]

A Diagnostic Controversy

It was syphilis more than other STDs that attracted the attention of the missionaries and medical experts. It appeared to early observers in Uganda that syphilis was excessively widespread. We now know in retrospect, however, that the medical experts of the time were misled in their diagnosis of syphilis. For my purpose, however, it is the contemporary understanding of the disease and the policies based on those perceptions that are relevant.

It is likely that the disease described as epidemic was not, in fact, venereal syphilis. It is very possible that what Cook, Lambkin, and others saw in central and southern Uganda early this century was non-venereal, endemic syphilis or even yaws, all of which are caused by the same pathogen. "The modern view is that syphilis is but one of the manifestations of infection with Treponema pallidum and that there is a group of diseases, differing considerably in their clinical features and geographical distribution, which are all caused by organisms which are indistinguishable and, therefore, probably the same species. The exact clinical picture in the treponematoses seems to depend upon climatic and social factors."[12] J.N.P. Davies described the possible confusion between sexually transmitted, or venereal, syphilis and endemic non-venereal syphilis.[13] Although agreeing that by mid-century true venereal syphilis was widespread in Buganda, he postulated that the so-called earlier epidemic was in fact endemic non-venereal syphilis. Endemic syphilis is not an STD but a contagious disease mainly of children that "evolves into venereal syphilis as civilization modifies the environment and factors of transmission."[14] Davies suggested that "there had been an endemic form of syphilis in southern Uganda with yaws common in other areas and that at the turn of the century this original endemic form of syphilis was replaced by true venereal syphilis."[15] The endemic form conveys a degree of immunity against the venereal form.[16] In agreement with this view, another expert, J. Orley, postulated that there had been an endemic form of syphilis or yaws present for many centuries in Uganda and that the so-called epidemic of the early century "may have been due to increased awareness of the disease and decreased immunity to sexually transmitted syphilis as endemic syphilis diminished."[17] In the 1950s yaws was virtually eradicated in most regions of the country.

Theories of Origin and Spread

Early theories of the origin and spread of gonorrhea and syphilis included a range of cultural, social, and economic factors. African societies were profoundly affected in the mid- to late nineteenth century, and for many there was a widening of scale resulting from new trade relations, opportunities for travel, introduction of world religions, and colonization. Rural cultivators were thrust into new economic relations with sometimes onerous labor and tax demands. All of these factors played a part in the introduction and spread of STDs.

Most informants agreed that gonorrhea was a very old disease and well known by the population, which had evolved linguistic terms to identify it. Population mobility is a classic feature in the epidemiology of STDs. There was popular consensus that although syphilis had been present for a long time it was not indigenous, but had been introduced by traders from the East Coast of Africa who first arrived in Uganda in the 1860s.[18] One African chief blamed the recent wars between Buganda and Bunyoro that ended with the arrival of the British. Medical investigators dated the beginning of the epidemic of syphilis to the mid-1890s and the increased mobility of population as a result of the completion of the Uganda Railway linking Kampala with Mombassa in 1899.

Major emphasis in causal explanations was placed on the issue of moral standards. Europeans and Africans (mainly male) agreed that the loss of social control and resulting immorality in Uganda was a major reason for the spread of STDs. Women were particularly singled out for blame as the transmitters of disease. The control of women and moral standards became the catchwords of the STD campaign. The introduction of Christianity and its impact on African cultural sanctions was implicated. At the time of their religious conversion and in line with European notions of gender relations, many Bagandan men emancipated their women, who had been formerly kept under strict surveillance and confinement. In addition, they often chose one of their many wives to be the true wife, thereby disclaiming responsibility for the other wives of their polygamous unions. Apolo Kagwa, a prominent Bagandan leader, added that the abolition of the punishments that used to be given to both men and women for crimes of immorality was yet another factor for the spread of STDs. The Church Missionary Society was deeply offended that Christianity was cited as a cause of STDs. At the insistence of his London superiors, Albert Cook published a statement in *The Lancet* in 1908. "I must give emphatic denial to the assumption that Christianity has been the chief cause of this epidemic. It has been all the other way round. Read 'civilization' for 'Christianity' and there may be some amount of truth in it."[19] Echoing the moral debate today in Uganda concerning the cause of AIDS, Cook added: "Christianity . . . is indeed, when intelligently accepted, the only true prophylaxis to this terrible scourge."

Cultural practices were cited as another factor in the spread of disease. Among the Bahima of Ankole, the practice of husbands sharing wives with their brothers was thought to explain widespread STD. (It is noteworthy that at present with AIDS this practice is still condemned and discouraged by health workers.) Other cultural practices included vaccination of infants with syphilitic discharge, wrapping infants in cloths soaked in discharge, or placing them to sleep in beds with syphilitic victims in an attempt to convey a form of immunity. Such practices argue long familiarity with a treponemal disease. The experts' chronology of the introduction and spread of syphilis taken together with the obviously very old cultural practices mentioned highlight a contradiction in Lambkin's analysis of a "virgin soil epidemic."[20]

The Venereal Diseases Campaign

In December 1908 a commission of three Royal Army Medical Corps officers headed by Captain W.M.B. Sparkes arrived in Kampala to begin the venereal diseases campaign as suggested by Lambkin.[21] Medical staff concurred that "the present state of civilization of the country does not permit any legislative measures with a view to prevention." Treatment rooms were to be established and staffed by African medical subordinates and visited weekly by a medical officer. Initially, treatment consisted of a 21-month course of painful intramuscular injections of 1-grain doses of mercury, together with the application of mercury ointment and calomel cream. At his first treatment session, to reassure the skeptics Sparkes had himself injected in the buttocks with a full dose of mercury in front of a large crowd that was reported to be greatly "impressed."[22]

Six months later the colonial secretary expressed concern that only 2,482 patients had attended the treatment center. "I cannot think that . . . represents anything like the number who require treatment round Kampala. The chiefs ought to have their attention drawn to this."[23] It soon became clear that Africans were avoiding the injections that in many caused mercury poisoning, manifested by profuse salivation, which had resulted in the death of eight or nine patients.[24] People simply refused to return for injections once visible signs of disease disappeared. Others were frightened away by rumors that the European medicine was an injection of fire that removed the blood and caused miscarriages.[25] In spite of the difficulties, there were 3,851 attendances at the Kampala treatment room, and during its first year the program was expanded to three treatment rooms. The centerpiece was the Venereal Diseases Hospital opened in 1913 in Kampala as the central treatment center and a teaching venereal clinic.

Control and Public Health: African Responses

As mentioned earlier, the history of STDs in Uganda provides a window on the tensions between a European model of prevention and indigenous models. African societies had their own ideas and practices for the preservation of well-being long before Europeans arrived. These were based on quite different conceptions of what constitutes and maintains well-being. Western notions of public health, with their emphasis on the group rather than the individual, require the sanction and organizing capabilities of a strong central authority. All pre-colonial African societies acknowledged some form of religious or political authority and the well-being of the community, the public, was traditionally a concern shared by political and religious authorities. African healers and leaders throughout the continent regularly supervised activities intended to protect and maintain the public well-being. In Buganda, which can serve as an example of kingdoms in Uganda, the king was the absolute authority. Authority flowed through the king to the powerful clan leaders in the *Lukiiko* (parliament), either directly appointed or ratified by him. Individual rights were subordinated to the well-being of the group.

The Bagandan king and other leaders supported the efforts of the colonial administration to control STDs. The Lukiiko promulgated strict, even

Draconian, laws to control people. When the foreign administrators implemented the Contagious Diseases Act there was little resistance from African leaders, who instead apparently sanctioned the harsh legislation. Explaining the use of the Contagious Diseases Act in Uganda, Major Keane said that "Compulsory examination owes its origin entirely to native wish and native conception as to how v.d. measures should be conducted. . . . In considering coercion it is essential to divest one's mind of European conditions. Coercion is recognized as the customary method of introducing new ideas and advancing progress in this country."[26] Keane's explanation that it was entirely native wish and native conception reveals the cooperation of Bagandan authorities. He implied that Bagandan leaders viewed STD prevention efforts as enforceable law with no question of individual rights. By "European condition" Keane was implying the irrelevance in Africa of the issue of individual rights; in Africa, he asserted, coercion was the rule.

Strong vestiges of these very different views of public health versus individual rights were clearly perceptible in many responses of African societies to HIV/AIDS. Some African leaders, like their early forebears, suggested harsh, repressive measures to prevent the spread of the virus. For example, in 1986 in Rakai District of southwestern Uganda, it was reported that "teenage girls and young women in their thirties are being arrested and deported from the area for fear they could be AIDS carriers."[27] Returning to the history of STDs, an episode early this century will illustrate the tensions between Western and local views toward public health, and, further, it will show how African men sought to utilize new public health legislation to control their women.

In 1923 the vertical campaign against STD was merged with general medical work. The change in policy arose from a number of factors including a scandal in 1921–22 that had drawn attention to Uganda to the embarrassment of the Colonial Office. The London *Daily News* on February 17, 1922, reported the Colonial Office's attempt to introduce contagious diseases acts in Uganda, based on the similarly contentious regulations attempted years before in England. The 1866 Contagious Diseases Act in England required compulsory medical examination of prostitutes, and it aroused enormous public opposition. Individual rights were fiercely defended over the expedient of public health legislation. The act was suspended in 1883 and later between 1913 and 1916 a Royal Commission examining the problem of widespread STDs advised against any legislation of compulsion in order to protect strict anonymity. The 1922 *Daily News* article drew public attention to events in the small, distant colony and awakened the old controversy over public health versus individual rights. At the request of a number of concerned organizations in Britain, the National Council for Combating Venereal Diseases began an inquiry into the matter. Interested parties included the Catholic Women's League, the Federation of Medical Women, the Association for Moral and Social Hygiene, and the International Woman Suffrage Alliance.

A female doctor sent to Uganda to treat women and children was sacked five months later after accusing senior Royal Army Corps medical officers of applying regulations unacceptable anywhere else in the world and of degrading and humiliating African women during physical examinations. "I found I was called upon to assist in working venereal disease laws and regulations which are far worse than any Contagious Diseases Acts ever in force in any country . . . [that] apply to the whole native population; they involve the compulsory examination and treatment of whole villages of people and this at regular intervals."[28]

The 1921 law was one of a number passed over the years in an attempt to legislate morality and health. The first venereal disease legislation was promulgated by Bagandan authorities in 1913 when the Lukiiko passed the Native Law. It required the chiefs to notify authorities of infected persons and to send them to government treatment centers for attention. The earlier colonial Township Rules of 1903 had sanctioned compulsory examination and detention of persons, male or female, thought to be infected with dangerous diseases.

The Lukiiko later implemented other laws including in 1918 the Adultery and Fornication Law and in 1931 the Law Preventing Movement of Women in Buganda. That action was a vivid indication of the pace of change occurring in African society and the ways in which the new economic opportunities and pressures were affecting gender relations. Again, the law illustrates that both European and African men regarded women as the primary reservoir and transmitters of STDs.

The scandal in Uganda was eventually forgotten and, although exonerated through the efforts of a large number of supporters of the STD campaign in Uganda, Lambkin and the small specialist STD establishment were soon amalgamated within a larger, unitary colonial medical establishment. The principal medical officer thought that the STD campaign had developed too rapidly between 1921 and 1923 and had become antagonistic, even detrimental, rather than complementary to other medical work in the Protectorate. This was in spite of the fact that the campaign operated within a circumscribed area of the Protectorate representing not more than 5 percent of the total population.[29]

THE COLONIAL MEDICAL DEPARTMENT

Restructured as a component of the new colonial medical department, the campaign continued, fueled by the perception of the impact of STDs on fertility and morbidity. With ever-increasing demands for laborers, this was a major concern to the authorities. New forms of labor organization and rural agricultural production disrupted African social systems profoundly. In Uganda by 1908 there was such a shortage of labor that Governor Bell introduced a scheme of obligatory labor, *kasanvu*. Chiefs were required to supply able-bodied men to work for one month each year, a system that functioned until 1922. The administration then followed recommendations to allow voluntary labor to evolve in response to wages and prices; nevertheless, there was such a shortage of labor that massive numbers of men from neighboring colonies of Rwanda, Belgian Congo, and Sudan were encouraged and recruited to work in Uganda. It was not long before the foreigners were accused of introducing new diseases including sexually transmitted ones.[30]

Over the next decades syphilis appeared to decrease in incidence while gonorrhea increased considerably. Other travelers and laborers and the veterans returning from duties in World War II were often cited as having introduced gonorrhea to new populations back home. Government and mission hospitals and dispensaries continued to offer treatments, but a very large proportion of Africans preferred to seek medical attention from either their own traditional practitioners or in the numerous private clinics and even more informal private injectors that by the 1970s proliferated. Thus, official statistics give us only an indication of the true scale of these diseases over the decades (see Table 5.1).

In spite of the repeated observations that STDs were a serious public health issue, by the mid-1950s there was not a single STDs expert present in the country. In a report to the World Health Organization, the Medical Department claimed, "Venereal disease in the form of syphilis and gonorrhea has constituted one of the most intractable problems which the Medical Department of Uganda has had to deal with during the last thirty years."[31] Of all hospital admissions, 8 percent were for STDs, mainly gonorrhea, syphilis, and granuloma inguinale, and, although prevalent throughout the country, the highest incidence was in the southern half. With the poor compliance of the vast majority of patients and the scarcity of staff, there is some question that most patients, in fact, were cured of their infections. It was particularly worrying to discover that "at Mulago Hospital, 15% of 2,763 patients were school children, and 70% were unmarried. Many had been 'cured' three or four times before."[32] Again, the poor compliance, particularly of young people, must be recalled before accepting the verdict of cured. Europeans had long argued that the primary cause of widespread STDs was the uncontrolled sexual activity of Ugandans that, coupled with their lack of social sanctions, was a recipe for disaster.

Half a century after the first missionaries and colonial administrators cited promiscuity and immorality as chief factors in the prevalence of STDs, the Medical Department complained, "The transmission of venereal disease is facilitated by lack of any marked social sanction against promiscuity . . . [making] the chances or reinfection within a short period

TABLE 5.1
Syphilis, Yaws, and Gonorrhea in Uganda
Reported in Government Hospitals 1926–69

Year	Syphilis	Yaws	Gonorrhea
1926	35,784	10,930	—
1927	52,032	26,629	—
1928	69,015	35,126	—
1929	74,722	37,378	8,609
1930	65,979	38,066	8,619
1931	64,591	47,598	8,931
1932	68,432	43,773	10,591
1933	72,218	49,546	10,702
1934	74,141	57,056	9,690
1935	72,361	64,715	11,849
1936	63,395	62,240	14,101
1937	67,621	65,359	16,236
1938	56,545	73,489	14,763
1939	57,542	76,427	16,465
1940	20,138	24,665	7,178
1941	18,951	22,942	7,347
1942	19,692	24,069	8,669
1943	23,599	26,769	11,415
1944	24,021	27,655	10,526
1945	31,549	33,697	14,936
1946	39,444	35,185	20,098
1947	45,464	37,803	30,111
1948	47,854	35,915	33,160
1949	41,089	—	30,900
1950	36,857	17,787	32,271
1951	29,760	17,852	23,381
1952	23,690	14,704	16,659
1953	20,090	14,436	19,388
1954	19,975	13,847	21,645
1955	17,224	10,880	25,707
1957	16,499	10,529	29,935
1958	13,279	8,557	34,704
1959	11,966	9,478	39,242
1960	6,430	9,594	39,150*
1961	7,689	—	39,363
1962	8,107	—	42,194
1963	9,247	—	45,835
1969	6,002	7,983	127,667

*Statistics from Uganda Protectorate, Medical Department *Annual Reports*, and Uganda National Archives. File GCW.3, April 30, 1955, Proposed Survey of Venereal Diseases.

Sources: Uganda Protectorate, Medical Department *Annual Reports*, and Uganda National Archives. File GCW.3, April 30, 1955, Proposed Survey of Venereal Diseases.

following cure of an infection . . . generally high."[33] This is a refrain that appears regularly throughout the history of STDs.[34] In light of the widely held European opinion that Africans were morally deficient and that this class of diseases was caused by weakness of character, it is not surprising that a large proportion of patients sought cures outside the formal health sector. Colonial records reiterated as a continuing problem the reluctance of patients to present at recognized treatment centers, preferring instead to see private practitioners, many of whom were only half trained or quacks. The result of misuse of drugs and underdosage is that in many instances the causative germs of the diseases have become resistant to the known drugs or antibiotics. For example, Table 5.2 illustrates resistance of *Neisseria gonorrheae* to antibiotics in 1997.[35]

In 1955 the Ugandan government requested the World Health Organization to conduct a nationwide survey of STDs and there were plans to launch a new prevention initiative through education and the use of radio. The plans included new STD clinics to be opened at each government and mission hospital in the country with free treatments. All schoolchildren were to be examined at the beginning of each term, and employers would be responsible for regular examinations of all employees. Prostitutes would be examined, and those found infected would be offered alternative forms of labor. The volatile political situation in the country forced a postponement of the survey together with the proposed new campaign.[36] The whole idea was dropped in 1956 with explanations from the World Health Organization that the continuing political difficulties in Uganda combined with the growing consensus that funds would be better spent on a "continental offensive against the endemic *treponematoses* in Africa" made such a survey unlikely.[37]

Such emphases on vertical campaigns rather than on more integrated approaches to public health had focussed undue attention on one cluster of diseases. Not all medical staff had concurred that STDs were the major

TABLE 5.2
Sensitivity of *Neisseria gonorrhea* to Antibiotics

Antibiotic	Percent Sensitivity	Level of Resistance
ampicillin	31.50	resistant
chloramphenicol	5.40	resistant
tetracycline	0.25	resistant
erythromycin	82.60	borderline resistant
augmentin	89.10	borderline resistant

Source: STD Unit Ward 12, Old Mulago Hospital, AMREF 1997.

health problem in Uganda, and some cautioned that there had been much misdiagnoses of other conditions as syphilis. For example one medical officer complained in 1951 that

Many people think that every sick child in this country is emaciated, pale and very irritable because of syphilis, and there is discontent on the part of parents when a doctor informs them that the child suffers from kwashiorkor. This department must plead guilty to over-facile diagnosis of "syphilis" and erroneous interpretation of hospital data in the past. In a pamphlet published in 1922 it was claimed that two-thirds of all pregnant women in Buganda suffered from syphilis and it is evident that many other diseases of childhood were in those days confused with syphilis. Enthusiastic concentration on a single disease is liable to override discrimination.[38]

SEXUALLY TRANSMITTED DISEASES: 1960 TO THE PRESENT

Syphilis was indeed not the problem by the late 1960s when gonorrhea was the most reported STD. One of its major sequelae was its impact on fertility because it led to sterility in females. Sterility was widespread among Bagandan women with estimates that 30 percent in 1948 were so affected,[39] and in 1963 the number had increased to a remarkable 50 percent.[40] Among other STDs, chancroid and trichomoniasis were particularly common. In spite of free government medical care considerable numbers of Ugandans were still attending private clinics and private injectors.

Studies in the 1960s and 1970s of STD among university students and the army provide further evidence of incidence rates. In 1966 23 percent of male attendances at the health clinic were related to STD, and by 1968 about 25 percent of male university students were infected.[41] Prevention advocates were sometimes a little more realistic than the earlier hard-line moralists. There were now calls for a modern health education program that would "fit the changing sexual mores of to-day rather than reliance on traditional and now unrealistic moral principles."[42]

War and Disintegration

Idi Amin is remembered by the West mainly for initiating the dramatic deterioration and decline of his country, but even Amin involved himself in campaigning against STD in Uganda. In 1971 in Masaka, one of the first districts later to be afflicted by HIV/AIDS, Amin urged the public that if "if anyone has gonorrhea, he or she should not fear to tell the doctor the truth because of fear."[43] He promulgated the 1972 "Decree to Prohibit the Wearing of Certain Dresses Which Outrage Decency and Are Injurious to Public Morals and For Other Purposes Connected Therewith" in an attempt to control the excitation of men by female attire.[44] Two years later he advised "all Ugandans to control themselves and to report to the doctors immediately they experience signs of the disease [gonorrhea]." In 1974 Amin ordered the ministers of Information and Broadcasting and of Health to "mount a big campaign against the disease . . . to introduce a special program on Radio and Television to explain to the people how to protect themselves against the disease."[45] Amin's opinions were clearly expressed in the introduction to his 1977 Venereal Diseases Decree: "This is a Military Government and a Government of Action. . . . The Life President wants to lead not only rich people but people who are literate, intelligent, peaceful, happy, healthy and strong. . . . He had fought the Economic War [evicted the Asian community] and won it. He has now set out to fight a war against all diseases."[46] The war against all diseases was considerably disrupted over the next decades by other kinds of wars and upheavals.

From the time of the expulsion of the Asians in late 1972 the economy, infrastructure, and all social services deteriorated rapidly. Between 1971 and 1975 the price of the major staple food in the southern half of the country, *matoke*, increased 413 percent.[47] The 1970s were years of destabilization with loss of security for life and property. The invasion of the country in 1972 by Ugandan forces based in Tanzania set off widespread tribal killing as Amin sought to eliminate all opposition inside the country. Many hundreds of Acholi, Langi, and prosperous Baganda were massacred, and by 1973 army units were stationed in "every village."[48] During the first two years of Amin's rule, the size of the army doubled from 6,700 to 12,600, and it is believed that by 1975 there were about 25,000 in the army.[49] "The inhumanity of the army extended to the economy from the *kondosim* [armed robberies] of the late 1960s to military business marauders, *mafuta mingi* of the 1970s and the rapist looters in the early 1980s."[50] In 1978–79 50,000 Tanzanian troops invaded and destroyed much of the districts of Masaka and Mbarara, and by 1981 they had marched the length and breadth of the land. It was widely held by many Ugandans and foreign observers that this invasion was responsible for much of the dissemination of the virus in Uganda. "It is also said that when AIDS was first seen in Uganda, it was the '*Bakombozi*' [liberating] soldiers from Tanzania who came with it."[51] Such blaming is reminiscent of accusations in history that syphilis was the French disease, the Italian pox, or introduced to us by them.

The omnipresence of the military interfered with nearly everyone and increased existing insecurity. The health care delivery system collapsed, and peasant farmers bore the brunt of the impact. Social welfare services disappeared as qualified people by the hundreds left the country, and the vacancies were often filled with mediocre, incompetent political appointees, thus ensuring total institutional collapse in the country.

Milton Obote returned in 1981 for a second term as president, but the bad times were not over, and many Ugandans insist that the next five years were far more brutal than the previous five years. Between 1981 and 1986 a bitter civil war ensued that gradually ousted Obote. The long war ended in early 1986, ushering in a long period of stability. The new government of Yoweri Museveni, like those before, highlighted the ever-present problem of STDs. In its political program published in 1988, the new regime described how during 1979 while fighting in central Uganda they had discovered that syphilis was rampant. "The most pathetic aspect, however, is the fact that the population are relatively unconcerned about it; you can find somebody with syphilitic skin marks completely unaware that he is still sick, arguing that this is due to the past sickness and that it is normal."[52]

Sexually Transmitted Diseases: 1980s

When HIV/AIDS was first noticed in Uganda in 1982 a range of STDs remained a major health problem. In spite of their presence, by 1997 there was only one government-run, dedicated STD clinic in the country: Ward 12 at Mulago Hospital (site of the original venereal diseases treatment room). A study of nine sites (hospitals located along the major east-west trade axis) in 1990 revealed that in some hospitals between 1986 and 1990 STDs had accounted for 16 percent of all admissions.[53] Antenatal screening for syphilis was initiated in 1991 in an attempt to track systematically the rates of STDs. Two of the major hospitals in Kampala, both voluntary (formerly mission), returned reports of high rates of infection. Nsambya Hospital reported 29 percent of women and Rubaga Hospital 22 percent of women reacted positively to serological tests for syphilis.

A national serosurvey was carried out in 1988 to determine the level of HIV in the general population.[54] At the same time syphilis was measured, and 17.5 percent of those tested were found to be antibody positive.[55] In addition, the serosurvey also revealed that in some areas of Uganda 15–30 percent of those infected with HIV had a history of genital ulcer disease (GUD) within the past five years;[56] for example, 30 percent of the outpatients at Mulago's STD clinic were presenting with genital ulcers. These were important clues concerning the relationship between other STDs and HIV. Bohenga Hospital in Fort Portal, western Uganda, reported that in 1989 24.3 percent of pediatric visits to outpatients were related to congenital syphilis.

HIV and AIDS

In November 1990 a team of U.S. demographers showed the president a glossy video in which a mathematical model of the epidemic was used to project the potentially devastating impact of HIV/AIDS on the population of his country.[57] Impressive graphics informed the president that if there were no HIV/AIDS, by the year 2015 there could be 32 million Ugandans.[58] However, if the dramatic AIDS epidemic continued unabated, the population would be only 20 million; a loss of 12 million people plus the added burden of 5–6 million orphans[59] resulting from the death of AIDS victims.

Soon after seeing the film the president announced that the AIDS epidemic was now "beyond the control of the medical experts" and what was needed was "a massive campaign to educate people to change their sexual behavior."[60] The following June Museveni set a precedent by opening the annual International Conference on AIDS in Florence, a clear indication of the importance accorded HIV/AIDS by the political leader.[61] Other speakers at the AIDS conference referred to the coming apocalypse in Africa with millions dying and economies and societies collapsing, while widening the discussion Museveni explained that "the AIDS epidemic has reached catastrophic proportions . . . by the year 2000, 80 per cent of all cases will be occurring in developing countries."[62] In June 1991 it was estimated that up to 6.5 million Africans were HIV positive. Teachers, engineers, businessmen, doctors, nurses and, as time passed, increasing numbers of rural cultivators were afflicted. AIDS was "not only a health problem but is a social, economic and political nightmare."[63]

There can be no doubt that the long history of STDs in Uganda is relevant to understanding the contours of the epidemic of HIV/AIDS in Uganda. It can be argued reasonably that the political upheavals and civil wars in Uganda from the mid-1970s until 1986 are implicated in the spread of an STD. By June 1991 it was estimated that nearly 1.5 million Ugandans were infected with HIV.[64] In urban hospitals like Mulago, up to 40 percent of beds were occupied by patients with AIDS-related infections.[65] The levels of infection, combined with the fact that treatment and prevention, while commendable efforts in Uganda, never achieved the scale necessary to eliminate STDs, help us to understand the wildfire spread of HIV in Uganda.

CONCLUSION

I have sketched the medical and scientific assessment of STDs in Uganda over most of this century. The medical authorities repeatedly admitted that these diseases were an intractable medical problem. Retrospective diagnosis is difficult and a dangerous exercise for the non-specialist, and I remind the reader that my concern is not the incorrect diagnoses caused by the confusion between endemic and venereal syphilis earlier this century. We must accept the contemporary perception that STDs constituted a demographic threat. The threat was expressed in medical and moral terms and it was believed that the solution would be found in science and moral teaching. Leaving aside the issue of early misdiagnoses of syphilis, clearly gonorrhea and other STDs increased in prevalence and incidence in Uganda over this century. Since mid-century STDs have been a major health problem, and recent studies such as the survey of nine sentinel sites between 1986 and 1990 remind us that these diseases remain widespread.

There was no cure for HIV/AIDS by 1997, although some effective drugs had been developed to suppress the virus and provided hope for the future. It was unlikely, however, that many Ugandans would have access to the expensive drugs. In the mid-1990s the national per capita spending on health was a little over $5.50. With no cure available during the first decades of AIDS, the only available weapon was information and education. For many Ugandans life would be forever changed by those efforts. Frank messages and discussions on hitherto repressed subjects put sexuality, sexual practices, and STDs on the agenda in ways never before known to most of the population. A major focus of much AIDS education was the introduction and use of condoms. In 1990 the majority of Ugandans professed to shun the condom, which was thought to be non-African or foreign. By 1997 the situation had been considerably changed with survey after survey showing high levels of knowledge about condoms and moderate levels of usage. In October 1996 the STD/AIDS Control Program published its report on declining trends in HIV infection rates in parts of the country. Uganda was one of the first countries in the world to record a significant decline in HIV among certain groups, for example, younger people.[66]

It is sobering, however, to recall that the other prevalent STDs, like gonorrhea, syphilis, and chancroid, have had cures for many decades, but public health campaigns in Uganda before HIV/AIDS that aimed at their control were limited or lacking. When there were public health efforts, much of the emphasis remained on the old view that these diseases are caused by immorality and promiscuity. In light of the very important role of STDs as potential co-factors, enhancing the transmission of HIV, this was a most unfortunate policy.

We can learn much more about the history of STDs in Uganda. Nevertheless, it remains clear that they were present when Europeans arrived in the last century, continued during the colonial period to afflict the health of significant numbers of the population, and remained widespread in the late 1990s.

NOTES

1. See M. Lyons, "The Point of View: Perspectives on AIDS in Uganda," in *AIDS in Africa and the Caribbean: The Documentation of an Epidemic*, edited by G. C.

Bond, J. Vincent, J. Kreniske, and I. S. Susser (Boulder, Colo.: Westview Press, 1997); Samuel V. Duh, *Blacks and AIDS: Causes and Origins* (Newbury Park, Calif.: Sage, 1991); John Comaroff and Jean Comaroff, *Ethnography and the Historical Imagination* (Boulder, Colo.: Westview Press, 1992).

    2.   Wilson Carswell, R. Mugerwa, N. Sewankambo, Fred Kigozi, and R. Goodgame, "AIDS in Africa: A Special Report by the Clinical Committee on AIDS," Kampala, unpublished manuscript, January 24, 1986.

    3.   Maryinez Lyons, "The Bible or the Condom: Implications for Women in Uganda," in *Ringvorlesungen zu Frauenspezifischen Themen*, edited by Dagmar Eissner (Mainz: Universitat Mainz, 1995).

    4.   E.M.K. Muwazi, H. C. Trowell, and J.N.P. Davies, "Congenital Syphilis in Uganda," *East African Medical Journal* 23 (1947): 152.

    5.   President Museveni's opening speech at the Seventh International AIDS Conference in Florence, June 16, 1991.

    6.   J.N.P. Davies, "The History of Syphilis in Uganda," *Bulletin of the World Health Organization* 15 (1956): 1041–55.

    7.   *Buganda* is the country, *Baganda* is plural for people, and a *Muganda* is an individual. Many Bantu languages employ a similar pattern of prefixes.

    8.   Albert Cook, "The Medical History of Uganda: Part II," *East African Medical Journal* 13 (1936–37): 99.

    9.   F. J. Lambkin, *Prevalence of Venereal Diseases in the Uganda Protectorate*, Africa No. 917: Uganda, Colonial Office.

    10. Congenital syphilis was called euphemistically *munnyu*, or salt, by the Baganda. They believed that too much salt taken during pregnancy caused miscarriage.

    11. F. J. Lambkin, "Syphilis in the Uganda Protectorate," *Journal of the Royal Army Medical Corps* 11 (1908): 153. A. Cook, who had practiced medicine for years in the country, disagreed with Lambkin's statistics. According to Cook's records for 1903–7, 14.8 percent of outpatients and 11.4 percent of inpatients were syphilitic, and complications occurred in about 25 percent of pregnancies.

    12. W. D. Foster, *The Early History of Scientific Medicine in Uganda* (Kampala: Uganda Literature Bureau, 1970), p. 82.

    13. J. A. Carman, "The Relationship of Yaws and Syphilis: Are They Two Diseases or One?" *The East African Medical Journal* 12 (1935–36):135–49.

    14. R. R. Willcox, *Textbook of Venereal Diseases and Treponematoses* (London: William Heinemann Medical Books, 1964), p. 263.

    15. J.N.P. Davies, "The History of Syphilis in Uganda," p. 1041; F. J. Bennett, "Venereal Diseases and Related Spirochaetal Infections," Occasional Paper No. 12, in Ministry of Health, East African Community Medical Research Institutes, and Makerere University College Medical School, *Uganda Atlas of Disease Distribution* (Kampala: Makerere University, Department of Geography, 1968), pp. 66–68.

    16. Some Ugandan peoples inoculated their babies by "wrapping them in a cloth which had on it the discharges from secondary syphilitic ulcers." J. Orley, "Concepts of Infectious Disease amongst the Rural Ganda — with Special Reference to Yaws and Syphilis," in *Nkanga: Special Edition on Medicine and Social Sciences in East and West Africa*, edited by F. J. Bennett (Kampala: Makerere Institute for Social Research, 1973), p. 62.

17. J. Orley, "Concepts," p. 62. He suggests the high child mortality witnessed by the early STD investigators was probably due to malnutrition, malaria, and other parasitic diseases and not congenital syphilis.

18. L.J.A. Loewenthal, "Syphilis in Natives of Uganda: A Brief Review," *The Urologic and Cutaneous Review* 43 (1939): 182.

19. A. Cook, "Syphilis in Uganda," *Lancet*, December 12, 1908, p. 1771. See Megan Vaughan, "Syphilis in Colonial East and Central Africa: The Social Construction of an Epidemic," in *Epidemics and Ideas*, edited by T. O. Ranger and P. Slack (Cambridge: Cambridge University Press, 1992); Carol Summers, "Intimate Colonialism: The Imperial Production of Reproduction in Uganda, 1907–1925," *Signs: Journal of Women in Culture and Society* 16 (1991): 787–807.

20. J.N.P. Davies, "History of Syphilis in Uganda," p. 1048.

21. The policy of implementing a campaign to investigate and control an epidemic disease had been established as a result of human trypanosomiasis, or sleeping sickness. This disease initiated in the newly established colonies of Sub-Saharan Africa the fear that laborers and potential taxpayers would be lost.

22. W.M.B. Sparkes, "Report on the Treatment of Syphilis in Kampala for the Month of January 1909," Uganda National Archives, File A45/29 Secretariat Minute Paper 165/09, February 13, 1909.

23. Uganda National Archives, Secretariat Minute Paper No. 165/1909, Venereal diseases medical staff, memo of June 29, 1909.

24. A. Cook, "The Medical History of Uganda, Part I," *The East African Medical Journal* 13 (1936–37): 78.

25. W.M.B. Sparkes, "Report on Treatment of Syphilis in Kampala for the Month of June 1909, "Uganda National Archives, File A25/29, Secretariat Minute paper 165/09, July 10, 1909;

26. Major Keane to Principal Medical Officer, Entebbe, "Venereal Disease in Uganda," Draft report, Uganda National Archives, File No. C.637, July 14, 1922. In Britain the Contagious Diseases Act of 1866, which required compulsory medical examination of prostitutes, aroused enormous public opposition and was suspended in 1883. Between 1913 and 1916 a Royal Commission examined the problem of widespread venereal diseases and advised against any legislation of compulsion in order to protect strict anonymity.

27. *Weekly Topic* (Kampala), March 1986.

28. Uganda National Archives, File No. C.637, 1922, "Abstract Made by the Association for Moral and Social Hygiene from Mrs. ___ — Letter, Now Being Circulated by Them to Members of Parliament and Others."

29. R. H. Reford, Principal Medical Officer, Entebbe, to Chief Secretary, Uganda National Archives, File No. C.637, March 28, 1923.

30. M. Lyons, "Foreign Bodies: The History of Labour Migration as a Threat to Public Health in Uganda," in *African Boundaries: Barriers, Conduits and Opportunities*, edited by A. I. Asiwaju and Paul Nugent (London: Pinter-Cassell, 1996).

31. World Health Organization, "Proposed Venereal Disease Survey," Uganda National Archives, File GCW.3, November 10, 1952–January 2, 1963.

32. Ibid.

33. "Application for Venereal Disease Survey by WHO in 1955," Uganda National Archives, File No. GCW.3.

34. See for example Allan M. Brandt, *No Magic Bullet: A Social History of*

Venereal Disease in the United States since 1880 (New York: Oxford University Press, 1987).

35. S. Fitzgerald interview and report to Centers for Disease Control, April 20, 1990. In the United States, penicillin resistance is in the region of 99 percent.

36. G. B. Cartland, The Secretariat, Entebbe, to Dr. Cambournac, Director, Regional Office for Africa, WHO, Brazzaville, Uganda National Archives, File GCW.3, June 4, 1955.

37. G. B. Cartland to Dr. Pierre P. Clement, Uganda National Archives, File GCW.3, June 20, 1956.

38. Uganda Protectorate, Medical Department, "Annual Report for 1951."

39. A. Richards and P. Reining, "Report on Fertility Survey of Buganda and Bahaya," (Kampala: East African Institute of Social Research 1952), p. 35. The estimates of fertility were based on the 1948 census, which also indicated that 18 percent of women in the entire colony were childless (calculated as a percent of all women over 45 years). During this survey it was not possible to persuade every adult to be examined for venereal disease. Audrey Richards said "Venereal disease is openly discussed by the Baganda and little stigma is attached to infection. All the women were asked if they had had syphilis or gonorrhea and twenty-nine per cent reported that they had had one or the other of these diseases but the figures are not reliable because the women tended to call an undiagnosed illness, especially those producing skin rashes by the general name of kabotongo or syphilis" (p. 30).

40. H. B. Griffith, "Gonorrhea and Fertility in Uganda," *Eugenics Review* 55 (1963): 103–8. W. D. Foster, Professor of Medical Microbiology at Makerere University College between 1963 and 1967, found that specific serological tests for syphilis were positive for some 15 percent of apparently healthy adults, the incidence of acute gonorrhea was very high, and late complications of this disease were one of the commonest causes of death. Foster, *The Early History of Scientific Medicine in Uganda*, pp. 78–79. Interview with W. Carswell, June 10, 1993. New Mulago Hospital was built by the British who left it as a gift in 1963 at the time of independence; the new hospital had no STD clinic..

41. O. P. Arya and F. J. Bennett, "Attitudes of College Students in East Africa to Sexual Activity and Venereal Disease," *British Journal of Venereal Disease* 44 (1968): 160. The rate of gonorrhea per 100,000 people in Denmark was 319, in Sweden 514, and in the United States 308. Based on his research he estimated that Kampala had 15,000 cases. O. P. Arya, "The Greatest Hazard of Sexual Pollution — VD," *Tropical Health* (Quarterly review of the Department of Preventive Medicine, Makerere University) 4 (October 1972): 1–4.

42. O. P. Arya and F. J. Bennett, "Venereal Disease in an Elite Group (University Students) in East Africa," *British Journal of Venereal Disease* 43 (1967): 276, 279. A study of the military in 1968 revealed that a third of the cohort of 712 individuals gave a history of venereal diseases. V. L. Ongom, "Prevalence and Incidence of Venereal Diseases in Military Communities in Uganda," *East African Medical Journal* 47 (1970): 481.

43. "Our Rural Riches Not Yet Fully Utilised," *Uganda Argus,* November 3, 1971.

44. Idi Amin Dada, The Penal Code Act (Amendment) Decree, June 6, 1972.

45. "V.D. Rate Worries General," *Voice of Uganda,* April 6, 1973.

46.   Idi Amin Dada, The Venereal Diseases Decree, September 17, 1977.

47.   Jan Jelmert Jorgensen, *Uganda: A Modern History* (London: St. Martin's Press, 1981), pp. 298, 303.

48.   H. B. Hansen, *Ethnicity and Military Rule in Uganda*, Research Report No. 43 (Uppsala: Scandinavian Institute of African Studies, 1977), pp. 97, 107.

49.   T. Avigan and M. Honey, *War in Uganda: The Legacy of Idi Amin* (New York: Lawrence Hill, 1982), p. 7.

50.   T. B. Kabwegyere, "The Politics of State Destruction in Uganda since 1962: Lessons for the Future," in *Beyond Crisis: Development Issues in Uganda*, edited by P. D. Wiebe and Cole P. Dodge (Kampala: Makerere Institute for Social Research and the African Studies Association, 1987), p. 18.

51.   F. Bakanyebomera of Lira, "New Vision," July 28, 1989.

52.   NRM Secretariat, "Political Programme of the NRM: Two Years of Action," Uganda National Archives, 1988, pp. 16–17.

53.   S. A. Fitzgerald, "Report of Short-Term Consultancy: AIDS Control Programme, Republic of Uganda, 16.1.90–20.4.90," May 1990 (unpublished). Sentinel HIV surveillance is the serial collection of HIV prevalence data over time and place in selected groups of the population in order to monitor trends in HIV infection using an anonymous unlinked procedure. Sites included: antenatal clinics, Kampala area; HIV among blood donors, Nakasero Blood Bank, Kampala; STD clinical syndromes in Mbale (Eastern Uganda); Lacor (North); Ft. Portal (West); and Mbarara (Southwest).

54.   Insecurity in the northern region precluded surveying the entire country. A total of 3,426 adults representing 61 percent of the population were tested. The weighted prevalence rate of positivity was 9 percent with much variation among regions: central urban rates = 21 percent; western urban rates = 29 percent; West Nile urban rates = 8 percent.

55.   Findings in 1994 from the Rakai Project, a collaborative, long-term study by Columbia University and Makerere University revealed very similar statistics for syphilis in a rural population where 17.5 percent of men and 17.5 percent of women, all aged 15–59, tested positive. The HIV rates in the same study were 16.4 percent men and 20.9 percent women.

56.   Fitzgerald, "Report," April 20, 1990. GUD has been identified as an enhancing factor for HIV transmission rates. GUD occurs with diseases such as syphilis and chancroid. On GUD and HIV transmission, see R. M. Greenblatt, S. A. Lukehart, F. A. Plummer, T. C. Quinn, C. W. Critchlow, R. L. Ashley, L. J. D'Costa, J. O. Ndinya-Achola, L. Corey, and A. R. Ronald, "Genital Ulceration as a Risk Factor for Human Immunodeficiency Virus Infection," *AIDS* 2 (February 1988): 47–50.

57.   The AIDS Impact Model (AIM) computer program for presenting information about AIDS was prepared by John Stover for the Futures Group in collaboration with AIDSTECH/Family Health International and presented to the president by the U.S. ambassador, William A. Burroughs, Jr.

58.   Uganda's population increased from approximately 5 million in 1948 to 9.5 million in 1969 and by 1997 had exceeded 18 million. About 49 percent of the population is under the age of 15, and working age adults comprise some 47 percent of the population.

59.   There is much to say about the assumptions and definitions upon which

the models are based. In AIM, for instance, the definition of an AIDS orphan is a child under 15 who has lost its mother to AIDS. In many Ugandan societies, an orphan is a child who has lost either a mother or a father, and some feel that an orphan is a child who has lost a father and not a mother. More careful social research is required before we can accept unquestioned the results of mathematical models for projecting the impact of AIDS in Africa. John Stover, *AIM: AIDS Impact Model — a Computer Program for Presenting Information about AIDS* (Washington, D.C.: Futures Group, 1991), p. 69; See Elizabeth A. Preble, "Impact of HIV/AIDS on African Children," *Social Science and Medicine* 31 (1990): 671–80.

60.   *Weekly Topic* (Kampala), December 1990.

61.   Y. Museveni, "AIDS and Its Impact on the Health and Social Service Infrastructure in Developing Countries," International Conference on HIV/AIDS, Florence, Italy, June 16, 1991.

62.   *The Guardian*, June 17, 1991.

63.   Warren Namaara, "Progress on the AIDS Epidemic in Uganda." (Entebbe: Ministry of Health, AIDS Control Programme, 1991). The sex ratio of cases reported to the AIDS Control Programme is 1:1.

64.   Warren Namaara, "AIDS Control Programme," *AIDS Newsletter*, July 19, 1991.

65.   See W. Namaara, "Progress on the AIDS Epidemic in Uganda."

66.   Anonymous,, "A Report on Declining Trends in HIV Infection Rates in Sentinel Surveillance Sites in Uganda." (Entebbe: Ministry of Health, STD/AIDS Control Programme, 1996).

6

Local Histories of Sexually Transmitted Diseases and AIDS in Western and Northern Tanzania

Philip W. Setel

Through the mid-1990s Tanzania remained one of the most severely AIDS-affected countries in sub-Saharan Africa; by 1995 it had reported more cases of AIDS to the World Health Organization than any other country in the region (53,247).[1] That year according to government projections 1.6 million Tanzanians were infected with HIV. Despite its severity, the first decade of Tanzania's AIDS epidemic has been characterized by great diversity in its local manifestations. This chapter charts the vicissitudes of HIV epidemiology in two regions, Kagera and Kilimanjaro. The shifting (and often ambiguous) scientific and popular epidemiologies of sexually transmitted diseases (STDs) and AIDS in these locations have revolved around socio-geographic networks[2] in subgroups of the population. These networks arose in the context of colonialism, the encroachment of cash economies, population growth, urbanization, and stratification in rural areas. Although these forces of social change and development were not unique to Kagera and Kilimanjaro, they evoked particular cultural responses in these places that local actors and epidemiologists alike tied to the emergence of AIDS.[3]

THE SCIENTIFIC EPIDEMIOLOGY OF SEXUALLY TRANSMITTED DISEASES AND AIDS

Sexually Transmitted Diseases in Tanzania before the Age of AIDS

The diagnosis of the first cases of AIDS in Tanzania signalled the beginning of biomedical awareness of HIV's arrival in the country and the end of decades of lack of attention to research on STDs and sexuality. Little can be deduced epidemiologically about the overall prevalence of STDs in Tanzania prior to the advent of AIDS, and extensive research would be required to reconstruct a history of STDs for Tanzania as a whole. Although epidemic outbreaks of STDs were chronicled (as in the case of the Haya of Kagera discussed here) and medical journals of the time may yield some clinic- or hospital-based figures, these data alone would not be sufficient to assemble a historical or social epidemiology. The lack of reliable census data until the late 1970s (and some would argue up until the present day) and the unknown biases of selection for those who encountered the colonial health care system would make the numerators and the denominators in any prevalence equation extremely difficult to estimate.

Aside from some scant archival material on the anti-venereal disease campaign among East African troops during and after World War II,[4] there are few sources of data on the topic of STDs prior to the 1980s. Anecdotal descriptions and estimates of the prevalence of syphilis, gonorrhea, and chancroid before the 1940s are too scanty to weave into any broad picture, and some estimates, such as the claim in the 1930s that 90 percent of Maasai had syphilis or gonorrhea, were clearly implausible (and were dismissed as such by Medical Department staff at the time). Whatever the overall prevalence, STDs were of some concern to British health officials after their takeover of Tanganyika from the Germans in the early twentieth century but became more central to colonial medical policy after World War II.

In the late 1940s the STD control strategy in the territory centered on coercive measures to confront an expected invasion of syphilitics — African soldiers returning from duty in Ethiopia and Somaliland. The Medical Department prepared for the imagined onslaught by invoking the Imperial Emergency Powers Defence Act. This legislation included provisions for the compulsory treatment of syphilis, gonorrhea, genital ulcerative disease, lymphogranuloma, and granuloma venereum. In addition, fines and jail sentences could be meted out to anyone suspected by authorities of loitering or engaging in prostitution and who refused physical examination. The medical establishment was not unanimous, however, in adopting a law-and-order approach to the control of STDs. In the early 1940s one medical officer urged a destigmatizing and nonmoralizing approach to the treatment of those with STDs. He stated quite pragmatically that the "remnants of the old idea that sufferers were sinners more deserving of punishment than sympathy must be abolished"; that STDs should be treated in general medical practice, not in specially designated clinics; and that a measure of prevention could be achieved by "improving conditions in brothels."[5]

With the exception of outbreaks of syphilis and gonorrhea in the western part of the territory, very little was published or written about STDs in Tanzania between the mid-1940s and the early 1980s. For most of the twentieth century records of cases seen at government and voluntary health facilities provided most of the quantitative data on STDs in Tanzania.[6] These data must be interpreted cautiously and cannot be assumed to reflect the history of STD patterns in the general population.[7]

The First Cases of AIDS in Tanzania

The first three cases of AIDS in Tanzania were diagnosed in 1983 by a surgeon in the Kagera region of Western Tanzania. In the following two years, AIDS cases were identified in 7 more of Tanzania's 20 mainland regions. By 1986, after the establishment of the National AIDS Task Force, the National AIDS Control Programme, and the issuance of national clinical case notification guidelines, every mainland region had reported its first cases. In the mid to late 1980s the heavily affected areas of East and Central Africa, including southern Uganda, Western Tanzania, and Rwanda and Burundi, were subject to intense international interest. Within this zone the Kagera, Tanzania-Rakai, Uganda border region appeared to be especially heavily affected, and during the first decade of the epidemic in Tanzania, Kagera, along with Mbeya, Dar es Salaam, Coast, and Kilimanjaro, reported the greatest numbers of AIDS cases.[8]

Epidemiologic surveillance of sentinel groups of blood donors and pregnant women attending antenatal clinics began in the mid-1980s and continued into the 1990s. In addition, HIV prevalence estimates were made of numerous demographic, geographic, and occupational subpopulations. Between 1983 and 1995 hundreds of HIV-1 and HIV-2 prevalence figures were published for such groups as blood donors, pregnant women, healthy adults, family planning and STD clinic attenders, tuberculosis patients, truck drivers, and bar workers.[9] In addition, population-based serosurveys were conducted in several locations.[10] This type of study offers the most complete picture of disease conditions in a location or population subgroup. In general, results of population-based serosurveys gave epidemiologists the impression that the highest HIV prevalences were to be found in urban areas and along transport routes. At best, however, community-based studies can serve only as snapshots, and because they are extremely costly and labor-intensive exercises there is rarely the opportunity to perform repeat or follow-up studies in a single location. Hence, the presence of higher rates of HIV infection in towns and peri-urban areas raised a question that epidemiologists have been not able to answer: "whether seroprevalence is higher in towns because HIV-1 infection was introduced earlier, or because risk behaviour is different."[11] Many epidemiologists believed that the latter was the case,[12] a belief that also informed much of what Muhondwa called the folk epidemiology[13] of AIDS among Tanzanians. This notion of different risk behavior in towns (that is, higher rates of sexual networking), has been part of popular perceptions of African sexuality on the part of both Africans and Europeans for decades.[14] Yet more recent demographic survey research in Tanzania calls such suppositions into question and indicates that levels of sexual networking and partner change may well be higher in rural than urban areas in the country as a whole.[15]

The only clarity to emerge from the testing frenzy of the 1980s and 1990s was that the epidemic in Tanzania was anything but "a monolithic blight."[16] Rather, an enormous degree of heterogeneity characterized the early manifestations of the epidemic across the country. By 1995 it had become fairly well established that HIV was concentrated among adults and that young women were especially at risk in East Africa.[17] Rates were particularly high among young adults in urban areas and among women engaged in marginal occupations, such as commercial sex work or bar work. Between 1987 and 1993, cumulative regional seroprevalence rates among blood donors (whom the government felt were a reliable indicator group) ranged from a low of 2.0 percent in Kigoma to a high of 10.5 percent in Iringa and Kagera. Kilimanjaro ranked seventeenth out of 20 regions with cumulative seroprevalence of 2.7 percent. The surveillance of sentinel populations and the targeted testing of high risk occupational groups began to fill an information vacuum about the status of the HIV epidemic. Nevertheless, questions remained about the interpretation of HIV prevalence data. How representative of the general population were the sentinel groups?[18] What general significance should be given to HIV rates among risk groups, such as female bar workers?

Although rates among women engaged in high risk occupations were of immediate practical significance for targeted interventions, important contextual issues remained unstudied. These included topics such as the rate of turnover among bar workers, the percentage of the female population engaged in this occupation, and, perhaps most importantly, whether bar workers in Tanzania shared structural risks for STDs and HIV with women in other occupational categories.[19]

From early on, the sentinel surveillance in more heavily AIDS-affected regions revealed a great deal of subregional diversity in HIV epidemiology. For example, HIV seroprevalence rates reported among antenatal clinic attenders at five rural locations in the southern region of Mbeya fluctuated dramatically over time and differed drastically within a small geographic area (Table 6.1). The factors that account for this variation are probably not limited to changes in risk or behavior among the tested populations. Passive, non-random sampling procedures for sentinel surveillance of blood donors and pregnant women and small sample sizes may have influenced the accuracy and consistency of reported rates over time within these relatively small geographic areas. Undoubtedly, many estimates of rates of HIV infection among healthy Tanzanians have suffered from these (and other) technical and methodological problems and may not have represented the actual HIV seroprevalence rates among sampled populations.[20]

The interpretation of HIV epidemiology under these conditions should be seen in the context of anthropological analyses of the social and geographic networks that can account for the observed variation in patterns of infection.[21] In Tanzania, for example, forces related to the cultural organization of productive and reproductive life, demographic trends in fertility and migration, and socio-geographic networks of sexual relations have contributed to a heterogeneous epidemic, a web of interconnected and shifting micro-epidemics. This is not to say that each location has had an entirely unique experience with AIDS, that there are no commonalities in the way AIDS manifests in sub-Saharan Africa, but that the social history and epidemiology of HIV within Tanzania can fruitfully be thought of as a heterogeneous process.

However, the social experience of an epidemic is not determined by its epidemiology, particularly so in the case of the nebulous plague that is

TABLE 6.1
HIV Prevalence for Rural Ante-Natal Clinic Attenders,
Mbeya Region, 1988–91
(percent HIV positive)

	1988	1989	1990	1991	1992	1993
Chimala	4.17	6.25	8.80	9.50	8.0	10.8
Isoko	2.94	2.00	2.40	6.60	18.0	8.5
Itete	1.72	9.09	6.40	3.90	5.3	15.5
Kyela	—	21.21	14.60	17.50	30.4	27.2
Mwanbani	—	12.00	8.50	12.90	8.0	10.7

Sources: Center for International Research, *HIV/AIDS Surveillance Data Base* (Washington, D.C.: Center for International Research, United States Bureau of the Census, 1994); National AIDS Control Programme, *National AIDS Control Programme HIV/AIDS/STD Surveillance Report No. 8* (Dar es Salaam: United Republic of Tanzania, Ministry of Health, 1994).

AIDS. From the very start there has been a dialectic between the epidemiology of the disease and the perceptions of local actors as to who was vulnerable to infection and who was spreading the disease. The social experience of AIDS has largely been contingent upon this dialectic. Furthermore, perceptions have changed over time as the epidemic has moved into and among sexual networks that fluctuate, overlap, and dissolve, according to the actions and movements of their participants. In this sense, both the epidemiology and history of HIV in Tanzania have never been fixed among a single social class or category of person.

To illustrate this phenomenon, I shall examine the scientific and popular epidemiologies of AIDS in Kagera and Kilimanjaro between 1983 and 1993. These cases serve to highlight this diversity of cultural meaning and epidemiologic manifestation. Early on, the disease generated the impression for some that AIDS would "kill all the people with a certain lifestyle and leave the rest of us alone," as a Tanzanian AIDS researcher once asserted.[22] Yet over time, the historical similarities and differences in Kagera and Kilimanjaro regions show that there has not been one overall pattern in the epidemic and that the histories of AIDS in Tanzania have been innately plural, a succession of "travelling waves of HIV infection."[23]

MOBILITY, SEXUAL STRATIFICATION, AND AIDS IN WESTERN TANZANIA

Kagera region, which lies in the far West of Tanzania and borders Rwanda, Burundi, and Uganda, is perhaps the only area of the country for which it is currently possible to construct a general history of STDs from written sources before the era of AIDS.[24] The Haya are the primary inhabitants of Bukoba and Muleba districts in Kagera region. Other main ethnic groups in Kagera include Hangaza in Ngara and Subi in Biharamulo. This discussion of AIDS and STDs in Kagera focuses on Haya experience and perspectives because these are much better documented than for other groups. Periodic epidemics of STDs among Haya, the mobility of Haya women, and the seemingly large numbers of women engaged in commercial sex work have been a focus of medical, social scientific, and missionary concern throughout the century.[25] Themes in colonial medical inquiries into STDs in western Tanzania from the 1930s to the 1950s resurfaced half a century later in scientific explanations for the high prevalence of AIDS among Haya.

In the 1930s and 1940s the East African medical establishment thought that syphilis and gonorrhea were afflictions of urban migrants and the African soldiery. As Africans moved out of traditional contexts, it was thought, the strength of cultural constraints on their sexual lives diminished. Yet colonial medical staff and social scientists also vilified local traditions that were presumed to promote disease and ill health.[26] These

European explanations of disease among Africans were evident in comments made by the medical director of the Tanganyika Territory. Noting the high levels of syphilis in Western Tanzania, he stated, "I believe it is correct to say that the highest incidence in the Territory is among the Haya, who neither live in large towns, nor work. The prevalence of the disease . . . is primarily due to the fact that when a man is married, all his brothers have the same rights immediately after the wedding as he has."[27]

There is little doubt that STDs were extremely common in Kagera; syphilis and gonorrhea were so prevalent among Haya in the first half of the twentieth century that they accounted for up to 31 percent of cases at native dispensaries.[28] Such figures must be interpreted with caution. As discussed above, figures based on clinic records may not accurately reflect the relative place of STDs in the overall disease burden in Haya communities. Nevertheless, in absolute terms most sources concur that STDs have been a serious source of morbidity in Kagera since the 1930s. Indeed, a district medical officer reckoned that having an STD was seen by Haya as part and parcel of entry into adulthood (we do not know, however, how systematic was his investigation into Haya perspectives on the topic).

In the late 1940s and 1950s colonial medical discourse refined the theories of urban vulnerability and unhealthy traditions by focusing on the mobility of adults and what was perceived to be a loosening of cultural controls over female sexuality. To medical authorities it appeared that Africans were readily turning to selling and buying sex. Rising prostitution was seen as central to the rapid spread of syphilis across the border in Uganda during the 1940s and 1950s.[29] Sociologists and anthropologists suggested that high rates of STD infection in Kagera also stemmed from the effects of an increasing sex trade compounded by weakening marital stability. Because there was presumed to be a social basis for the scourge, government officials prescribed social remedies, such as anti–venereal disease clubs, in an attempt to foster a new medico-moral ethos of sexual health. However, changes in patterns of sexual life among young Haya adults should not be seen merely as an adaptation to urban contexts.[30] The forms of sexual and material reciprocity that emerged among Haya in the twentieth century (and the attendant high prevalence of STDs) were part of sexual and economic stratification in the history of western Tanzania.

In the pre-colonial era Haya men, particularly those in high social positions or from powerful clans, used the sexuality and fertility of female relations (usually daughters) in political and economic exchange.[31] Although oral historical data suggest that the earliest prostitutes in Haya areas may have been Ganda women (from Uganda), other accounts indicate that Haya women selling sex were popular among the very first German and African colonial forces in Bukoba in the 1890s.[32] As early as the 1930s the number of women engaging in commercial sex work became of concern to at least one indigenous African organization. The African Association explicitly acknowledged that women, who could not by custom inherit land, were structurally vulnerable to becoming involved in prostitution; the group unsuccessfully petitioned the Council of Chiefs that women be allowed equal inheritance rights with men.[33]

The movement of Haya women engaged in commercial sex work throughout East Africa, some have argued, contributed substantially to high rates of STDs and, later, of HIV infection in the predominantly Haya districts of Kagera region.[34] Indeed, the far-flung Haya prostitute became a stereotype in many urban areas. Women's networks spread out and away from Haya areas of Kagera. During the 1950s, for example, Haya women outnumbered Haya men in Dar es Salaam by three to one. Many involved in prostitution stayed closer to Kagera and followed long-established seasonal patterns of movement, staying in Bukoba town during the coffee season and moving to Mwanza and across Lake Victoria to Uganda during the cotton season.

Over time there were various push and pull factors that accounted for increasing numbers of Haya women becoming involved in sex work. These included parental support that ranged from tacit approval to facilitation, recruitment by mothers or older female relations, and personal desire for economic and social independence. Such findings indicate that Haya realized that: "Prostitution everywhere has always been a socioeconomic phenomenon. Resentment of sexual oppression was an important dimension but the quest for economic opportunity in a society deeply penetrated by the cash nexus was an even more crucial factor in Haya prostitution."[35] Women engaging in commercial sex work were likely to be the structurally disadvantaged wives and ex-wives of economically disenfranchised men. There appears also to have been a connection between infertility (some of it presumably STD-induced) and prostitution: Among 15 prostitutes from one Haya village, one researcher found that 8 of the women gave the social consequences of childlessness as a primary motivating factor for their commercial sex work.[36]

Thus, contrary to some of the more popular theories of the day, Haya prostitution cannot be easily attributed to the entrepreneurship of women who exploited a cultural linkage of sex and exchange for personal gain or to the loosening of traditional constraints on sexual life; many of the women who entered this profession did so to escape their marginal positions in local sexual hierarchies. Haya women have not been alone in Africa in confronting such circumstances and in responding through wide scale participation in sex trade. In West Africa the circular migration of Ghanaians to Abidjan in Côte d'Ivoire has been dominated by women selling sex who have come from one particular district and who have found themselves increasingly disenfranchised in their home communities.[37]

The Arrival of AIDS in Kagera

In terms of culturally informed medical understandings of STDs in East Africa, little had changed by the time AIDS emerged in the region.[38] Instead, much of the early medical literature about AIDS in Africa relied upon the familiar assumptions that the spread of the disease stemmed from maladaptations to development in urban settings and from pathological traditions in rural areas. To what extent, however, were such medical presumptions shared in African perceptions about disease and changes in productive, reproductive, and sexual life? As the Kagera and Kilimanjaro cases show, AIDS was indeed configured as a disease of development by local actors, albeit along very different lines from its construction as such in epidemiologic narratives and medical supposition. The local knowledge and experience of the AIDS epidemic in Kagera, as in Kilimanjaro, derived from an awareness of an intersection of disease with persons belonging to particular social networks, not an inherent cultural proclivity or vulnerability.

In addition to the forces acting upon Haya women, men faced imperatives to adopt itinerant lifestyles. The combined effects of long-standing generational and interlineage hierarchies and land pressures resulting from population growth impelled them to become more mobile in seeking economic security. By the 1970s many young men had found a niche that their mobility enabled them to exploit: smuggling. Juliana traders, who got their name from a particular brand of clothing popular among successful smugglers, rapidly became a mobile *nouveau riche* in Bukoba and Muleba districts. "Restrictions on foreign-currency exchange and imports and the scarcity of essential household commodities as well as luxury goods in the 1970s and early 1980s increased incentives for people to travel and trade with countries where goods were in greater supply. . . . Unlike the majority of the population, whose subsistence activities and cash-crop production were disrupted in the late 1970s and early 1980s, the Juliana traders had cash and access to valued goods that could not be obtained locally for any price."[39] Cross-border trade was associated with risk, reward, and sexual and material desire for both the rich and the poor. Border posts became centers of trade and also of conspicuous consumption of liquor and sex. As one Haya historian has put it, "money was made and money was spent on pleasure."[40] Trading centers in Haya areas within Kagera, in turn, became the foci of socio-geographic networks revolving around mobile young men and women and commerce. As the first cases of AIDS in Tanzania were being diagnosed by physicians, a cultural awareness of this fatal wasting syndrome afflicting these businessmen also emerged.

Early on there was a strong cultural association of the materialism of Juliana traders with the new and devastating syndrome. Although STDs had remained prevalent, becoming the second most common diagnosis in outpatient clinics in Bukoba district during the early 1980s,[41] the sexual transmission of AIDS was not initially recognized. Instead, the syndrome was thought to have either been imported somehow with the smuggled Juliana shirts themselves or to have resulted from the unscrupulous business practices of the traders; having cheated their Ugandan trading partners, they were thought to be suffering from witchcraft attacks.[42] However, over time this popular epidemiology of AIDS in Kagera began to shift. Many Haya began to recognize the sexual transmission of AIDS, but others rejected this theory. Some of those who were not perceived to be at risk fell ill, but others who seemed to be extremely promiscuous remained healthy.[43]

A population-based study of HIV prevalence by Killewo and colleagues revealed a great deal of subregional diversity in HIV epidemiology in Kagera during the 1980s, countering the popular perception of the entire region being devastated by the AIDS epidemic (Table 6.2).[44] For example, even among the wards of Bukoba town (Kagera's main urban center and predominantly Haya in population), there were large variations in HIV rates. The study also pointed to the association of HIV with poverty, contradicting the predictions that African urban elites were those most at risk. Residence in lower socioeconomic status urban wards correlated much more strongly with risk of being HIV infected than did residence in the most modern and urbanized ward, which actually had the lowest prevalence rate in the town.[45] More in line with popular and epidemiologic expectations, it was found that a ward's distance from Bukoba town was a strong correlate of lower rates of HIV infection. These less affected wards were also those with more of the population engaged

TABLE 6.2
HIV Prevalence Rates for Adults in Districts of Kagera Region, 1987

Location	Percent Prevalence
Bukoba Town	
high socio-economic status ward	16.1
low socio-economic status ward	42.0
Bukoba Rural/Muleba Districts	10.0
Karagwe District	4.5
Ngara/Biharamulo Districts	0.4

Sources: J. Killewo, L. Dahlgren, and A. Sordström, "Socio-Geographical Patterns of HIV-1 Transmission in Kagera, Tanzania," Social Science and Medicine 38 (1994): 131–32 ; Center for International Research, HIV/AIDS Surveillance Data Base (Washington, D.C.: Center for International Research, U.S. Bureau of the Census, 1994).

in agricultural production and had lower measured rates of extended sexual networking and less travel.

Among Haya, the demographically and economically circumscribed movements of networks of sexually active men and women fostered a popular epidemiology of AIDS that echoed some, but not all, of these findings. Early popular epidemiologies of the origin and spread of HIV centered on connections among new forms of material and sexual desire, the modern contexts in which they emerged, and an uncontrolled transmission of disease.[46] Local perceptions, however, were not fixed, and people were well aware of how the epidemic could confound expectation as it traveled across the social landscape.

DEVELOPMENT, DISPLACEMENT, AND DISEASE IN KILIMANJARO

Sexually Transmitted Diseases and Models for the Emergence of AIDS

Kilimanjaro region lies on the Kenyan border in Northeast Tanzania and comprises a range of ecosystems and productive regimes that encompasses the permanent banana and coffee cultivation of the Chagga on Kilimanjaro, the Pare in the Pare Mountains, and the semi-nomadic pastoralism of the Maasai on surrounding low-lying plains. This account will deal with the northern part of the region, comprising the Kilimanjaro mountain system, and the regional capital of Moshi. It focuses on Chagga social and cultural history.

STDs have a much scantier written history in Kilimanjaro than in Kagera. However, it does appear that STDs were present and culturally acknowledged among Chagga since at least the late nineteenth century.[47] STDs were specifically included among the misfortunes that could be called down upon malefactors who were the objects of publicly uttered curses in marketplaces, and warnings about STDs figured in initiation lessons given to young women. During the era of British rule Chagga proposed the formation of their own Medical Executive Committee, which was to take on the job of advising government health officials on the control of STDs as one of its primary tasks. Beyond this, however, there is little to suggest how prevalent STDs may have been or what kinds of contexts local actors associated with them. Although STDs were present in Kilimanjaro, they do not ever seem to have reached the prevalences of Kagera earlier in the century.

The first case of AIDS in Kilimanjaro region was diagnosed in 1984, the year after the disease was identified in Kagera. By 1988 scientific and popular explanations of the presence of the disease in the region began to emerge. Both of these explanatory frameworks of the epidemiology of

AIDS were built around versions of an urban disease model. The model was based upon a familiar urban-rural dichotomy and its attendant assumptions about African responses to city life — less social control and more sexual risk. The model was inaccurate or misleading in two regards. The first problem was that researchers focused primarily on rates and not on the distribution of the population; with 80 percent of the regional population of 1 million resident in rural areas, rural prevalence rates a fraction of those in the regional capital of Moshi (population 95,000) represented a far greater total number cases. In addition, there was little appreciation of the fact that young adults in many rural districts of Kilimanjaro led mobile, itinerant lifestyles similar to those that produced high rates of HIV and STD infection in Kagera.

These problems with the urban disease model become clearer when examining the prevalence of STDs among roadside and rural populations in Kilimanjaro from the 1990s. Prevalence data on STDs are available from two population-based studies for 1991–92 and 1995 (Table 6.3). These studies revealed that lower genital tract infections were very common among women (mostly caused by *Trichomonas vaginalis*) regardless of urban or rural residence and that chlamydia rates among urban bar workers and roadside women were comparable.[48] Overall STD rates were much higher among bar workers in the regional capital of Moshi than among women in the roadside village of Kahe about 60 kilometers away, and women engaged in bar work had significantly higher rates of syphilis and gonorrhea than their male co-workers.[49] However, syphilis and gonorrhea rates among young adults in Moshi Rural District in 1995 were as high or higher than those among male and female bar workers in Moshi in 1991–92. Although the data were collected several years apart, such a finding points to some of the shortcomings of an urban disease model. Indeed, the STD burden among youth in Moshi Rural District was frequently heavier than that found in studies from the most severely HIV-affected regions in Tanzania and in urban populations elsewhere in Tanzania and East Africa.[50]

Interestingly, among Chagga many aspects of the epidemiologic iteration of the urban disease model resonated with cultural interpretations of risk for AIDS and of the origin of the epidemic in Kilimanjaro. As we shall see, however, there was not a complete fit between cultural and medical views of the epidemic. One of the most profound gaps was because the scientific epidemiologic outlook was generally not a historical one and seldom problematized social contexts for risk and infection with much depth. Nevertheless, for Tanzanians, this deeper, more retrospective consciousness of transformations of patterned reproductive and sexual action was inextricable from cultural epidemiologies of AIDS.

TABLE 6.3
Prevalence Rates for Sexually Transmitted Diseases among Urban Bar Workers and Roadside and Rural Village Populations, Kilimanjaro Region
(in percent)

Population Subgroup	Syphilis	Gonorrhea	Chlamydia	Lower Genital Tract Infection
Urban Bar Workers in Moshi				
Female (1991–92)	15.0*	4.0*	8.0*	44.0*
Male (1991–92)	6.0*	0.3	7.0*	—
Roadside Village (Kahe)				
Women (1991–92)	4.7	—	6.8	33.0*
Men (1991–92)	2.6	—	9.7	—
Youth in Moshi Rural District				
Women aged 15–24 (1995)	14.2	6.3	—	19.1†
Men aged 15–24 (1995)	8.6	4.0	—	9.1†

*figures rounded to nearest whole percent in original.
†trichomoniasis only.

Sources: Elise Klouman, Elisante J. Masenga, Noel E. Sam, and Zebeda Lauwo, "Control of Sexually Transmitted Diseases: Experiences from a Rural and Urban Community," in Knut-Inge Klepp, Paul M. Biswalo, and Aud Talle (Eds.), *Young People at Risk: Fighting AIDS in Northern Tanzania* (Oslo: Scandinavian University Press, 1995), pp. 207–10; Anna Tergia Kessy, "Risk Factors and Prevalence of Sexually Transmitted Diseases among Youths in Moshi Rural District, Kilimanjaro Region, 1995," paper presented at Workshop on Youth and Related Problems, Dar es Salaam, 1995, p. 12.

The Urban Disease Model and Scientific Epidemiologies of AIDS in Kilimanjaro

Clinicians and epidemiologists working in Kilimanjaro derived their urban disease model from research in capital cities elsewhere in sub-Saharan Africa. They then adapted it to their own perceptions of local conditions. They suggested that HIV was spreading into the region through a combination of "infected pools of people and mobile transmitters. The infected pools which are established in major towns or affected countries include the prostitutes and barmaids. . . . The mobile transmitters mainly include the truck drivers and young businessmen."[51] This model emerged from the results of a cross-sectional serosurvey in which the rate of HIV infection in blood samples was highest in Moshi town and progressively lower in sampled populations resident on the mountain at increasing distances from the city.[52] Researchers acknowledged that the geographic cross section was not comprehensive, but pointed out that their results showed "that adjacent groups chosen on the basis of their geographical location may show enormous variation in seropositivity."

This model for AIDS in northern Tanzania began to evoke the notion of socio-geographic networks to account for heterogeneity in the manifestation of the epidemic. The model implied a historical and gendered character to the movement of the disease across the social landscape; the fixity of largely female pools of infection and the mobility of mostly male transmitters. This particular formulation of the spatial role of young men and women in HIV transmission oversimplified matters somewhat. Although some women who engaged in full-time or occasional commercial sex in sub-Saharan Africa may be more or less permanent urban or roadside residents, many are not. The Haya case and studies from Dar es Salaam[53] and Kilimanjaro[54] indicate that women in these occupations are peripatetic, usually by necessity rather than choice. Furthermore, it is not at all clear that women who fall into the occupational category of barmaid have an inherently or substantially greater risk of exposure to HIV than, for example, itinerant market women,[55] although no seroepidemiology has been conducted in Kilimanjaro on the basis of this occupational subgroup to argue the case one way or another.

The most thorough assessment of longitudinal HIV prevalence data in northern Tanzania has been made by Klepp and colleagues.[56] Their analysis indicates that between 1987 and 1993 prevalence increased rapidly among sentinel populations, such as pregnant women in Moshi, and more slowly among male blood donors (Table 6.4). Between 1991 and 1993, increases were also noted among female blood donors in urban and rural areas. For other groups, longitudinal data are either unavailable or sample sizes too small to derive stable prevalence estimates.[57] Although the prevalence among blood donors at rural hospitals steadily increased,

TABLE 6.4
HIV Prevalence Rates for Adults in Northern Kilimanjaro Region, Selected Years 1987-95

(in percent)

	1987	1991	1992	1993	1995
Pregnant Women					
Moshi	1.1	7.6	10.4	15.1	—
Blood Donors (all ages)					
Men (urban, regional hospital)	3.9	3.7	3.0	4.6*	—
Men (rural)	—	2.6	—	3.9	—
Women (urban & rural)	—	3.2	—	5.4	—
Population-Based Figures					
Kibosho (rural, both sexes, all ages)	0.2	—	—	—	—
Kahe (roadside, men, all ages)	—	0.7	—	—	—
Kahe (roadside, women, all ages)	—	2.0	—	—	—
Moshi Rural Dist. (men, 15–24)	—	—	—	—	5.0
Moshi Rural Dist. (women, 15–24)	—	—	—	—	9.7
Prostitutes and Bar Workers					
Male bar workers (urban)	4.9	—	6.8	—	—
Female bar workers (urban)	11.1	—	32.6	—	—
Self-identified prostitutes (urban)	58.0	—	—	—	—

*composite figure for the zonal and regional hospitals.

Sources: Knut-Inge Klepp, Kagoma Mnyika, Naphtal Ole-King'ori, and Per Bergsjø, "The Local AIDS Epidemic in Arusha and Kilimanjaro," in Knut-Inge Klepp, Paul M. Biswalo, and Aud Talle (Eds.), Young People at Risk: Fighting AIDS in Northern Tanzania (Oslo: Scandinavian University Press, 1995), pp. 4–13; Philip W. Setel, Bo'n Town Life: Youth, AIDS, and the Changing Character of Adulthood in Kilimanjaro, Tanzania, doctoral dissertation, Boston University, 1995, p. 252; Anna Tergia Kessy, "Risk Factors and Prevalence of Sexually Transmitted Diseases among Youths in Moshi Rural District, Kilimanjaro Region, 1995," paper presented at Workshop on Youth and Related Problems, Dar es Salaam, 1995, p. 12.

HIV rates among the blood donors at urban hospitals and among pregnant women showed few discernible trends between 1987 and 1993. Prevalence data from targeted studies are difficult to interpret because Moshi was the only location in the region where risk groups, such as male and female bar workers, were tested. Thus, the relatively high rates of HIV infection among them are not easily comparable to data from elsewhere in the region. A cohort study in the village of Kahe, however, seemed to confirm the earlier picture of geographic heterogeneity in HIV infection. In this village, which lies along a major highway, women aged 25–30 had higher rates of HIV infection than antenatal clinic attenders in

Moshi. Although Kilimanjaro was one of the least HIV-affected regions in Tanzania in terms of prevalence rates among sentinel groups, it had one of the highest cumulative totals of AIDS cases. This anomaly is probably explained by the facts that the formal health care sector has been more active in diagnosing and reporting cases of AIDS and HIV disease than have the medical services in other regions, and that many Chagga resident elsewhere in Tanzania have returned home to die upon learning of their sero-status.[58]

Population Dynamics and Cultural Explanations of AIDS in Kilimanjaro

How did Chagga perspectives on the origin and spread of HIV in and around Moshi mesh with the epidemiologic version of AIDS as an urban disease? Again, the most profound difference stemmed from the fact that popular epidemiologies of AIDS were inextricably linked to oral histories of demographic process on the mountain, to gendered views of the development process, and to the embodiment of these forces in two types of networks, one male-dominated, the other the province of young adults of both sexes. The first type of socio-geographic network was that of long-term male migrants who maintained links with their mountain homes. They appeared to be a significant proportion of the first wave of AIDS-ill in the region, returning from their usual places of residence elsewhere in the country after having been diagnosed with HIV disease. The second network included the mobile young adults who quickly came to epitomize risk and contagion in the epidemic. Although the prevalence of HIV and AIDS was clearly increasing through the 1980s, it was not until 1989 that many people in Moshi and nearby areas believed that AIDS was affecting those who were not long-term residents outside of the region.

The group experience of profound changes in productive and reproductive life during the twentieth century anchored explanations of the local origin and manifestation of AIDS. The history is one of displacement of cohorts of young men, and, more recently, of increasing numbers of young women. During the nineteenth and early twentieth centuries, Chagga life courses were oriented around the irrigated, permanently cultivated *kihamba* (pl. *vihamba*) gardens that lie on Kilimanjaro's southern slopes at elevations of 3,000–7,000 feet. Passed from fathers to their first- and last-born sons, during the nineteenth century *vihamba* housed families, held their stall-fed cattle, and contained the staple-producing banana groves. With the introduction of coffee cash-cropping in the twentieth century these lands acquired a new, monetary value; unclaimed lands in the *kihamba* zone were quickly appropriated by more powerful lineages. At the same time Kilimanjaro experienced spectacular population growth. Halfway through the twentieth century the Northern Province (which included Kilimanjaro) was the fastest growing area in the Territory. Based on calculations of rural carrying capacities for all districts of Tanzania, Kilimanjaro was said to be the most overpopulated region in the country by 1967.[59]

The combined effect was such that on one part of the mountain the majority of young men were under threat of landlessness within a single generation. After World War II, emigration picked up considerably and reached its peak in the 1960s and 1970s. At this time Kilimanjaro had the highest migration rates among young men in Tanzania. Educated young men in particular seemed to leave Kilimanjaro en masse, with migration rates of 80 percent for men between 20 and 34 with a year or more of secondary education.[60] In the 1970s most of a sample of 400 farmers in the former Chagga chiefdom of Marangu were born on the *kihamba* land on which they were living; yet 62 percent of the men in these households reported having two or more sons who had no access to land. The rapid movement of the productive lives of adult men away from the mountain (whether on a long-term or temporary basis) was the origin of the networks through which HIV was thought to have arrived in Kilimanjaro.

The predicament of the long-term migrants and the women whom they often left behind to hold their places on the *kihamba* land, however, set apart the popular histories of AIDS in the two regions under discussion. The wives of long-absent men often expressed deep anxiety about their vulnerability to HIV infection at their husbands' annual visits home. Over the years many of these men had established other lives and other wives in such cities as Dar es Salaam, Mwanza, Morogoro, and Mbeya. In the 1980s AIDS was seen by many in Kilimanjaro as a disease of the city and of Kagera; the return of husbands from these areas in particular provoked appeals at church-run AIDS prevention seminars for religious leaders to support women in putting into practice the AIDS education that they had been given.[61]

Several years into the epidemic in Kilimanjaro there was, as in Kagera, an awareness that the character of the epidemic had shifted. Many of those seen to be falling ill were not among the long-term male migrants or their spouses, but were local folks who had not travelled extensively. Increasingly, AIDS was associated with the much more restricted patterns of movement of small businessmen and businesswomen, many of whom spent only a day or so away from their homes every week as they made the rounds of the main regional markets.

As economic growth and opportunity stagnated through the 1970s and into the 1980s, increasing numbers of women were also caught up in itinerant lifestyles. Some of these phenomena resonated with the Kagera experience. For example, one informant dated the beginnings of an era of risk to the early 1970s when business became a way of life for many young people in Chagga areas:

The people of Moshi are engaged in business . . . nearly the whole region . . . young people, adults . . . they do business and they don't stay in Moshi. They travel around to Kagera, to Dar. . . . This is the way that AIDS was brought to Kilimanjaro. . . . They come home from the border areas with Kenya. During the 1960s and 1970s, the Chaggas did not have much prostitution. It wasn't their nature, but by the end of the 1970s, many Chagga women were engaged in business and started travelling. They got influence and became promiscuous through their business contacts. Those women came from Moshi and traveled to Dar, Nairobi, and Mombassa to buy cloth, soap, cooking oil. There were many involved in this trade, this smuggling, and even today many of them engage in sex at the Kenyan border in order not to be arrested.[62]

As in Kagera, the confluence of these new forms of desire and the lack of fixity in the young adult phase of the life course were often represented as especially cogent aspects of the local context of HIV transmission.

In the absence of community-based studies, the exact consequences of shifting arrangements in productive and sexual life for the local epidemiologic manifestations of HIV/AIDS will remain a subject of speculation. Regardless of the now unknowable biological trajectory of HIV in Kilimanjaro in the 1980s and early 1990s, there were some initial parallels between the scientific and popular urban disease models; both narratives of the arrival of AIDS revolved around the themes of gendered vulnerability and mobility. Because so many socio-geographic networks among Chagga link Moshi and surrounding rural areas or bypass the city altogether, it seems reasonable to hypothesize that AIDS has been moving throughout the northern part of the region in ways that have not been readily apparent from the epidemiologic surveillance of HIV through the mid-1990s.

CONCLUSIONS

The diversity in epidemiologic manifestations and cultural meanings of AIDS in Tanzania has resulted in part from local contexts for productive and reproductive life. The concept of socio-geographic networks has been used in this account as a heuristic for describing the inherently unstable spatio-temporal crossing points of specific categories of persons and disease within varying social and cultural contexts. In Kagera and Kilimanjaro these networks were comprised of people who had bonds of sociality and sexuality in various locations — some simultaneously, some serially. The historical development of these networks in each region had to do with processes of political economy, demography, and cultural hierarchies of generation and gender. In Kagera Haya gained a great deal of wealth through small holder coffee and tea production, as did Chagga in Kilimanjaro through a focus on coffee cash-cropping. Other similarities among Haya and Chagga included a productive system that once revolved around inherited, family-farmed garden plots. Increasing involvement in cash economies seemed to exacerbate rural stratification within and between the sexes, accelerating regional urbanization and the dislocation of young men and women in both areas.

In spite of the fact that development, disease, and dislocation figured in the histories of AIDS in each location, the tenor of the popular narratives differed. In Kagera the overriding themes were the movements of women and young Juliana-type traders; the narrative did not focus as much on the regional urban center of Bukoba as it did upon the travel of young adults across borders and out of the region altogether. In Kilimanjaro, an early focus on the visits home of long-term migrants gave way a few years into the epidemic to concerns about the mobility of young adults, many of whose movements crosscut the urban-rural dichotomy.

These local histories demonstrate that the overall story of the epidemic has not, in essence, been one of an infectious disease becoming rampant among individuals with high degrees of risk behavior before spreading to other, low risk members of the population. Rather, the disease has followed along the connecting links of social and sexual networks. These networks have centered on the fluctuating circumstances of young men and women. Their economic, demographic, and structural positions within their own social landscapes provided an "ecology of risk"[63] in which cultural hierarchies of generation and gender, HIV, demography, and political economy have all intersected to create a tragic epidemic.

In terms of the disparity in the severity of AIDS in the two regions, one may speculate about the factors that may have contributed to Kagera apparently having had a much heavier involvement than Kilimanjaro from 1983 to 1993. Based on current knowledge about the synergistic effects of STDs and HIV infection in Africa,[64] it seems possible that relatively high prevalence of STDs in Kagera compared with Kilimanjaro played a significant role. In addition, large numbers of young women have been displaced from agrarian livelihoods relatively recently in Kilimanjaro, compared to Kagera. Last, it seems possible that there may have been a differential effect of various AIDS prevention activities in the two regions. By the early 1990s at least five distinct AIDS prevention and service organizations were operating in northern Kilimanjaro.[65] People there had what one physician there called "a window of opportunity";[66] while HIV prevalence climbed in Kagera, people in Kilimanjaro had the chance to internalize and act upon AIDS prevention messages before the prevalence of infection had reached very high levels, perhaps preventing some degree of transmission in the region. The AIDS epidemic, however, is far from over, and there is no way to predict what a comparison of regions five years hence may reveal.

NOTES

Field research was conducted with the approval of the Tanzanian Commission for Science and Technology (COSTECH) and the Tanzanian Ministry of Health, National AIDS Control Programme. I am grateful to Eustace Muhondwa, M. T. Leshebari, and George Lwihula of the Department of Behavioral Sciences, Muhimbili University College of Health Sciences, Dar es Salaam; to William Howlett and Watoki Nkya of KCMC; to others in Kilimanjaro who gave so generously of their time during the course of this study; and to Jo Healy-North for editorial advice on drafts of this chapter. Research was supported by grants from the Joint Committee on African Studies of the Social Science Research Council and the American Council of Learned Societies with funds provided by the Rockefeller Foundation and from Health in Housing, a World Health Organization Collaborating Center at the State University of New York at Buffalo.

1.   World Health Organization, "Acquired Immunodeficiency Syndrome (AIDS): Data as at 15 December 1995." *Weekly Epidemiological Record* 70 (1995): 353–54.

2.   Roderick Wallace, "Travelling Waves of HIV Infection on a Low Dimensional 'Socio-Geographic' Network," *Social Science and Medicine* 32 (1991): 847–52.

3.   See, for example, Brooke G. Schoepf, "Women, AIDS, and Economic Crisis in Central Africa," *Canadian Journal of African Studies* 22 (1988): 625–44; Brooke G. Schoepf, "Political Economy, Sex and Cultural Logics: A View From Zaire," *African Urban Quarterly* 6 (1991): 94–106 for an analysis of these forces at work in the AIDS epidemic among women in Kinshasa, Zaire.

4.   Tanzania National Archives (hereafter, TNA), "Venereal Disease — Anti-Venereal Disease. Volume I (1930); Volume II (1940–1944)," accession no. J.9.19153.

5.   Dr. Scott, Report to Medical Department, Tanganyika Territory, March 1943. TNA J.9.19153.

6.   Eustace P. Y. Muhondwa, "Social Aspects of Sexually Transmitted Diseases in Tanzania," paper presented at 1986 Medical Association of Tanzania Symposium on STDs, Dar es Salaam, 1985.

7.   This is particularly because the patterns of usage of Western medical clinics for the treatment of STDs and other prevalent ailments are unknown and entirely unquantifiable. Africans have long relied upon traditional practitioners for treating all types of illness, including STDs and infertility. More recently therapeutic resources outside the formal health care sector have included commercial pharmacists and faith healers.

8.   National AIDS Control Programme, *HIV/AIDS/STD Surveillance Report No. 8* (Dar es Salaam: United Republic of Tanzania, Ministry of Health, 1994), p. 22.

9.   Center for International Research, *HIV/AIDS Surveillance Data Base, December 1994* (Washington, D.C.: Center for International Research, United States Bureau of the Census, 1994).

10.   Longin R. Barongo, Martien W. Borgdorff, Frank F. Mosha, Angus Nicoll, Heiner Groskurth, Kesheni P. Senkoro, James N. Newell, John Changalucha, Arnoud H. Klokke, Japhet Z. Killewo, Johan P. Velema, Richard J. Hayes, David

T. Dunn, Lex A. S. Muller, and Joas B. Rugemalila, "The Epidemiology of HIV-1 Infection in Urban Areas, Roadside Settlements and Rural Villages in Mwanza Region, Tanzania," *AIDS* 6 (1992): 1521–28; Japhet Killewo, Klinton Nya-muryekunge, Anita Sandström, Ulla Bredberg-Raden, Stig Wall, Fred Mhalu, and Gunnel Biberfeld, "Prevalence of HIV-1 in the Kagera Region of Tanzania: A Population-Based Study," *AIDS* 4 (1990): 1081–85; Kagoma S. Mnyika, Knut-Inge Klepp, Gunnar Kvåle, Steinar Nilssen, Peter E. Kissila, and Naphthal Ole-King'ori, "Prevalence of HIV-1 Infection in Urban, Semi-Urban and Rural Areas in Arusha Region, Tanzania," *AIDS* 8 (1994): 1477–81.

    11.   Barongo et al., "The Epidemiology of HIV-1 Infection," p. 1526.

    12.   See, for example, Ona A. Pela and Jerome Platt, "AIDS in Africa: Emerging Trends," *Social Science and Medicine* 28 (1989): 1–8.

    13.   Eustace P. Y. Muhondwa, "Contending with Unbelief and Fatalism among the Youth Concerning HIV/AIDS Control in Tanzania," *AIDS and Society Bulletin*, 1991, p. 3.

    14.   Megan Vaughan, *Curing Their Ills: Colonial Power and African Illness* (Stanford, Calif.: Stanford University Press, 1991), pp. 1–28; Callahan and Bond, Chapter 8, this volume.

    15.   See Naomi Rutenberg, Ann K. Blanc, and Saidi Kapiga, "Sexual Behaviour, Social Change, and Family Planning among Men and Women in Tanzania," in *AIDS Impact and Prevention in the Developing World: Demographic and Social Science Perspectives*, edited by John Cleland and Peter Way (Canberra: Health Transition Centre, Australian National University, 1994), pp. 173–96.

    16.   Barbara O. de Zalduondo, Gernard I. Msamanga, and Lincoln Chen, "AIDS in Africa: Diversity in the Global Pandemic," *Daedalus* 118 (1989): 165–204.

    17.   Knut-Inge Klepp, Kagoma Mnyika, Naphtal Ole-King'ori, and Per Bergsjø, "The Local AIDS Epidemic in Arusha and Kilimanjaro," in *Young People at Risk: Fighting AIDS in Northern Tanzania*, edited by Knut-Inge Klepp, Paul M. Biswalo, and Aud Talle (Oslo: Scandinavian University Press, 1995), p. 12.

    18.   Martien Borgdorff, Longin Barongo, Ellen van Jaarsveld, Arnoud Klokke, Kesheni Senkoro, James Newell, Angus Nicoll, Frank Mosha, Heiner Grosskurth, Ronald Swai, Henri van Asten, Johan Velema, Richard Hayes, Lex Muller, and Joas Rugemalila, "Sentinel Surveillance for HIV-1 Infection: How Representative are Blood Donors, Outpatients with Fever, Anaemia, or Sexually Transmitted Diseases, and Antenatal Clinic Attenders in Mwanza Region, Tanzania?" *AIDS* 7 (1993): 567–72.

    19.   Kilimanjaro is one of the few settings in which such issues have been clarified. See Elise Klouman, Elisante J. Masenga, Noel E. Sam, and Zebedia Lauwo, "Control of Sexually Transmitted Diseases: Experiences from a Rural and an Urban Community," in *Young People at Risk: Fighting AIDS in Northern Tanzania*, edited by Knut-Inge Klepp, Paul M. Biswalo, and Aud Talle (Oslo: Scandinavian University Press, 1995), pp. 204–21; Aud Talle, "Bar Workers at the Border," in *Young People at Risk: Fighting AIDS in Northern Tanzania*, edited by Knut-Inge Klepp, Paul M. Biswalo, and Aud Talle (Oslo: Scandinavian University Press, 1995), pp. 18–30.

    20.   Borgdorff et al., "Sentinel Surveillance for HIV-1 Infection," p. 567.

    21.   J. Killewo, L. Dahlgren, and A. Sandström, "Socio-Geographical Patterns of HIV-1 Transmission in Kagera Region, Tanzania," *Social Science and Medicine*

38 (1994): 129–34; Christine Obbo, "HIV Transmission Through Social and Geographical Networks in Uganda," *Social Science and Medicine* 36 (1993): 949–55. Also see Ann Larson, "Social Context of Human Immunodeficiency Virus Transmission in Africa: Historical and Cultural Bases of East and Central African Sexual Relations," *Reviews of Infectious Diseases* 11 (1989): 716–31.

22.   Author's fieldnotes.

23.   Wallace, "Travelling Waves," p. 847.

24.   This account of STDs, AIDS, and sexuality in Kagera draws heavily upon de Zalduondo, Msamanga, and Chen, "AIDS in Africa," pp. 181–86; Fred J. Kaijage, "The AIDS Crisis in Kagera Region, Tanzania, in Historical Perspective," in *Behavioral and Epidemiological Aspects of AIDS Research in Tanzania: Proceedings from a Workshop in Dar es Salaam*, edited by Japhet Z. Killewo and George K. Lwihula (Dar es Salaam: SAREC, 1989), pp. 52–61; Brad Weiss, "'Buying Her Grave': Money, Movement, and AIDS in North-West Tanzania," *Africa* 63 (1993): 19–35.

25.   Weiss, "'Buying her Grave'," p. 19.

26.   Randall M. Packard, *White Plague, Black Labor* (Berkeley: University of California Press, 1989), pp. 33–66; Vaughan, *Curing Their Ills*, pp. 1–28.

27.   Dr. Scott, Report to Medical Department, Tanganyika Territory, March, 1943, TNA J.9.19153, p. 13.

28.   Kaijage, "The AIDS Crisis," p. 53.

29.   Vaughan, *Curing Their Ills*, p. 134.

30.   W. A. Rushing, *The AIDS Epidemic: Social Dimensions of an Infectious Disease* (Boulder, Colo.: Westview Press, 1995), pp. 59–91.

31.   Marja-Liisa Swantz, *Women in Development: A Creative Role Denied?* (London: C. Hurst, 1985), pp. 48–52. As Swantz recounts, these exchanges revolved around systems of tribute and status seeking among cattle-owning and cultivating clans and later among land-owning and tenant farming clans.

32.   Ibid., p. 51.

33.   Ibid., p. 52.

34.   de Zalduondo, Msamanga, and Chen, "AIDS in Africa," p. 182.

35.   Kaijage, "The AIDS Crisis," p. 57.

36.   Swantz, *Women in Development*, p. 72.

37.   John Anarfi, "Sexual Networking in Selected Communities in Ghana and the Sexual Behavior of Ghanaian Female Migrants in Abidjan, Côte D'Ivoire," in *Sexual Behavior and Networking: Anthropological and Socio-Cultural Studies on the Transmission of HIV*, edited by Tim Dyson (Liège: Editions Derouaux Ordina, 1992), pp. 243–44.

38.   See Richard Chirimuuta and Rosalind Chirimuuta, *AIDS, Africa, and Racism* (London: Free Association Books, 1989), pp. 23–34; Randall M. Packard and Paul Epstein, "Epidemiologists, Social Scientists, and the Structure of Medical Research on AIDS in Africa," *Social Science and Medicine* 33 (1991): 771–94.

39.   de Zalduondo, Msamanga, and Chen, "AIDS in Africa," pp. 183–84.

40.   Kaijage, "The AIDS Crisis," p. 60.

41.   Gernard I. Msamanga and K. J. Pallangyo, "Characterization of Tanzanian Outpatients Presenting with Sexually Transmitted Diseases," *East African Medical Journal* 64 (1987): 30–36.

42.   George K. Lwihula, "Social Cultural Factors Associated with the Transmission on HIV Virus in Tanzania: The Kagera Experience," paper presented at

Workshop on Counselling of AIDS Patients, Morogoro, October 31–November 4, 1988, pp. 2–3.

43. de Zalduondo, Msamanga, and Chen, "AIDS in Africa," p. 184; Muhondwa, "Contending with Unbelief," p. 3.

44. Killewo, Dahlgren, and Sandström, "Socio-Geographical Patterns," p. 129.

45. Ibid., pp. 130–31.

46. See Weiss, "'Buying Her Grave'," pp. 24–27.

47. Bruno Gutmann, *Das Recht der Dschagga* (Munich: Felix Kreuger, 1926), p. 563.

48. Anna Tengia Kessy, "Risk Factors and Prevalence of Sexually Transmitted Diseases among Youths in Moshi Rural District, Kilimanjaro Region, 1995," paper presented at Workshop on Youth and Related Problems, Dar es Salaam, October 19–21, 1995, p. 12; Klouman et al., "Control of Sexually Transmitted Diseases," p. 207.

49. Klouman et al., "Control of Sexually Transmitted Diseases," p. 210.

50. Kessy, "Risk Factors and Prevalence of Sexually Transmitted Diseases," p. 21.

51. W.M.M. Nkya, W. Howlett, C. Assenga, and B. Nyombi, "AIDS in Northern Tanzania: An Urban Disease Model," paper presented at the Fourth International Conference on AIDS, Stockholm, 1988, p. 6.

52. Nkya et al., "AIDS in Northern Tanzania," pp. 1–5.

53. Fred Mhalu, Karim Hirji, Petrida Ijumba, John Shao, Ephraim Mbena, Davis Mwakagile, Caroline Akim, Paul Senge, Hussein Mponezya, Ulla Bredberg Raden, and Gunnel Biberfeld, "A Cross-Sectional Study of a Program for HIV Infection Control among Public House Workers," *Journal of Acquired Immune Deficiency Syndromes* 4 (1991): 290–96.

54. Klouman et al., "Control of Sexually Transmitted Diseases," pp. 213–14; Talle, "Bar Workers at the Border," pp. 21–22; author's fieldnotes.

55. I. O. Orubuloye, Pat Caldwell, and John C. Caldwell, "The Role of High-Risk Occupations in the Spread of AIDS: Truck Drivers and Itinerant Market Women in Nigeria," *International Family Planning Perspectives* 19 (1993): 43–48, 71.

56. Klepp et al., "The Local HIV/AIDS Epidemic," pp. 4–13.

57. Ibid.

58. This should not imply, however, that a high percentage of those infected with HIV are aware of their sero-status; the vast majority are not (see Philip Setel, "The Effects of HIV and AIDS on Fertility in East and Central Africa," *Health Transition Review* 5 (supplement) (1995): 179–90.

59. J. E. Moore, "Rural Population Carrying Capacities of the Districts of Tanzania," BRALUP Research Paper No. 18 (Dar es Salaam: Bureau of Resource Allocation and Land Use Planning, 1971).

60. H. N. Barnum and R. H. Sabot, *Migration and Urban Surplus Labour: The Case of Tanzania* (Paris: Development Centre of the Organization for Economic Co-operation and Development, 1976), p. 108.

61. For example, women asked priests for formal support in either refusing to have sexual relations with their husbands or in demanding that the men use condoms (author's fieldnotes).

62. Author's fieldnotes, interview with Samuel H., October 13, 1991.

63.   Tony Barnett and Piers Blaikie, *AIDS in Africa: Its Present and Future Impact* (New York: Guilford Press, 1992), p. 68.

64.   Heiner Grosskurth, Frank Mosha, James Todd, Ezra Mwijaribu, Arnoud Klokke, Keshini Senkoro, Philippe Mayaud, John Changalucha, Angus Nicoll, Gina ka-Gina, James Newell, Kokugonza Mugeye, David Mabey, and Richard Hayes, "Impact of Improved Treatment of Sexually Transmitted Diseases on HIV Infection in Rural Tanzania: Randomised Controlled Trial," *Lancet* 346 (1995): 530–36.

65.   In addition to the display of posters in many public locations and private businesses, methods of prevention education included: a drop-in information center located in Moshi, individual AIDS counselling, classroom and worksite seminars and video screenings, day-long parish-based workshops, drama festivals, and a travelling AIDS awareness puppet theatre.

66.   Author's fieldnotes, interview with W. P. Howlett, December 12, 1991.

7

Sexually Transmitted Diseases in Colonial Malawi

Wiseman Chijere Chirwa

Of late, "the HIV/AIDS crisis in sub-Saharan Africa has stimulated renewed interest in the social, cultural, and epidemiological history of sexually transmitted diseases (STDs) under colonialism."[1] Scholars from various disciplines "have challenged the evidence behind colonial era narratives on syphilis and sexuality by noting that European observers often vastly overestimated the incidence of this STD among Africans."[2] This chapter aims to contribute to this debate in relation to the epidemiological history of STDs in colonial Malawi. However, it departs from analyses that focus on African sexuality and official misconceptions of STDs by discussing the connections between the capitalist economy and its creation of the STD-vulnerable cohort groups. It argues that African sexuality was not created in a material vacuum, and the official colonial misconceptions of it were influenced by both local and external developments. In a variety of ways, the constellations of sociocultural and socioeconomic factors at the local level had an impact on the pattern of STDs and on the collective official and community responses to them.

The chapter focuses mainly on the period from the early 1920s to the early 1960s. The material relating to the period prior to the 1920s is included to provide a background against which to understand the developments in the subsequent decades. Of particular importance is the development of the colonial economy during this period, its labor demands, and the effects on people's mobility. These were socioeconomic factors that affected the sexual morality of the local communities and, thus, created an environment in which STDs rapidly spread. Three themes are analyzed in this chapter: the relationship between people's mobility and the spread of STDs, the socioeconomic environment in which these diseases spread, and the official and non-official responses to them. The first two were intrinsic parts of the capitalist system. The labor demands of the colonial economy and the social conditions in which the workers lived created high risk of exposure to STDs. The various categories of workers were STD-susceptible populations, and the risk spread from these to all those who sexually serviced them, both at the work place and at home. The spread of STDs in colonial Malawi, as in Africa in general, should, therefore, be understood as a result of a combination of economic and social forces associated with the capitalist economy. The responses of the African communities, those of the white settlers and the colonial administrators, varied according to these groups' respective knowledge of the diseases, their cultural and religious backgrounds, and their ideological commitments. The colonial medical and health policies relating to these diseases changed from time to time depending on pressure and resources.

Viewed in relation to the current rapid spread of HIV/AIDS in the country, this chapter throws some light on risk factors in a historical context. It attempts to provide insights into, and knowledge of, the economic and social context within which risk behaviors are set and how vulnerable populations are created. It will be noted that the co-factors of STDs during the colonial period and the official and community responses to these diseases are similar to those of HIV/AIDS in the present period. At the beginning of the 1990s STDs were listed as the ninth commonest communicable disease in the country. Studies done in some selected district hospitals showed an STD prevalence of 4.7 percent of patients in the 12-and-above age group.[3] More recent studies show a close connection between STD patterns and those of HIV/AIDS. Many, although not all, HIV/AIDS–positive patients tend to have a history of STDs. The high risk groups for HIV/AIDS are the same as those of STDs. They include prostitutes (commonly known as bar girls), truck drivers, itinerant traders, migrant workers, and teenage school children.

These observations suggest that STDs are possible co-factors of HIV/AIDS in the country. This, however, is not to suggest that the STD prevalence is the only or the major factor for the rapid spread of HIV/AIDS. A lot of socioeconomic and health factors contribute to this. The STDs are also not the major cause of illness and death, but they are, surely, a health problem deserving medical and scholarly attention. The account herein is based on information derived from colonial administrative and medical reports, coupled with reports of white settlers in the Shire Highlands, the southern part of the country, the center of the colonial economy. Because the settlers employed large numbers of male workers who were vulnerable, and often victims of STDs, they had firsthand information on the patterns of the spread of these diseases.

THE ARAB DISEASE

The commonest STD in colonial Malawi was syphilis, caused by the spirochete *Treponema pallidum*. Gonorrhea, caused by the bacterium *Neisseria gonorrhoeae*, although known from quite an early period, became widespread from the 1920s, but at a much lower rate than syphilis. Accounts of early missionaries suggest that syphilis was brought into the country by slave traders, hence popularly known as the Arab disease.[4] It spread slowly along slave trade routes during the last half of the 1800s. The most affected areas were along Lake Nyasa and especially the slave centers of Karonga in the north, Nkhota-Kota in the center, and Mponda (now Mangochi) at the southern end of the lake. The concentration of traders, slaves, and slavers in these areas contributed to the fast spread of the disease.

As was the case with gonorrhea in Ghana, syphilis in Chad, and venereal disease in general in West and Central Africa,[5] trade routes, labor movement, and communication networks influenced the pattern of the spread of syphilis in colonial Malawi. From the lake areas the disease spread inland following portage routes. With the coming of the colonial economy in the 1880s, porters became the major vectors of syphilis. It is not surprising, therefore, that the disease is said to have been associated with the Chikunda, who were professional porters. Porters were therefore the first STD-susceptible group created by the colonial economy. Portuguese traders and travellers employed porters and crews for ships and boats along the Zambezi-Shire trade route from as early as the mid-1800s, if not much earlier. They paid their workers in trade goods and *kachaso*, a strong gin.[6] With colonial penetration, portage became the commonest mode of transportation. It existed in two forms: *mtenga-tenga* for goods and *machila* for human beings. Early European settlers, travellers, missionaries, and colonial administrators travelled by *machila*, a hammock carried by porters in turn. The *machila* and *mtenga-tenga* bands were large, especially where they carried trade goods.[7] They would camp for several days in a village to rest and to get enough food supplies before proceeding on their journey. Through camping en route the porters came into contact with village women, and, in turn, the contacts became avenues for the spread of the STDs to both the villagers and the porters themselves.

The local people's responses to these diseases at this time are difficult to determine. Most likely they treated the diseases as one of the ordered conditions of existence. However, there is evidence that the local people became aware of the new diseases. For example, syphilis was given the name *chizonono*, and gonorrhea became *chindoko*. The origins and meanings of these words are unclear, but they indicate growing awareness on the part of the local communities who must have developed an understanding of the etiologies of these diseases. However, there is no evidence that the diseases received special attention and no evidence of attempts to isolate the victims. Treatment and care must have been provided within the family.

A major difficulty in dealing with syphilis was that the local people could not make a clear distinction between it and yaws, which was common at this time. The latter is caused by a spirochete, *Treponema pertenue*, that is closely related to the pathogen for syphilis. Often those who suffered from yaws developed partial immunity to syphilis. The two diseases were treated in the same manner by applying various forms of herbs to the sores and affected areas to make them dry and by washing with water mixed with herbs or salt to reduce levels of bacterial infection. The treatment was for the sores and not for the pathogen for the disease itself.

Colonial officials developed awareness of syphilis from quite an early period. In 1897 David Kerr Cross, Nyasaland's first medical officer, included elaborate treatment guidelines for the disease in his medical handbook for European travellers and residents.[8] The treatment involved destroying the pimple by fuming it with nitric acid or strong sulfuric acid. This would be followed by washing the sore or chancre with soap and water and applying 10 grains of mercury-based calomel lotion and 2 tablespoonfuls of lime water to produce what was known as the famous black wash. Another way was to dust the sore with pure iodoform or iodoform ointment, followed either by 3 grains of blue pill or 4 grains of blue powder (hydrarg C. creta or mercury compound in chalk) or by 2 grains of green iodide of mercury three times a day.

To the patients the treatment procedure was clumsy and long. It took anywhere between a few weeks and several months. In fact, it was designed for white patients and travellers who had access to medical facilities. Given the absence of these in most areas of the country during the early colonial period, the majority of the African victims of the disease depended on their traditional forms of treatment. Only those who had access to mission hospitals benefited from the treatment. Throughout the early colonial period the treatment of syphilis was confined to treating the wounds rather than dealing with the pathogen and its mode of transmission. There were no special venereal disease clinics and no campaigns aimed at changing the victims' and potential victims' sexual behavior.

MIGRATIONS, SEXUAL COMPETITION, AND SOCIAL REPRODUCTION

The period between 1900 and the early 1920s saw two developments that created a conducive environment for the spread of STDs in Nyasaland. The first was the massive immigration of what are now known as Alomwe (formerly Anguru) ethno-linguistic communities from Mozambique.[9] The second was the expansion of the colonial plantation and estate economy. The combination of these two resulted in increased sexual competition and lax sexual morality or high levels of sexual networking. The immigrants, running away from the brutality of the Portuguese colonial regime across the border and from the harsh conditions on the plantations there, had "many destitute women amongst them, who [found] husbands or protectors amongst the local natives."[10] The women were exchanged for access to land and for physical and social protection. "Various sums" of money and other favors were given to those who brought them in; the majority of whom were "just relatives" or "chance friends." A gift or payment called *chikole*, some form of price or ransom, was given for every woman brought in. Through this practice local chiefs, village head men, labor overseers, and various influential and enterprising men had access to many of the destitute women, giving rise to sexual competition and lax sexual morality. A group of men who pursued sex and the acquisition of women for purposes of sexual and emotional gratification thus emerged. It was also a form of social reproduction. The more women these men had access to, the greater was their status. Given their vulnerability, the women's volition is said to have been "so very small that it [was] probably a matter of complete indifference whether they [were] attached to one man or another."[11] This, however, does not mean that the women were in total consent with the practice. It is because they were socially and economically vulnerable. The immigrant groups were also interested in their own social reproduction, to maintain relations with those they were attached to and from whom they got their protection. Giving out women to outsider groups or individuals was a traditional gesture of healthy political and social relations, as well as a way of asking for peace and reconciliation after hostilities. The side effect of the practice was that it gave rise to competition for the immigrant women by influential individuals and groups.

With the coming of the colonial economy from the 1880s, the labor demands and mobilization strategies of the white settler community contributed to sexual competition. The major sources of labor were the lakeshore districts, parts of the central province (Central Angoniland, now Ntcheu), the villages contiguous to the plantations, the villages across the political borders in Mozambique, and within the plantations themselves.[12] The lakeshore and the central Angoniland districts were areas where syphilis was already prevalent. The majority of the workers were recruited as single men on a seasonal basis and housed in temporary shelters known as *chitando* or *misasa*. The concentration of single men at the point of production — the estates and plantations — resulted in competition for local women. The single workers often moved in with the local women on the estates and in the neighboring villages partly for leisure, emotional satisfaction, and social reproduction, and partly also as a way of claiming permanent residence in the area. Accounts of the early settlers indicate that large numbers of women running away from slave raiders and traders and some running away from marital and other problems took refuge on the settler estates, especially those belonging to the African Lakes Corporation and those of the members of the Blantyre Mission of the Church of Scotland.[13] These women became a pool of casual wage workers. Like the immigrant single male workers, they were housed in *chitando* shelters on the estates. The mixing of the single male and female workers at the point of production was accompanied by the emergence of a lax sexual morality characterized by a culture of multipartnered sexuality. This created a favorable atmosphere for the spread of STDs.

It can, therefore, be argued that STDs derived more from the social conditions on the estates than from the natural moral behavior of the African people. This was a common feature of capitalist enterprises that involved the concentration of single men at the point of production. The mining centers of South Africa and Southern Rhodesia (now Zimbabwe) are good case examples of this.[14] In both cases "syphilis derived from social conditions in the compounds rather than from conditions underground" because prostitution was a common feature of compound life. Because the services of prostitutes "did much to attract and stabilize labor, mine management and state alike were unwilling to eliminate it, in spite of its direct contribution to the spread of a deadly disease through the black work force."[15] The same applied to Nyasaland. Because of the mixing of recruited single workers with local women, elements of prostitution emerged quite early on the Nyasaland estates and plantations and in the villages neighboring them. There is no doubt, therefore, that the labor demands of the plantation economy contributed to the spread of STDs during the first three decades of the colonial period.

INCREASED OFFICIAL AWARENESS

The outbreak of World War I further aggravated the health problems of the Nyasaland protectorate. Colonial reports for the war period indicate that "the health conditions of the protectorate [had] not been satisfactory, owing to the extensive movement of natives into and within the protectorate, necessitated by the military operations."[16] Among the communicable diseases, malaria had the largest number of cases. In order of frequency, the other diseases were dysentery, syphilis, gonorrhea, pneumonia, chicken pox, whooping cough, and yaws. It was from this time that gonorrhea began to spread more rapidly, but still not to the extent of syphilis, which was among the major causes of illness. Medical facilities were still poor, with only 5 government hospitals with a total of 52 beds, 8 dispensaries, and few mission hospitals and dispensaries. These could not cope with the massive flow of patients because of the poor health conditions of the protectorate during the war period. The majority of the STD victims, thus, continued to rely on the traditional palliatives.

A positive development of the poor health conditions of the war period was that colonial officials became more conscious of the need to report on venereal diseases. Although fragmented, figures on cases of syphilis and gonorrhea treated at government hospitals and dispensaries began to appear in official reports. For example, in 1923 some 72 cases of gonorrhea were reported. The figure rose to 183 in 1924 and 263 in 1925. Those of syphilis were 576 in 1924 and 528 in 1925. Large numbers of these were treated in poorly equipped rural dispensaries, which gives the impression that the STDs were widespread in rural areas. The treatment had greatly improved with the introduction of novarsenobillon and bismuth, which were more effective than the mercury and iodoform treatment previously used. Even so, most patients continued to rely on the traditional cures.

Colonial officials blamed the poor health of the protectorate and the spread of STDs on poor working conditions on the estates, low industrialization, low productivity, and poor nutrition. They were particularly concerned with the health conditions of Africans on the plantations of the Shire Highlands, where the health care and treatment of workers during sickness was, on the whole, "very far from satisfactory."[17] Distance from medical facilities and unavailability of medical staff also mattered. Government hospitals and dispensaries were few in numbers and the medical staff were inadequate and often poorly trained. On the estates and plantations, few employers would go so far as to employ a half-trained African dresser. The government urged them to improve the living conditions of their workers: "apart from the economic necessity for keeping all employees in a good state of health, it should be made compulsory that all employers of labour make adequate provision for the medical treatment of their labourers."[18] Unfortunately, the government could not go beyond this appeal. There was almost nothing it could do to force the employers to make medical facilities available to their African workers. In fact, the government itself was poorly equipped in the areas of medical facilities and health care provision.

Available statistical data suggest that there was no decline in the cases of either syphilis or gonorrhea in the late 1920s and early 1930s. If anything, the pattern was generally toward increase in the incidence. In 1930 917 cases of syphilis were treated. The figure rose to 1,267 in 1931 and 2,063 in 1932. Gonorrhea cases were 368 in 1930, 855 in 1931, and 1,020 in 1932. The incidence per thousand among patients for the period 1927–32 is shown in Table 7.1. If compared to the incidence of other communicable diseases, syphilis accounted for 7.5 percent of the total 17,102 cases in 1932 and gonorrhea was 2.92 percent. Malaria had the highest incidence with 23.41 percent, schistosomiasis was second with 12.43 percent, followed by

TABLE 7.1
Incidence of Sexually Transmitted Diseases per 1,000 Patients

Year	Syphilis	Gonorrhea
1927	4.1	1.5
1928	4.3	2.7
1929	4.2	2.7
1930	3.9	1.5
1931	4.6	3.1
1932	6.5	3.2

Source: Nyasaland Protectorate, Annual Medical Records, 1927–1933.

ankylostomiasis with 18.62 percent and influenza with 11.97 percent. This means syphilis ranked fifth among the communicable diseases. Of a total of 36 inpatient deaths from communicable diseases in that year, syphilis accounted for 11.86 percent, compared to 16.95 percent for both tuberculosis and malaria and 13.56 percent for ankylostomiasis.

Two developments contributed to the fast spread of venereal diseases during the 1930s. The first was the expansion of the tea estates, and the second was the increase of outward labor migration to Southern Rhodesia and South Africa. After the depression of the late 1920s and early 1930s, well capitalized settlers in Nyasaland abandoned tobacco, which had been the main crop, and switched to tea. The tea industry expanded rapidly from the 1930s up to the time of independence in the early 1960s.[19] What was particular about tea production in Nyasaland was that it depended to a large extent on three categories of socially vulnerable groups of workers: immigrants from Mozambique, women and children from within and outside the estates, and casual male workers from neighboring villages.[20] The immigrants and children were the most dependable. The majority of the former were single men coming to work on a seasonal basis or for periods ranging from six months to one year. Only those who decided to settle permanently in the area worked longer periods. The tea labor force was thus highly unstable, constantly moving in and out.

Recent studies show that the rapid turnover of male workers had serious implications for the social lives of women in the tea-producing areas. On average, three out of every five adult women over 30 years of age would have married more than twice and would have had more than five sexual partners outside marriage in their lifetime. Most of their marriages were informal and temporary. To them, marital breakdowns and multi-partnered sexual life were regarded as normal.[21] The reason is that the majority of these women married men who were on the estates only for short periods because of the temporary nature of their work. Large numbers of adult single women, widows, and abandoned wives also took refuge in the estates, partly for social and economic protection and partly also to have access to men who came there to work. After short periods of temporary marriages, the women were abandoned, as the landowners were aware: "During the past 18 months I have had some unfortunate experience with the abandoned families of men who have left here without leaving trace of their whereabouts. I have had to buy feeding bottles for infants, supply milk and look after the old women, and I do not propose, nor do I admit any obligation to continue to assist the families whose menfolk choose to abandon them. . . . The houses of the abandoned families must be pulled down and the women and the children go elsewhere."[22]

Such social conditions were not without benefits to the estate owners. The single women, widows, and abandoned wives were a major attraction to the single male workers. A floating population of women on the estates was, in itself, a reserve labor force in addition to being a bait for male workers. The concentration and mixing of single women and men on the estates increased sexual competition, which created a favorable environment for the fast spread of STDs. In 1942 the district commissioner for Cholo (now Thyolo), one of the tea-producing districts, observed that syphilis was "definitely increasing" and most of the cases that came for treatment were from the estate *chitando*. He attributed this to the fact that estate laborers were mostly unmarried, thus, STDs were "common amongst these boys."[23] A total of 266 cases of syphilis and 39 cases of gonorrhea were treated among this group in the district in that year.

The seriousness of STDs at this time can be measured in terms of the effects on labor. Between 1936 and 1938 medical officials carried out an exercise to determine which diseases had the greatest effect on workers' attendance at work in government departments. The results (shown in Table 7.2) indicated that STDs accounted for more off duty days than malaria, which was the leading cause of illness. The figures are only for workers in government employment. They do not include other sectors of the colonial society. It should also be noted that not every sick person took days off work. However, the data suggest that there were more cases of malaria but with fewer days off duty. Fewer cases of STDs accounted for more days off duty. Because there was always the possibility that many more unrecorded cases of both malaria and STDs resulted in workers being off duty, the above figures give an incomplete picture of the situation, but they provide insights into the seriousness of the problem.

From the 1930s the state began to deal with STDs and other health problems of the country with some degree of seriousness. For example, in 1930 the Colonial Development Fund provided some £101,410 for the improvement of hospitals and rural dispensaries, infant welfare centers,

TABLE 7.2
Loss of Work Days because of Illness

	Malaria	Sexually Transmitted Diseases
1936		
Cases	158	69
Days off	1,033	2,022
1937		
Cases	169	49
Days off	930	1,119
1938		
Cases	183	92
Days off	1,096	2,256

Source: Nyasaland Protectorate, *Annual Medical Records*, 1938, p 20.

mortuaries, and staff quarters. In the following year, there were 13 native hospitals and 91 rural dispensaries in the country. Two years later, two new native hospitals and two rural dispensaries were added. The older hospitals and dispensaries were renovated with brick walls and iron roofs, increased bed space, and additional staff. Between 1931 and 1934 the government annually provided a special medical grant of £1,400 for drugs, plus other medical supplies, to improve the health conditions of the country. The first STD clinics were established during this period. Unfortunately, "it was found that the natives avoided them and few cases of venereal diseases were being seen. It was then decided to treat these in the general hospitals."[24] The reason for the natives avoiding the clinics was that they were a source of embarrassment. The STD patients disliked the idea of being isolated from other patients and in the process their status being known by the public because there was very little privacy in the clinics. In some urban hospitals separate wards were provided for STD patients throughout the 1930s.

A campaign to educate the native population on STDs began in 1936. Pamphlets were printed in English and in vernacular containing information on the modes of transmission, risks, and effects of these diseases and emphasizing that cure was possible through free, "modern European" treatment available at government hospitals and dispensaries.[25] The pamphlets were supplemented with public lectures by the staff of the health department. The Public Health Ordinance included clauses on the compulsory treatment of venereal diseases. The government was, however, aware that all these efforts were "of little practical value" because the Africans had "their own so-called cures and [were] averse to the long-continued attendance at hospital which European treatment involve[d]."[26] The penalties of the Public Health Ordinance could seldom be enforced, because the government had very little capacity to do so. It lacked financial resources and adequate personnel to enforce the law. After all, the majority of the reported STD cases were those who had already voluntarily submitted to treatment. The law would, therefore, not have any meaningful effect.

There were three other problems to deal with: the incomplete treatment of cases, diagnostic handicaps, and the sociocultural orientations of the Africans themselves. Medical officers often complained that it was difficult to get the African patient to attend for regular courses of treatment. The patients invariably stopped attending when symptoms disappeared, but the disease was still transmittable. Such patients, mostly men with syphilis, were the most dangerous, because, confident that they were cured, they could not restrain themselves sexually. In the case of gonorrhea, the danger was greater with female patients, because the disease did not easily show physical signs in them. Only in the advanced stages did the signs come out vividly. Health officials frequently misdiagnosed syphilis, especially in the poorly equipped and grossly understaffed rural dispensaries. Often the disease passed as yaws and vice versa. This was a common cause for both under- and over-reporting of the disease. Wrong diagnosis often resulted in wrong treatment and patients carrying and passing on the disease for a long time before they were cured.

The general attitude and the socio-cultural orientation of the Africans to the STDs also mattered. The attitude was one of fear, shame, and loss of face and at times a good deal of indifference.[27] There was fear of sterility and of being accused of infidelity, especially on the part of women who would be taken to court by their husbands if found with an STD. Married women who revealed their STD status risked divorce or fine, unless they showed very concrete proof that they got it from the husband. There was a double standard here. While the women could be divorced or fined, the men usually got away with it; but they were equally afraid of being accused of infidelity and losing face. The reason is that culturally men were allowed to have more than one sexual partner. For unmarried young men, contracting STDs was regarded as a sign of "manhood," an indication that they were sexually alive and active for reasons of procreation, which was their prescribed role in society. Not surprising therefore that a young man with an STD was jokingly referred to as a "wounded soldier." Society and individuals were thus indifferent to the young men's risk of STDs. For both married men and women, fear and shame resulted in the disease being too often concealed, or resorting to African palliatives rather than to the more public method of attending hospital. Another dangerous cultural practice was sexual contact with an unaffected person with a view to "passing on" the disease as a necessary condition to completing the "cure" after receiving treatment from the herbalist. The practice is said to have been "very common."[28]

THE MORAL PANIC

Official colonial administration reports suggest that by the late 1930s STDs had reached epidemic levels in some districts of Nyasaland, especially in the Shire Highlands where the demands of the colonial economy provided an environment for the spread of the diseases. Elsewhere in the country increased labor migration to South Africa and Southern Rhodesia might have contributed to the spread. From 1936 Nyasaland legalized the recruitment of labor for the mines and farms of the Rhodesias and South Africa. This and independent clandestine migration increased the mobility of the Nyasaland men.

The relationship between labor migration and the spread of STDs was in two ways. The first was in the process of the migration itself, the actual journey. It involved traveling on foot for several days through villages where food could be obtained. The men camped several times on their way, and in the process some if not many of them had sexual contacts with local women. Through these the STDs could be spread to both the men and the women. In 1936 the Health Department reported that venereal diseases were commonest in townships and in the northern districts from which most of the male migrant workers derived. The second way was through the social conditions in the mining compounds where prostitutes were a common feature of compound life. By 1938 medical officers in Nyasaland were of the strong belief that "syphilis and gonorrhea are rapidly spreading in our native areas due mainly to the introduction of new strains of infection by laborers returning to this country after working abroad where males, separated from village control, are liable to contract infection."[29] Another reason suggested was the "separation of wives from their husbands over long periods, tending to immorality amongst the former especially with the younger men returning from abroad or with strangers passing through their villages."[30]

It was common for colonial officials to sensationalize and moralize the effects of labor migration. The above account, although factually grounded, might have been over-sensationalized. Colonial reporting on STDs and African sexuality reflected the general moral panic of the time.[31] It was influenced by the belief that "Africans were irreducibly 'different' in their attitudes to sexuality."[32] Their distinct sexuality accounted for the spread of STDs and other social and moral evils, such as frequent marital breakdowns, polygamy, and the disintegration of tribal and family life. Based on such beliefs, colonial administrators and white missionaries constructed what they regarded to be the African sexual morality and immorality. As Martin Chanock has observed, "African sexual morality and the position of women were severely condemned. . . . Some African people appeared to have no sexual morals at all."[33] Different ethnic groups had different moralities. For the Lomwe, it was of "so low a standard that adultery [was] not considered as an offense . . . they had their women in common." Among the Mang'anja, "the chastity of women, or their feelings on the subject . . . [was] not considered; it [was] their custom to loan their wives to a friend or for money value to a stranger." The Yao were generally and distinctly immoral. "No man . . . dare[d] trust his wife out of sight for any length of time."[34] Both colonial administrators and missionaries, thus, gave themselves the responsibility to liberate the African women and to reconstruct, improve, and control the Africans' sexual morality.

However, the belief that STDs were rapidly spreading in the country was shared by the Africans themselves. In 1938 chiefs in West Nyasa (now Nkhata Bay) district expressed concern "at the spread of venereal disease infections amongst their people." They suggested that "every native returning to their areas [from work abroad] should be compelled to submit to a medical examination prior to being permitted to enter."[35] In a way, the chiefs shared the moral panic of the colonial officials, but the latter's response was rather negative: "Although this is a policy of perfection, the [health] department could not undertake the examinations required, as there is no staff competent to perform them stationed in the area. The desirability of giving effect to this policy therefore does not need immediate consideration."[36]

In addition to inadequacy of staff, there were several other problems. The migrants entered the area and the country itself from several points. It would require stationing medical personnel at all of them. The exercise would be expensive given the large numbers of returning migrants. Given that the diseases were already prevalent in the local communities, testing and treating the returning migrants would not provide any guarantee that the incidence would be reduced. In fact, there was always the possibility of the returned migrants contracting the diseases in their areas of origin after returning home. After all, the returning migrants were neither the sole nor the major vectors of STDs. Porters, immigrant estate workers, and other STD-vulnerable groups within the country were equally responsible.

SEXUALLY TRANSMITTED DISEASES IN THE COLONIAL EMPIRE

After the outbreak of World War II, STDs became an empire-wide problem. The 1940s, thus, saw increased state interest in control programs, most of them originating from the Colonial Office in London. At the local level the programs and policies were designed to fit into the wider imperial initiative from which they received support. This was based on two reasons: the spread of these diseases in Britain itself and the effects of the war conditions on public health. Records of the debates of the House of Commons suggest that Britain experienced a rapid spread of STDs from the late 1920s. The *British Medical Journal* of the British Medical Association published alarming figures on the incidence of these diseases in the country. About 16,000 expectant mothers were said to have been infected by 1928. The numbers increased during the 1930s. In 1941 70,000 new cases of venereal diseases were said to have applied to civilian clinics for treatment, and there must have been "thousands more" who were not obtaining treatment or who had not been traced.[37] The movement of soldiers and other war personnel was responsible for this situation. Britain's colonies were affected in the same manner.

In March 1942 and in April 1943 Oliver Stanley, the secretary of state for the colonies, sent circular dispatches to the colonies outlining the policy on STDs:

I feel that there is one aspect of medical activities which is of special importance, particularly under war conditions, namely the occurrence and spread of venereal disease. I have learned with concern how the incidence of this disease has assumed serious proportions in many colonies. . . . It is now the accepted principle that questions of health education and treatment, together with the prevention of venereal disease, should be part of the normal responsibilities of the medical and education departments of colonial governments. This principle is in accord with the recommendation contained in the Statement of Medical Policy . . . drawn by my Colonial Advisory Medical Committee.[38]

In May 1943 he set up a standing subcommittee of the Advisory Medical Committee "to keep the venereal disease situation under review and to advise [him] on the application of the approved policy." He requested all the colonies to report to him within six months on the action taken in relation to the matter because "unless measures can be planned successfully to check the incidence of the disease, the consequent results will be serious."[39]

The Nyasaland governor responded to the secretary of state's request by appointing a committee "to enquire into the social and medical aspects of the problem of venereal disease in Nyasaland and to advise on the preventive and curative measures to be taken to control the spread of this group for diseases."[40] The committee submitted its report in January 1944. The document was divided into five parts dealing with the civil conditions influencing the spread of the diseases, medical aspects, preventive measures, curative measures, and the contribution of war conditions to the spread of these diseases.

Out of the recommendations made emerged four important policy proposals. The first was the proposal for a legal framework for the control of the spread of the diseases. It was recommended to confer power on native courts to administer the provisions of section 34 of the Public Health Ordinance (chapter 73/74), which read: "Every person who wilfully or by culpable negligence infests any other person with venereal disease, or does or permits, or suffers any act likely to lead to the infection of any other person with any such disease shall be guilty of an offense, and shall be liable to a fine not exceeding £200 or to imprisonment for a period not exceeding six months or to both."[41] It also became illegal for employers to engage servants and other categories of workers suffering from venereal diseases "in communicable form." The targets of this were not the employers but their workers: domestic servants, truck drivers, railway crew, and all those regarded as being in the categories of high risk.

The second proposal was to mount propaganda aimed at changing the behavioral attitudes of the African population. This included pamphlets, sex education in schools, radio programs on STDs, press coverage, and explanations of the forms of the diseases. The colonial officials were aware that for propaganda to be successful it needed to have guidance of the chiefs, village headmen, parents, and guardians and custodians of tradition and customs, such as those who performed initiation and other rites of passage, coupled with the cooperation of missionaries for their close contact with village communities. The inclusion of mission health centers in the scheme for the extension of treatment facilities would also be mandatory. The involvement of the Christian missions, traditional leaders, and other players was the state's tacit admission that it could not deal with the problem on its own. It was also a realization of the complexity of the social issues involved in the topic.

The third, and related to the others, was the proposal to improve social services, including organized sport and leisure, especially for the younger generations. The reasoning was that "immorality following public beer drinks which continued after dark [was] one of the factors encouraging the spread of the disease. In several areas it [was] alleged to be the main factor."[42] There was, therefore, need to organize the Africans' leisure to control the immoral practices arising from the effects of public beer drinking. There were some dangers in this. The traditional beer industry, which expanded very rapidly in the areas affected by the colonial estate economy, and especially in the Shire Highlands districts, was part and parcel of the totality of the relations of production.[43] On the one hand, it was a reliable source of income for the beer-brewing women, the majority of whom were poor wives of estate workers or single or divorced and widowed rural village women. On the other hand, it provided the estate workers with a form of leisure and entertainment. In beer drinking and in the dancing and the sex that often accompanied it the poorly paid estate workers ironed out their emotional peaks and troughs and found their social fulfillment. The estate owners liked this social environment because it provided them with a socially-controlled labor force. The other beneficiaries were chiefs. They collected fees for the beer brewed and sold in their areas. The fees were a major source of revenue for the chiefs' treasuries.[44] It was, thus, very difficult to control beer brewing and drinking.

The committee's report also recommended to the government to urge employers of labor to improve housing for their workers, especially on the estates. The thinking was that the inadequacy of housing impeded and denied the natural movement of African workers with their families to places of employment. This was a cause of family instability leading to lack of sexual restraint, loose sexual behavior, and high risk of STD transmission and contraction. As a long-term policy, it was important to raise the status of women because the migration of male workers had resulted in the breakdown of native moral codes, and the worse affected were women. The improvement of the latter's status would also help solve the problem of prostitution, which was "generally due to poverty and to the instability created by the absence of the males." The aim of most so-called prostitutes was "to secure a man to live with, or to make ends meet during the absence of the neglectful husband."[45]

The other important policy proposal was to provide free supplies of STD drugs — bismuth, neoarsphenamine, sulphapyridine, and penicillin — to all nongovernmental medical centers staffed by either a qualified medical practitioner or a competent hospital assistant. These drugs would be administered to patients free of charge. In addition to the provision of the drugs was the recommendation to extend to rural areas improved medical services by establishing "as rapidly as possible" an adequate number of rural health units suitably disposed throughout the country.

The above proposals covered both preventive and curative measures. Unfortunately, some of them were difficult to accomplish. The legal framework was put in place between 1944 and 1946. The Native Courts Ordinance and the Public Health Ordinance were accordingly amended to include sections on STD protection. However, it was not easy to enforce them. No chief would risk his position by rounding up and fining STD victims in his area, and in the process creating a bad name for himself. The law would be effective only where the disease was revealed, but the reality was that a lot of people were unwilling to reveal their STD status. As for the propaganda, the director of Medical Service thought it could only be effective if it was constant and suited to local requirements. There was always a danger that film exhibitions, drama, and radio programs would become forms of entertainment rather than tools for useful propaganda. The director of Medical Services emphatically warned that "the roots of sex hygiene lie deep in social structure and social customs. The provision of better staff and adequate supplies of special drugs are not going to solve the problem."[46] He further observed that some of the drugs listed were rated as group one poisons; their circulation was restricted.

Both arsenical and sulfonamide drugs were very expensive. They could not be cheaply and easily procured for free distribution.

The above proposals encouraged the Nyasaland government to apply for funding to mount a campaign against STDs. In 1945 it received a grant of £42,000 from the Colonial Development and Welfare Fund for the campaign. The grant was for five years, meant for the procurement and free distribution of drugs to both government and nongovernment health centers and for the general improvement of medical and health facilities in the country. The expenditure on drugs amounted to approximately half of the total funds granted, and by 1949 it was decided to extend the period of the scheme for another five years. The success of the program was in the number of cases treated rather than in the reduction of the incidence of the diseases. Official figures (shown in Table 7.3) suggest that the cases continued to increase.

The majority of the cases were treated in government hospitals and dispensaries, especially in the Southern Province. The tea-producing districts of Mulanje and Thyolo and the urban and peri-urban areas of Blantyre, Limbe, and Zomba in this province accounted for the highest numbers of STDs. The situation in the tea-producing districts was blamed on

TABLE 7.3
Cases of Sexually Transmitted Diseases Treated

Year	Syphilis	Gonorrhea	Other	Total
1940	3,231	1,131	—	4,326
1941	4,932	1,382	—	6,314
1942	6,219	1,585	—	7,804
1943	—	—	—	—
1944	—	—	—	—
1945	5,681	—	—	5,618
1946	8,555	2,056	39	10,650
1947	14,143	5,638	103	19,884
1948	13,088	5,054	35	18,177
1949	15,407	6,671	172	22,250
1950	19,403	4,304	1,892*	25,599

*The 1950 figure of 1,892 for the "other" category is said to have been because of "faulty testing," and the absence of complete figures for 1943–45 is because of the unavailability of records for those years. The "other" STDs included soft chancre and other infections arising from sexual contact.

Sources: Nyasaland Protectorate, *Annual Medical Reports*, 1940–49; Colonial Office, *Annual Reports on the Nyasaland Protectorate*, 1945–50; National Archives of Malawi, S40/1/8/4, Venereal Disease, 1943–45.

immigrant workers from Mozambique in particular and on *chitando* workers in general. In 1943 there were eight estate dispensaries, one mission hospital, one government hospital, and three rural dispensaries in Thyolo. All of them reported treating large numbers of STD cases. The government hospital had an STD ward with nine beds, but because of the large number of patients, doctors "had to tell patients to go away as soon as the open sore is closed . . . thus there [was] a big number of out-patients attending the clinic for further treatment."[47] The same applied to the Malamulo hospital of the Seventh Day Adventists in the district. The urban and peri-urban areas of Blantyre, Limbe, and Zomba also reported high levels of STD incidence. In Blantyre, large numbers of Africans were said to have suffered from venereal diseases. Those attending hospital represented "only a fraction of those who actually had the diseases."[48]

There are four possible explanations for the very high figures presented in Table 7.3. The first is that the 1940s saw increased labor movement into and out of the country. Large numbers of seasonal workers from Mozambique came to work on the Shire Highlands tea plantations. At the same time large numbers of Nyasaland men left for employment in the South African mines and on the Southern Rhodesian tobacco estates. This was a period of intense competition for Nyasaland labor in the Southern Africa regional economy. The second was the movement of soldiers and carriers during the war and their return from the war beginning in 1945. This was identified as the major factor in the spread of STDs in the post-war period. The high rise in the numbers of cases between 1945 and 1947 was most likely caused by this. The third explanation relates to the medical advancement and effects of the campaign started in 1945. The use of penicillin, which was a more advanced cure, created confidence in STD victims. Many of them came forward for treatment. The free distribution of this and other drugs from 1945 increased patient confidence and the desire to receive treatment at the hospital and dispensaries. The rise in the numbers of syphilis cases after 1949 could be caused by this and by the continuation of free distribution of drugs from that year, which further increased patient confidence. Last, the post-war STD campaign resulted in more efficient reporting than had been the case before. The figures in Table 7.3 could, thus, be more of a reflection of reporting than of increased incidence.

With the coming of the federation of the Rhodesias and Nyasaland in 1953, the Medical Department came under the jurisdiction of the Federal Ministry of Health. Reporting on STDs at the local level became rather irregular. The 1953 report indicates that venereal diseases were rife, and the curative services available became more and more thinly spread over increasingly populated areas that lacked even the economic ability to provide adequate preventive facilities and services. Within the federation, the state continued to run STD campaigns between 1955 and 1958. The largest of these was in the Namwala district in Northern Rhodesia (now Zambia) where STDs were very common, especially along the railway line from Livingstone to Ndola. The campaign was launched in 1946 and continued during the federation period until 1958. Mobile units of medical staff and field officers were deployed in a number of rural districts. In Southern Rhodesia (now Zimbabwe) the largest campaign was in the towns of Salisbury (now Harare) and Bulawayo. If official figures are to be believed, the campaign in these towns must have paid off. There was considerable decline in the numbers of patients treated in the late 1950s. In Salisbury STD admissions dropped from 1,972 in 1948 to 690 in 1958. Outpatients' attendance for the same period also dropped from 29,967 to 1,096. New cases of syphilis were 1,693 in 1948 and 435 in 1958 and those of gonorrhea were 2,200 and 256, respectively. In Bulawayo, 2,937 cases of STDs were admitted to hospital in 1948. The figure dropped to 1,085 in 1958. Outpatients' attendance was 90,737 in 1948 and 2,740 in 1958. New cases of syphilis recorded were 1,790 in 1948 and 827 in 1958, and those of gonorrhea were 4,572 and 1,459, respectively.[49]

Although the figures declined considerably, STDs were still rife and the population at risk is said to have more than doubled. The figures above suggest that there were major variations between the two cities. The situation was more contained in Salisbury than in Bulawayo. This could have resulted for two reasons: the former had more medical facilities than the latter because of the difference in the size of the white population and because Salisbury was the federal capital for the two Rhodesias and Nyasaland. The other reason could be that the African population of Bulawayo grew at a much faster rate than that of Salisbury. The estimates were 33,867 in 1948 and 121,000 in 1958 for Bulawayo, compared to 56,660 in 1948 and 122,000 in 1958 for Salisbury. It is, therefore, most likely that the risk population was larger in Bulawayo than in Salisbury.

The STD campaign in the federation was a continuation of the imperial initiative, based on both the exaggerated accounts of the problem in Africa and the genuine health effects of World War II. There is no doubt that the war had a major effect on the pattern of the spread of STDs in Britain's African colonies in the late 1940s and throughout the 1950s. Although the imperial campaign officially came to an end in the 1950s, in Nyasaland the government continued to supply mission hospitals with drugs for the free treatment of these diseases up to the time of independence in 1964.[50]

CONCLUSION

The colonial experience discussed here provides some useful insights into how STD-vulnerable groups are created. The socioeconomic conditions that facilitated the spread of STDs during the colonial period are similar to those that facilitate the spread of HIV/AIDS in present Malawi. Over the last five to ten years, the country has experienced a rapid spread of the disease.[51] The cultural orientations of traditional communities, poverty and lack of economic opportunities for women leading to prostitution, expansion in the tourist industry, improvements in road networks that increase mobility of people, labor migration, and the movement of refugees across political boundaries have been cited as among the major causes of the HIV/AIDS pandemic in the country.[52] However, few studies have explored the linkages between HIV/AIDS patterns and the socioeconomic changes in the country in a historical perspective. The tendency has been to understand the HIV/AIDS etiology from purely a behavioral (sexual) point of view, without linking it to the wider socioeconomic factors that shape sexual behavior. As Randall Packard and Paul Epstein have rightly observed, "sexual activity involves not only pleasure, but social reproduction,"[53] and the latter has economic, political, and cultural foundations. In a capitalist economy, sexual activity is part and parcel of the totality of the social and productive relations. The current HIV/AIDS pandemic, as was the case with STDs during the colonial period, "may prove to have a complex ætiology involving a combination of political and economic [as well as cultural] forces . . . which have brought together particularly susceptible populations, subject to high background levels of viral, parasitic, and bacterial infections, within a social setting marked by high levels of separation and multiple sexual partners."[54] The above account shows that sexual behavior is socially constructed and that there is always an environment in which people's sexuality is set. When planning HIV/AIDS containment programs, it is important to have precise "knowledge of the social and economic context within which risk behaviors are set. If a primary risk factor is being poor and unemployed, then the proposed interventions must address the causes of this condition."[55] The focus of the Malawi AIDS control program is on behavior modification, which does not address the socioeconomic conditions that shape people's sexual behavior. The colonial experience discussed here shows the dangers of the approaches that focus narrowly on causes and cures without looking at the wider context within which the causes are set.

NOTES

1. Bryan Callahan, "'Veni, V.D., Vice'?: Reassessing the Ila Syphilis Epidemic," *Journal of Southern African Studies* 22 (September 1997): 412.

2. Ibid., p. 421.

3. Ministry of Health, *Sexually Transmitted Diseases: A Treatment Guideline* (Lilongwe: Ministry of Health, 1989); Lillian R. Kamtengeni, "An Overview of Sexually Transmitted Diseases in Malawi," paper prepared for the Parent

Education Project in the Ministry of Community Services, Ministry of Community Services, Lilongwe, 1991.

4. Michael King and Elspeth King, *The Story of Medicine and Disease in Malawi: The 130 Years Since Livingstone* (Blantyre: Montfort Press, 1992), p. 54; Oliver Ransford, *"Bid the Sickness Cease": Disease in the History of Black Africa* (London: John Murray, 1983), p. 174.

5. See Mario J. Azevedo, "Epidemic Disease Among the Sara of Southern Chad, 1890–1940," in *Disease in African History: An Introductory Survey and Case Studies*, edited by Gerald W. Hartwig and K. David Patterson (Durham, N.C.: Duke University Press, 1978); K. David Patterson, *Health in Colonial Ghana: Disease, Medicine, and Socioeconomic Change, 1900–1955* (Waltham, Mass.: Crossroads Press, 1981).

6. See Fredrick Moir, *After Livingstone: An African Trade Romance* (London: Hodder and Stoughton, 1924), pp. 41–43.

7. See H. L. Duff, *Nyasaland Under the Foreign Office* (London: George Bell, 1906), pp. 51–54.; A. Colville, *One Thousand Miles in a Machilla: Travel and Sport in Nyasaland, Angoniland, and Rhodesia with Some Account of the Resources of These Countries* (London: Walter Scott, 1911).

8. David Kerr Cross, *Health in Africa* (London: James Nisbet, 1897), pp. 108–10.

9. See Robert B. Boeder, *Silent Majority: A History of the Lomwe in Malawi* (Pretoria: African Institute of South Africa, 1984); Alifeyo Chilivumbo, "On Labour and Alomwe Immigration," *Rural Africana* 24 (Spring 1974): 49–57; Wiseman Chijere Chirwa, "Alomwe and Mozambican Immigrant Labour in Colonial Malawi," *International Journal of African Historical Studies* 27 (1994): 525–49.

10. Colonial Office, *British Central Africa Annual Report* (London: His Majesty's Stationery Office, 1905), p. 22.

11. Ibid.

12. See Wiseman Chijere Chirwa, "'Theba is Power': Rural Labour, Migrancy and Fishing in Malawi, 1890s–1985," doctoral dissertation, Queen's University, Kingston, Ontario, Canada, 1992; Wiseman Chijere Chirwa, "Child and Youth Labour on the Nyasaland Plantations, 1890–1953," *Journal of Southern African Studies* 19 (December 1993): 662–80; Wiseman Chijere Chirwa, "Alomwe and Mozambican Immigrant Labour," pp. 525–49.

13. Such accounts are found in Moir, *After Livingstone*.

14. See Charles van Onselen, *Chibaro: African Mine Labour in Southern Rhodesia, 1900–1923* (London: Pluto Press, 1976); Charles van Onselen, *Studies in the Social and Economic History of the Witwatersrand, 1886–1914*, Vol. 1: *New Babylon* (Johannesburg: Ravan Press, 1982).

15. van Onselen, *Chibaro*, p. 49.

16. Colonial Office, *Annual Report on the Nyasaland Protectorate*, 1915, p. 17.; Colonial Office, *Annual Report on the Nyasaland Protectorate*, 1918, p. 8.

17. Nyasaland Protectorate, *Annual Medical Report on the Health and Sanitary Condition of the Nyasaland Protectorate* (Zomba: Government Printer, 1926), pp. 10–11.

18. Ibid., p. 11.

19. See Robin H. Palmer, "The Nyasaland Tea Industry in the Era of International Tea Restrictions, 1933–1950," *Journal of African History* 26 (1985): 215–39.

20.   See Chirwa, "Child and Youth Labour," pp. 662–80; Chirwa, "Alomwe and Mozambican Immigrant Labour," pp. 525–49; Robin H. Palmer, "Working Conditions and Worker Responses on Nyasaland Tea Estates, 1930–1953," *Journal of African History* 27 (1986): 105–26.

21.   See Edna Msungu, "Women on the Tea and Tobacco Estates of Thyolo District, 1923 to 1953," Seminar Paper No. 5, Chancellor College, University of Malawi, (1993–94); Wiseman Chijere Chirwa, "Women on Private Estates in Colonial Malawi," paper presented at a Workshop for the Winners of the Sixth OSSREA Research Competition on Gender Issues, Karen, Kenya, May 10–14, 1994; Wiseman Chijere Chirwa, *Women, Gender and Production on Colonial Malawi's Estates: A Report for the Organization of Social Science Research in Eastern and Southern Africa* (Zomba: Chancellor College, 1995).

22.   National Archives of Malawi (hereafter, NAM), NSE 2/1/8, Manager, Gontha Tea Estates, Ltd. Reports, 1940–1949, cited in Msungu, "Women on the Tea and Tobacco Estates," p. 9.

23.   NAM NSE 5/1/7 Cholo District Annual Report, 1942.

24.   Colonial Office, *Annual Report on the Nyasaland Protectorate*, 1933, p. 9.

25.   NAM PCS 3/5/19 Health Pamphlet No. 1. Venereal Diseases: Nthenda Zoopsya Ziwiri: Chindoko ndi Chizonono (Two deadly diseases: gonorrhoea and syphilis). Issued by the Medical Department, Zomba (Zomba: Government Printer, 1936).

26.   Colonial Office, *Annual Report on the Nyasaland Protectorate*, 1936, p. 8.

27.   NAM PCS 3/5/19 Report submitted by the Committee Appointed to Consider and Make Recommendations on the Problem of Venereal Disease in Nyasaland, 1944.

28.   NAM PCS 3/5/19/ and S40/1/8/4, Report submitted by the Committee Appointed to Consider and Make Recommendations on the Problem of Venereal Disease in Nyasaland, 1944.

29.   Nyasaland Protectorate, *Annual Medical Report*, 1938, p. 15.

30.   Ibid.

31.   See Megan A. Vaughan, *Curing Their Ills: Colonial Power and African Illness* (Stanford, Calif.: Stanford University Press, 1990); Megan A. Vaughan, "Syphilis, AIDS, and the Representation of Sexuality: The Historical Legacy," in *Action on AIDS in Southern Africa: The Maputo Conference on Health in Transition in Southern Africa, April 1990*, edited by Zena Stein and Anthony Zwi (New York: Committee for Health in Southern Africa and the HIV Center for Clinical and Behavioral Studies, Columbia University, 1991), pp. 120–27.

32.   Vaughan, "Syphilis, AIDS, and the Representation of Sexuality," p. 151.

33.   Martin Chanock, *Law, Custom and Social Order: The Colonial Experience in Malawi and Zambia* (Cambridge: Cambridge University Press, 1985), p. 146.

34.   NAM, J2/4/1, Correspondence, 1903–4, cited in Chanock, *Law, Custom and Social Order*, p. 146.

35.   Nyasaland Protectorate, *Annual Medical Report*, 1938, p. 15.

36.   Ibid., p. 16.

37.   House of Commons, *Parliamentary Debates: House of Commons Official Report* (London: Her Majesty's Stationery Office, 1943), p. 1807.

38.   NAM S40/1/8/4, Colonel Oliver Stanley, Secretary of State for the Colonies, Circular Dispatch, July 4, 1943.

39. Ibid.

40. NAM S40/1/8/4 and PCS 3/5/19, The Committee Appointed to Consider and Make Recommendations on the Problem of Venereal Disease in Nyasaland, 1944.

41. NAM PCS 3/5/19, Public Health Ordinance Section 34 Amendment, 1944.

42. NAM PCS 3/5/19 and S40/1/8/4, Report of the Committee on Venereal Disease, 1944.

43. See Chirwa, *Women, Gender and Production.*

44. See NAM NSE 5/1/6 Cholo District Report, 1939; NSE 5/1/7 Cholo District Reports for 1940–43; NSE 5/1/8 Cholo District Report, 1944–46.

45. NAM PCS 3/5/19 and S40/1/8/4, Report by the Committee on Venereal Disease, 1944.

46. NAM S40/1/8/4, Director of Medical Services to Chief Secretary, May 28, 1943; also in his comments on the Report by the Committee on Venereal Disease.

47. NAM NSE 5/1/7 Cholo District Annual Report, 1943.

48. NAM PCS 3/5/19, District Commissioner, Blantyre, to Provincial Commissioner, South, October 6, 1949.

49. Federation of Rhodesia and Nyasaland, *Annual Report of the Public Health of the Federation of Rhodesia and Nyasaland* (Salisbury: Government Printer, 1958).

50. Malawi Government, *Ministry of Health Annual Report* (Zomba: Government Printer, 1964), p. 22.

51. See William House and George Zimalirana, "Rapid Population Growth and Poverty in Malawi," *Journal of Modern African Studies* 30 (1992): 141–61; C. Carr, ed., *Technical Analysis of HIV/AIDS Situation in Malawi* (Lilongwe: U.S. Agency for International Development, 1992); I. Chirwa, "AIDS Epidemic in Malawi: Shaking Cultural Foundations," *Network* 13 (1993): 31–32; John Cuddington and John D. Hancock, "Assessing the Impact of AIDS on the Growth Path of the Malawian Economy," *Journal of Development Economics* 43 (1994): 363–68; Anne V. Akeroyd, "HIV/AIDS in Eastern and Southern Africa," *Review of African Political Economy* 60 (1994): 173–84; The AIDS Secretariat, *Malawi AIDS Control Programme: Medium-Term Plan II, 1994–1998* (Lilongwe: AIDS Secretariat, 1994).

52. See Paul A. K. Kishindo, "High Risk Behaviour in the Face of the AIDS Epidemic: The Case of Bar Girls in the Municipality of Zomba, Malawi," *Eastern Africa Social Science Research Review* 11 (June 1995): 35–43; Paul A. K. Kishindo, "Sexual Behaviour in the Face of Risk: The Case of Bar Girls in Malawi's Major Cities," *Health Transition Review* 5 (supplement) (1995): 153–60; Wiseman Chijere Chirwa, "Malawian Migrant Labour and the Politics of HIV/AIDS, 1985 to 1993," in *Crossing Boundaries: Mine Migrancy in a Democratic South Africa,* edited by Jonathan Crush and Wilmot James (Ottawa: International Development Research Council, 1995): 120–28; Wiseman Chijere Chirwa, "Migrancy, Sexual Networking and Multi-partnered Sexuality in Malawi," *Health Transition Review* 7 (supplement 3) (1997): 5–16; Wiseman Chijere Chirwa, "Aliens and AIDS in Southern Africa: The Malawi-South Africa Debate," *African Affairs* 97 (December 1997): 53–79.

53. Randall Packard and Paul Epstein, "Epidemiologists, Social Scientists, and the Structure of Medical Research on AIDS in Africa," in *Action on AIDS in Southern Africa: The Maputo Conference on Health in Transition in Southern Africa,*

April 1990, edited by Zena Stein and Anthony Zwi (New York: Committee for Health in Southern Africa and the HIV Center for Clinical and Behavioral Studies, Columbia University, 1991), p. 132.

54.   Ibid., p. 133
55.   Ibid.

8

The Social, Cultural, and Epidemiological History of Sexually Transmitted Diseases in Zambia

Bryan T. Callahan and Virginia Bond

Zambia has emerged as one of the nations most seriously affected by the HIV/AIDS epidemic in sub-Saharan Africa. Estimates of HIV infection among the sexually active stabilized in 1997 at approximately 26 percent for urban areas and 15 percent for rural areas.[1] As a new disease condition, HIV/AIDS provides a potent metaphor for the dangers of modern life, yet strong continuities link the long-term history of sexually transmitted diseases (STDs) in colonial and post-colonial Zambia with the contemporary history of HIV. These continuities include the influence that socioeconomic changes — particularly transformations in human mobility patterns — have exerted over disease transmission patterns; the central role that so-called parallel economies have played in reshaping household dynamics in response to the emergence of capitalist market relations; the impact that economic development priorities have had on the formulation of state level health policy; and the impact that popular discourse on the relationship between sexuality and pathology has had on shaping definitions of sexual risk arenas within Zambian society. This discourse has tended to blame women for the promiscuity of African men and the spread of STDs.

However, at other levels it is difficult to link the broader history of STDs in Zambia with contemporary issues surrounding HIV/AIDS. This chapter argues that colonial authorities commonly overestimated the prevalence of syphilis by confusing its clinical symptoms with manifestations of endemic yaws, a treponemal disease condition that was once common throughout colonial Zambia (formerly Northern Rhodesia).

Since the 1970s, however, a prolonged economic decline has created spiraling poverty and shifted the epidemiological landscape of STDs. Although we can argue that colonial period concerns with STD prevalence often reflected little more than the anxieties of British officials, it appears that the social and demographic consequences of the HIV crisis may indeed be catastrophic for the near future.

SEXUALLY TRANSMITTED DISEASES IN COLONIAL ZAMBIA: 1890–1964

Health Policy, Labor Concerns, and Sexually Transmitted Diseases in the Early Colonial Period, 1890–1924

Because of limitations in source materials, it is difficult to develop a clear analysis of STD incidence patterns for the early colonial period. Before the emergence of its own mining industry in the mid 1920s, Northern Rhodesia produced little more than cheap migrant labor for the mines and commercial farms of neighboring territories. Prospectors initially deemed the territory's copper deposits unworkable, and high transport costs from the landlocked protectorate made agricultural exports uncompetitive. Despite initial expectations that Northern Rhodesia would become an integral part of White Africa, the total European population still numbered less than 2,000 by World War I.[2] There were probably no more than 20 qualified doctors resident in the territory at any given time, and, with the exception of a handful of medical missionaries, most of these health professionals devoted their practices to the settler population.[3] Recorded commentary on African health for this period is, thus, incidental at best.

Northern Rhodesian officials also showed little initial interest in or regard for the health of their African subjects. From the 1890s to 1924 the territory was ruled on behalf of the Colonial Office by the British South Africa Company (BSAC), a chartered corporation that received its policy directives from a board of private investors based in London. Profit was the BSAC's bottom line, and its administration imposed stiff taxes on rural African communities to force adult men into the region's nascent labor market.[4] Most of these men worked in Southern Rhodesia's gold mines, and prior to 1910 about 5 percent of all "Zambezi boys" died each year from a combination of industrial accidents, infectious diseases, and dietary deficiency syndromes. Many others perished on their journeys to and from work. The mines generally refused to subsidize travel costs for migrants, leaving their workers to walk hundreds of miles without the aid of rest camps, food allowances, preventive medical care, or other basic amenities.[5] Rather than intervene in this exploitive dynamic, Northern

Rhodesia's native commissioners actively abetted it by burning the huts of tax evaders and by publicly flogging African headmen who refused to call out their young men for work. Only in 1907, when the Colonial Office threatened to ban interterritorial labor exports entirely, did the BSAC enact basic recruiting regulations.[6]

This callous attitude toward African health did not really begin to change until the early 1910s, when growing labor shortages prompted European authorities to reexamine the developing relationship between capitalist penetration and indigenous population dynamics.[7] Government medical officers began to note a high incidence of venereal disease (VD) in communities near the "Line of Rail,"[8] and reports from the western regions of the territory indicated that syphilis was assuming epidemic proportions among the Ila and the Lozi.

To assess the validity of these observations, the government asked Stanley Colyer, its medical officer for Barotseland, to conduct a formal epidemiological survey. The doctor's findings, summarized in the territory's annual medical report for 1912–13, defused anxieties by suggesting that previous commentators had misdiagnosed common clinical manifestations of endemic yaws as venereal syphilis. Colyer also pointed out that the Lozi did not make a verbal distinction between yaws and syphilis, but referred to both diseases by a single generic name, *manansa*. Etymological imprecision on the part of Lozi informants had thus contributed to etiological inaccuracy on the part of colonial medics. Colyer concluded his remarks by noting that the "gradual loosening of the tribal idea" was probably contributing to a breakdown in established social controls over sexuality, but he found no evidence to indicate that syphilis posed an immediate threat to African fertility.[9] Northern Rhodesia's Medical Department responded to this report by scaling down its VD estimates and by giving yaws a higher profile in succeeding annual reports. The Medical Department also began a long-term experiment on yaws treatment at its African clinic in Solwezi, and Northern Rhodesia became one of the first British territories to apply low-cost bismuth compounds to yaws therapy.[10]

This shift in opinion on the relative incidence of yaws and syphilis may have been nothing more than a byproduct of careful medical inquiry. However, it is also likely that shifts in regional labor dynamics played an important role in temporarily reversing official anxieties toward syphilis. The territory's first major syphilis scare had coincided with a severe manpower shortage. Newly established copper mines in the Katanga region of the Belgian Congo had drawn labor away from the BSAC's own prospecting operations at Kansanshi, and Northern Rhodesia's small contingent of white commercial farmers, eager to supply the growing Katanga consumer market, had demanded workers. The administration had also agreed to supply Southern Rhodesia's Native Labor Bureau with several thousand men annually, and agents of the Witwatersrand Native Labor Association had begun to tap directly into the territory's labor reserves by posting agents in northern Mozambique.[11]

These competing strains on labor gradually resolved in the early 1910s. The Kansanshi mine proved unprofitable and its operations closed; World War I disrupted commercial agriculture and forced many of Northern Rhodesia's farmers out of business; and the Witwatersrand Native Labor Association stopped actively recruiting central African labor because of appallingly high mortality rates among these workers, who commonly reached the Witwatersrand in a state of complete exhaustion and malnourishment, which rendered them highly susceptible to pneumonia and tuberculosis (TB).[12] Northern Rhodesia, thus, shelved its immediate aspirations for internal economic development and returned to a policy of encouraging long-distance labor migration as a way to generate much needed state revenue.[13]

In the final decade of BSAC rule, official concerns with STDs were episodic at best. The annual medical report for 1918–19 claimed that the demobilization of some 37,000 African veterans of the German East Africa (Tanganyika) campaign had spread gonorrhea and venereal syphilis into the eastern parts of the territory, namely the Fort Jameson and Kasama districts.[14] With the exception of minor treatments dispensed by Fort Jameson's medical officer, however, the government took no action on these reports of advancing rural infection. Then in 1923 the native commissioner of Mumbwa District, Frank Melland, attempted to invoke local chiefly authority to ban the migration of women to towns and mines along the Northern Rhodesian Line of Rail. Melland was especially concerned with the activities of Ila women, whom he described as thoroughly "syphilized" and naturally predisposed toward the practice of commercialized sex. He claimed that a large contingent of Ila women were pursuing lucrative careers as prostitutes in town and returning to their home areas to recruit their sisters and friends into the business.[15]

Melland's commentary reflected a common assumption among British officials that nearly every African woman in town was engaged in the exchange of sexual favors for cash, clothing, and other popular commodities. Indeed, there is evidence to indicate that many women gained entry to towns by engaging into short-term domestic partnerships with working men, but many of them practiced prostitution only until they could accumulate enough cash to move into petty marketing ventures. Other women came to town with the object of finding successful men from their home areas whom they could marry. Many temporary marriages, thus, became permanent ones, and they were recognized in many African communities as a modernistic variation on traditional forms of elopement.

Melland's attempt to impose controls over women's migration to commercial areas once again raised questions about the social and epidemiological effects of capitalist development on rural African communities,
but the government's chief magistrate declared that the native commissioner's travel restrictions exceeded the legal powers available to traditional leaders and struck them off the district's register.[16] Given Colyer's
earlier statements on the high prevalence of yaws in western areas of the
territory, it is possible that the administration treated Melland's comments on syphilis as nothing more than a case of amateur misdiagnosis,
but it is also probable that the government's response was tied into wider
concerns with regional labor dynamics.

Industrial Development and Medical
Intervention against Sexually Transmitted
Diseases in the Copperbelt, 1924–64

In the early 1920s rising prices on the world copper market had stimulated renewed interest in the productive potential of Northern Rhodesia's
mineral deposits. Geological explorations conducted in 1923 revealed that
rich secondary sulfide ores lay beneath the territory's relatively poor sur-
face outcroppings, a discovery that immediately led to the local formation
of two internationally financed mining conglomerates, the Rhodesian
Selection Trust, Limited (RST) and the Rhodesian Anglo-American Corporation (Anglo-American). Northern Rhodesia experienced its first real
economic boom as RST and Anglo-American set to work on developing
the ore bodies, and the administration once again found itself having to
balance its established role as a regional labor exporter with rising internal demands for a low-cost work force.[17]

Colonial officials, thus, worked with the mines to develop a strategy to
redirect regional migration patterns. Their task was complicated by the
inability of RST and Anglo-American to offer competitive wages because
of the financial constraints imposed by their basic capital investments.
The mines also had to deal with the hesitancy of African men to work in
a remote area where death rates from malaria were initially high and
where basic food and housing conditions were still quite poor.

Under these circumstances, RST and Anglo-American chose to adopt a
policy of temporary labor stabilization modeled on initiatives taken by
the Union Minière du Haut Katanga directly across the border in the Belgian Congo. They invited workers to bring women and children with
them to the residential compounds, a privilege that the segregationist
regimes of the south were unwilling to allow on a large scale. The new
mines, thus, gained a positive social advantage over regional competitors,
and early surveys indicated that married men did, in fact, sign on for
longer contracts than their bachelor counterparts.[18]

Mine management also realized that it could relieve itself of costs associated with the daily reproduction of its labor power by facilitating the relocation of African women's labor to the Copperbelt. The companies assigned garden plots to married women, and the produce from these holdings supplemented basic rations. Many women increased their household's average income by selling produce or by cooking meals for bachelor workers. Moreover, women who engaged in beer brewing often earned more from the proceeds of a single beer drink than their partners could secure from an entire month of underground toil. An informal economy thus developed through women's initiatives that contributed directly to the health and contentment of the male laboring population and supplemented household incomes in ways that reduced wage demands. This policy also provided women with vital access to urban spaces, where they could obtain new commodities and achieve a high degree of economic and social independence despite their technical reliance on marriage as a marker of legitimacy.[19]

Given this situation, both the mines and the colonial state were originally willing to turn a blind eye to casual domestic arrangements between their workers and migrant women. Melland's restrictions on women's mobility posed a direct threat to early capitalist development in the Copperbelt, where mine management soon recognized that its toleration of temporary marriages allowed it to purchase the labor power of an entire household for slightly more than a single man's wage. As a result, long-term concerns with the effect of STDs on African generational reproduction were put off in favor of immediate concerns with the day-to-day social reproduction of a stable male work force.

This attitude toward temporary marriages remained in place until the early 1930s, when the onset of the Great Depression closed all but two of the Copperbelt's mining operations. Thousands of unemployed men defied government orders to return home, fueling official anxiety that capitalist development was causing permanent ruptures in established African social controls, a decline in rural agricultural productivity through the displacement of male labor power, and the rise of a dangerous and uncontrollable class of detribalized natives. Northern Rhodesia's policymakers thus began to question the benefits of their laissez-faire approach to African social change, and they implemented a forced repatriation program. Managers at the RST's Roan Antelope Mine in Luanshya also tried to resurrect the power of customary law by appointing tribal elders to serve as local agents for rural chiefs.[20] Melland's 1923 policy initiative thus gained new credibility as Northern Rhodesian officials tried for the first time to regulate the social dynamics of migration and household formation.

As was the case in the rest of colonial Africa during the depression, policymakers turned to indirect rule to mitigate the impact of capitalist change. Officials voiced new concerns with the autonomous development of production and exchange networks over which they had very little direct control or that appeared contrary to the established frameworks of pre-colonial African social hierarchies. In this context, women's work in the informal economy — especially work conducted in urban areas outside the bonds of traditionally sanctioned marriages — became suspect.

There is strong evidence to indicate that African women were using surplus accumulation from consumer services and prostitution for reinvestment in the African rural economy. Several female entrepreneurs were key figures in the emergence of an independent African transport business in the 1940s, and women dominated the lucrative fish trade between the Luapula River and the mines of the Northern Rhodesian and Congolese copperbelts. There is also evidence from Kenya that women's earnings played an important role in cattle purchases and bridewealth subsidies for male family members in the early colonial period.[21] However, colonial officials generally regarded women's work in town and in long-distance trade as supplementary at its best and parasitic at its worst. They also feared that women's household demands were contributing to rising consumer aspirations that industrial capitalism was not yet prepared to meet. The dynamics of social reproduction in town were thus seen as a contributing factor in the rise of labor militancy, and when tax increases stimulated a general strike in the Copperbelt in 1935, the special commission dispatched to investigate the incident placed substantial blame on the influence of women and juveniles in stirring up discontent.[22]

In response, Northern Rhodesia's government adopted an official policy of stabilization without urbanization to meet the labor demands of industrial development while maintaining the rural economy's capacity to reabsorb male labor during recessions. Because women provided the backbone of rural agricultural production, the colonial state collaborated with rural chiefs and headmen to prevent unmarried women from leaving their home areas. In towns colonial officials began to crack down on unattached women by conducting late-night compound raids and by demanding proof of marriage from men who applied for residency in the family quarters.[23]

In theory these measures were meant to force young African men and women into traditionally sanctioned unions, but in practice they were relatively meaningless. Some native authorities erected roadblocks to check the marriage certificates of women in transit to the mines, but many women avoided these posts by disembarking and walking around them. Furthermore, men and women who were engaged in informal household arrangements often secured better compound housing by hiring "relatives" to certify the legitimacy of their marriages in the eyes of the tribal elders.[24]

Finally, as Northern Rhodesia's mining economy revived in the latter half of the 1930s, RST and Anglo-American lost interest in the stringent enforcement of the colonial state's new marriage regulations. Renewed economic expansion throughout southern Africa during the same period increased demands on local manpower reserves, prompting the mines of the Copperbelt to relax their marriage certification policy. However, this concession did not signal a return to laissez-faire social policy. To the contrary, the mines launched a sweeping program of medical surveillance to regulate the health and social hygiene of miners, miners' dependents, and other members of the local African community. The reasons for this initiative were two. First, the mines wanted to increase the stabilization of their skilled African workers by improving housing and sanitary conditions. Because these improvements could be effected through economies of scale, they represented less of an investment than wholesale wage increases. Second, the mines wanted to facilitate the reproduction and socialization of their own labor force by instituting maternal and child health care programs to increase the African live birth rate and by working with local Christian missionaries to create programs for African youth in education, sport, and scouting.[25]

The introduction of these measures helps to explain why, in sharp contrast to the mines of Southern Rhodesia and South Africa,[26] Northern Rhodesia's mining conglomerates never expressed serious worries over VD prevalence in their compounds.[27] During the 1930s a complex program of medical surveillance over African households in the Copperbelt took shape. Preliminary medical examinations became mandatory not only for male job seekers but for their female partners and child dependents as well. These inspections included an external genital examination for venereal lesions. The mines also developed a program of contact tracing for syphilis and gonorrhea cases discovered among their employees, who were required to parade naked before the company's medical staff once a month.

In 1937 the mines negotiated an agreement with the state that allowed them to take control of public health work in adjacent government townships. This pact permitted RST and Anglo-American to extend medical examination to both domestic servants and Africans employed by private contracting firms.[28] In 1938 the RST's chief medical officer, Charles Fisher, also convinced the government to add primary and secondary syphilis to its schedule of notifiable diseases. This amendment to the public health law empowered the mines to detain workers with infectious cases and force them to undergo treatment before returning to their rural homes.[29] In this way the mines sought to break the link between oscillating labor and the spread of syphilis between places of employment in the Copperbelt and rural labor reserves.

The mines also sought to effect profound social change within African households in the Copperbelt by implementing a wide-reaching maternal and child health program. This work began in 1936 under the initiative of Fisher, who drew on model programs pioneered by the Union Minière du Haut Katanga and on his own personal experience as the child of renowned Northern Rhodesian medical missionaries.[30] Between 1937 and 1957 annual attendances at Roan's maternal and child health clinics rose from fewer than 7,000 to more than 450,000. By the late 1950s Roan's clinics were supervising nearly 2,500 births annually, an impressive figure when one considers that the total African female population in the compounds was estimated at a little more than 6,000. Given the very high number of reported births, it is possible that women not normally residents of the mines were coming to town to have their deliveries.[31]

The mines used their growing control over the dynamics of African women's reproduction to conduct Kahn tests for syphilis among antenatal cases. This testing procedure complemented the monthly medical examination for male employees and helped to reduce VD incidence considerably. The widespread introduction of antibiotics in the early 1950s provided a further contribution to VD control by guaranteeing a relatively quick cure for syphilis and gonorrhea, thereby reducing chronic problems with lapsed treatment associated with long-term arsenic, bismuth, and sulfonamide therapies. These factors combined to reduce the recorded VD incidence at Roan to less than 1 percent per year by 1956 (that is, fewer than 200 total infectious cases for an estimated resident population of 20,000).[32]

Anglo-American was initially less willing to promote medical and social welfare programs in its compounds because its South African–based ownership was hesitant to encourage the long-term stabilization of African labor in areas officially designated for white settlement. Nonetheless, Roan's success with these programs increased its competitive advantage in securing skilled African workers, and by the late 1940s Anglo-American was following suit.[33]

The intensity with which the mines set about implementing medical and social welfare programs for resident Africans reflected a shifting climate of opinion in Northern Rhodesia on the general health and material status of the African community. Between the late 1930s and the mid 1950s, Northern Rhodesia faced chronic labor deficits that once again threatened to undercut the pace of its internal economic development. This problem was partly addressed through the negotiation in 1936 of a trilateral labor pact with the colony's two immediate neighbors, Nyasaland and Southern Rhodesia.[34] However, British officials in Northern Rhodesia remained concerned with long-term male absenteeism and its potential effects on village life. This anxiety was specifically expressed through increasingly detailed commentary on marital breakdown, declining agricultural production, and decreased fertility.[35]

Rural Campaigns against Sexually Transmitted Diseases, 1946–58

Growing political uncertainties in Europe during the 1930s raised the profile of this ongoing commentary on the changing dynamics of rural society and eventually prompted Northern Rhodesia's administration to take direct action against the spread of syphilis in rural areas for the first time. Tensions between Britain and Germany were forcing Britain to look beyond its traditional European metals markets and increase its reliance on southern Africa as a mineral supplier for its rearmament program. In this context, efforts to improve the quantity and quality of available African manpower became paramount. In 1938 a royal commission appointed to investigate economic and social conditions in Northern Rhodesia advised the administration to implement anti-VD campaigns among the Ila and Lozi as a central feature of the protectorate's first comprehensive development plan.[36] District officers stationed among these peoples were reporting alarming decreases in population, and their observations convinced the protectorate's Medical Department that its previous field surveys had seriously underestimated rural syphilis prevalence.[37] Colonial Office policymakers thus endorsed intensive VD treatment as a critical development priority.

The inauguration of rural VD treatment was temporarily postponed by World War II. Medical intervention against syphilis remained a key priority, however, and in 1946 Northern Rhodesia's Medical Department launched a compulsory screening and treatment campaign among the Ila of Namwala District. The financial and administrative scale of this exercise made it an unprecedented event in the history of VD treatment in British central Africa. In its first year the campaign examined nearly 8,000 people and treated 1,807 syphilis cases with a 20-week course of alternating neosalvarsan and bismuth sodium tartrate injections, at a total cost of £3,910.[38] By its conclusion in 1958 the campaign had treated more than 7,000 of Namwala's estimated 20,000 residents for syphilis.[39]

Concerns with the availability of African labor had thus stimulated a reconceptualization of Northern Rhodesia's epidemiological landscape, but it is unlikely that any dramatic change in syphilis prevalence had actually occurred since Colyer's 1912–13 report. There can be little doubt that labor migration created opportunities for the widespread introduction of STDs in rural areas between the 1890s and the 1940s, but basic immunological factors would have made it difficult for syphilis to supersede yaws as the dominant treponemal disease condition. Because syphilis and yaws are closely related, they confer a relatively strong cross-immunity to one another, and because yaws is normally contracted through casual contact during childhood, most of its presenters are immune to syphilis infection by the time they become sexually active.[40]

We should thus question the accuracy of colonial-era pronouncements on increasing syphilis prevalence in areas where yaws prevalence was already high, and Namwala was one of those areas. Until the 1920s disabilities caused by yaws infection formed the largest tax exemption category for Ila men, and the local Primitive Methodist mission hospital listed yaws as its most frequent complaint until the 1930s.[41] It is possible that the mission's treatment program created an opportunity for the local introduction of syphilis by interrupting the production of treponemal antibodies in its patients, yet most patients received a maximum of three neosalvarsan injections, so their potential for relapse was quite high.[42]

Moreover, the campaign's medical reports noted that the syphilis it encountered in Namwala was atypical. In 1947 the campaign's specialist, A. J. Evans, observed an extremely low incidence of congenital syphilis among newborns despite the fact that more than 20 percent of his adult patients were seropositive. Of the 1,459 babies that Evans examined, only 23 (1.5 percent) showed typical syphilitic lesions.[43] Evans also noted that the common late complications of syphilis — dementia, locomotor ataxia, and cardiovascular breakdown — were virtually absent in his adult patients. He explained this finding by arguing that chronic malarial fever had probably suppressed these sequelae, but his argument neglected the fact that medics were detecting neurological and coronary syndromes among Africans in urban areas where malaria was quite prevalent in many compounds. Evans was also puzzled by the relatively low incidence of STDs other than syphilis. Between 1952 and 1958 the campaign found 658 gonorrhea cases out of nearly 26,000 examinations, a 2.5 percent incidence rate (as opposed to a 23.1 percent incidence rate for syphilis). Evans tried to explain this anomaly by arguing that his patients had probably acquired a partial immunity to gonorrhea as a byproduct of their alleged culture of sexual excess. Finally, the campaign found primary genital chancres in only 6 percent of its syphilis cases, whereas the vast majority of cases were classified as latent. These cases had advanced beyond the infectious stage and were clinically and serologically indistinguishable from yaws.[44]

If, as this evidence suggests, syphilis was not the treponemal disease of note in Namwala, how do we account for colonial commentary on rural African population decline during this period? To answer this question we must draw on a wide variety of data. First, colonial observers were generally predisposed to associate perceived changes in demography with rising VD rates, but many other constraints on fertility operated within rural African society in Northern Rhodesia. Food scarcity and famine were chronic phenomena during the colonial period, and these factors may have limited fertility directly through nutrition deficiency or indirectly through increased morbidity and mortality from a wide variety of infectious diseases. There are also indications that Ila women may have used induced abortion and lactational anovulation as fertility control strategies. Furthermore, the Ila were known to observe periods of sexual abstinence between spouses following both childbirth and miscarriage, and the long-term absence of many husbands because of labor migration may also have reduced opportunities for conception.[45]

In contrast, oversights in colonial census methods may also have contributed to a significant underestimation of Ila population. Following the imposition of colonial rule, rural settlement patterns underwent a dramatic change as the Ila peoples took advantage of the relative peace imposed by British overrule to move out of stockaded villages and reoccupy abandoned lands.[46]

Nonetheless, colonial officials continued to tabulate Ila population according to those who reported to the chiefly villages for the annual census, although under the best of conditions this system was problematic. Because the census was directly linked to tax collection, many adult men fled to the woodlands until the district officer's party had passed. Moreover, because European officials were most interested in assessing the available male labor supply, other segments of the population were often ignored.[47]

Labor migration patterns may also have contributed to sizable distortions in rural census data. The introduction of waged labor in the industrial centers of Southern Rhodesia and South Africa provided a new avenue of wealth accumulation for many young Ila men, and there is strong archival and oral historical evidence to indicate that many Ila worked at the Wankie Colliery and in Bulawayo for periods of five to ten years as a way to accumulate bridewealth. Many migrated to these commercial centers as juveniles, which means that they would not have been registered on the tax rolls prior to their departure. Moreover, as Melland's 1923 commentary indicates, many young Ila women followed the path blazed by their male counterparts and established long-term residence in the towns.

Using the Ila case as a model, we can also question colonial commentary on the threat that syphilis posed to other endangered ethnic groups. For example, capitalist penetration in Barotseland caused a major shift in Lozi settlement patterns. Prior to the colonial period, the Lozi agricultural system had focused on cultivating the Zambezi flood plain's rich alluvial soils. This system was predicated on the labor-intensive maintenance of drainage canals, and it gradually broke down as an ever-increasing percentage of Lozi and "Wiko" left the area for commercial employment elsewhere.[48] Cultivation thus shifted to the forest margins of the Zambezi plain, where colonial officials experienced great difficulties in tracking down residents of the new garden settlements.[49]

Sexually Transmitted Disease Treatment Policy Reforms in Late Colonial and Post-Colonial Zambia, 1958–80

In the late 1950s the Medical Department abandoned its emphasis on rural anti-VD campaigns as a strategy for short-circuiting the transmission of venereal pathology within Northern Rhodesia's African population. The Ila syphilis campaign had provided a model for additional campaigns among the Ngoni of Eastern Province and among the Nkoya of Barotseland, but colonial officials gradually came to question both the political consequences and epidemiological relevance of these biomedical interventions. Each of the treatment programs had stimulated local resistance by insisting on the compulsory medical examination of African women, and this resistance had fed into the emerging rhetoric of African nationalism. Under the leadership of a former Ila schoolteacher, Harry Nkumbula, the African National Congress had mobilized resistance to a broad range of post-war development initiatives by characterizing them as attempts to expand white domination over the recently created Federation of Rhodesia and Nyasaland. The Medical Department thus revised its VD treatment policy by terminating the regional campaigns and by making voluntary antibiotic treatment widely available through its expanding rural clinic system.[50]

Northern Rhodesia's medical policymakers had also recognized that large numbers of urbanized Africans were actively seeking antibiotic treatment for syphilis and gonorrhea in urban areas. Indeed, it was acknowledged that private European practitioners had become the primary distributors of penicillin injections in towns. The Medical Department thus committed itself to building an urban clinic system to complement the rural dispensary network that it had initiated in the 1930s.[51] Government clinics made penicillin freely available, and by the end of the colonial period STD incidence along the Line of Rail had decreased measurably.[52] Ironically, however, it is quite possible that the colonial government's intensive anti-VD work during the 1940s and 1950s actually laid the groundwork for a subsequent geometric increase in venereal syphilis incidence by eliminating the cross-immunity that many people had acquired through childhood infection with yaws.[53]

Public access to STD treatment improved further following independence in 1964, but these gains ultimately proved short-lived. The new Zambian state under President Kenneth Kaunda committed a sizable percentage of its copper revenues to development programs on a socialist model known as Zambian Humanism, and medical services received a high priority. Between 1964 and 1974, the number of government-operated rural health centers rose from 187 to 376, and the number of urban clinics expanded from 39 to 111.[54] At a broader level, Kaunda stimulated general economic prosperity and sustained residential stability by expanding employment opportunities in the civil service sector. During this period Zambia's towns became magnets for persons seeking the benefits of well-paid government employment as well as state-subsidized food and housing.

With the collapse of the world copper market in 1974, however, Zambia entered a period of prolonged economic decline. The Kaunda regime's dependence on foreign aid increased dramatically, and by the late 1980s Zambia's national debt problem had spiraled out of control. Mismanagement and corruption in the public sector further eroded the nation's capacity for recovery, and Zambia was forced to implement an Economic Structural Adjustment Program in 1991 as a condition for continued foreign aid. The Economic Structural Adjustment Program has since compounded economic hardships by contributing to massive layoffs in the public sector, serious disruptions in state-sponsored marketing facilities, sizable increases in basic commodity prices, and the introduction of fees for many social welfare services, including attendances at hospitals and dispensaries.[55]

Sharp increases in reported STD incidence coincided with Zambia's economic downturn. In the first decade after independence, Zambian medical authorities paid relatively little attention to STDs. Given the widespread availability of antibiotics at government clinics, the Ministry of Health probably no longer regarded syphilis, gonorrhea, chancroid, and lymphogranuloma venereum as serious public health concerns.[56] This casual approach changed in the late 1970s, however, when government physicians began to report disturbing increases in all STD categories. Between 1973 and 1978 STD attendances at government clinics nearly doubled, and in 1978 the government documented 75,000 new cases of syphilis and gonorrhea alone.[57]

It is difficult to isolate the most important causes for this increase in STD incidence, and it is likely that numerous factors contributed to its resurgence between the late 1950s and the late 1970s. Deteriorating economic conditions led to a rapid decline in the availability of antibiotics, and Zambia's clinic system found itself in a poor position to fight the rapid spread of penicillin resistant strains of gonorrhea because of the high costs attached to newer, more effective drug treatments. The general mobility of the population also increased following a period of relative stabilization as many Zambians began to move back and forth between rural and urban areas, seeking material assistance from friends and kin. Because STD infection has been strongly associated with increased susceptibility to HIV, it is quite possible that the general economic downturn of the 1970s created new opportunities for increased STD incidence and contributed to the emergence of HIV at an epidemic level. As Zambia entered the 1980s its resources to fight infectious disease were at a low ebb.

THE HIV/AIDS CRISIS IN CONTEMPORARY ZAMBIA

In the early 1980s Anne Bayley, a surgeon at the University Teaching Hospital in Lusaka, recorded a marked increase in Kaposi's sarcoma incidence, changes in the disease's epidemiology and physical characteristics, and increasingly poor treatment responses among patients with the condition.[58] Bayley's findings reflected observations that physicians and surgeons were making elsewhere in central Africa at that time. The age and gender profile of Kaposi's sarcoma patients changed as young women replaced older men as the most common presenters of the malignancy, and the disease became characterized by widespread lesions on the trunk as well as lesions in the lymph nodes, mouth, and lungs. These atypical manifestations were eventually associated with the presence of HIV-1 antibodies, and in 1984 Zambia's Ministry of Health reported the nation's first AIDS cases.[59]

In the late 1980s medical researchers began extrapolating estimates of Zambia's HIV incidence and prevalence from a variety of select groups, namely new STD patients, blood donors, and pregnant women attending prenatal clinics. No national serological survey has ever been conducted, but medical researchers have carried out sequential sentinel surveys in at least two sites in every province since 1989, covering urban, peri-urban, and rural areas. In 1995–96 researchers conducted Zambia's first population-based samples of HIV incidence by performing a cross-sectional assessment of HIV incidence and prevalence around the cities of Lusaka and Kapiri Mposhi.[60] Data were also generated by medical studies on TB, other STDs, and fetal HIV transmission patterns.

Studies conducted on hospital inpatients indicated a high rate of HIV among recent mothers, newborns, and persons admitted with infectious diseases. A 1989 study of children born to HIV-positive mothers at University Teaching Hospital revealed that 39 percent of newborns remained infected with the virus, of whom just under 50 percent died by the age of two.[61] Other studies indicated a dramatic increase in HIV-related infectious diseases. Between 1987 and 1992 TB notifications rose by 20 percent each year to reach a total figure of 310 per 100,000 population. In 1989 73 percent of patients tested at the University Teaching Hospital chest clinic were HIV-positive, and these patients showed a much higher tendency toward mortality, reactions to TB treatment, and recurrent TB infections than their HIV-negative counterparts.[62]

Blood screening surveys also indicated a high prevalence of HIV within broader population samples. In 1989–91 the Zambia Consolidated Copper Mines examined serum samples from its recruits and found that 17 percent of its prospective workers (aged 20–29) were HIV-positive. Blood screenings conducted in 1991–92 showed that health workers, office workers, and teachers had an HIV prevalence of around 30 percent, and a 1995 survey of 516 mothers and their children in Lusaka showed that 23 percent of mothers and 18 percent of children under one year had HIV.[63] These statistics suggest that HIV has attained a high prevalence and incidence within most sectors of Zambia's population.

Although localized serological surveys have provided partial insight into the probable prevalence of HIV in Zambia, national statistics on blood screening for HIV and other STDs generated by the Ministry of Health have remained very unreliable. For example, between 1983 and 1987 the number of nationwide notifications for STDs rose from 46,726 to 109,496. In 1991, however, only 56,937 STD cases were reported, a number that probably reflected the deteriorating quality of government medical services and public health reporting procedures more than anything else. STD care at public clinics had deteriorated markedly by the early 1990s, and many people were beginning to seek alternative treatment options through private clinics and self-medication with herbal compounds and illegally marketed antibiotics.

A 1994 sentinel site survey indicated that HIV prevalence in Zambia's sexually active population ranged from a low of 1.6 percent to a high of 31.9 percent. Rural prevalence rates averaged about 10–15 percent and urban and peri-urban areas averaged about 25–30 percent. Incidence still appears to be rising in rural areas, but it may be stabilizing in urban areas. Indeed, preliminary findings from a 1996 sentinel site survey have supported this conclusion. HIV prevalence in Lusaka leveled off at around 26 percent between 1990 and 1996. AIDS mortality and HIV infection have contributed to an overall reduction in the annual population growth rate (from 3.7 to 3.1) as well as a decrease in total fertility (from 6.7 to 6.1), but epidemiologists are now predicting that the number of AIDS-related deaths will peak in the next decade.[64] In 1997 it was estimated that 800,000 Zambians (17 percent of the adult population) were HIV positive, of whom about 150,000 were symptomatic.[65]

The 1995–96 population-based survey suggested that there were striking differences in the age distribution of HIV infection by both gender and residence, with the highest HIV prevalence rates among urban women aged 20–29 (50 percent) and urban men aged 30–39 (42 percent). Young men in the 15–29 age group had a much lower prevalence than women of the same age, and evidently more women were infected at a younger age than men.[66]

The 15–19-year age group provides an important category of analysis because it may reveal the influence of behavioral changes on HIV incidence. A 1996 sentinel survey monitored a pronounced drop in HIV incidence among urban adolescent women since 1993 (from 28 percent to 17 percent), and the survey indicated that girls who were attending school were four times less likely to be infected on average. These findings may indicate that many younger girls had begun taking steps to protect themselves from HIV.[67]

Numerous socioeconomic factors appear to influence HIV prevalence in contemporary Zambia. People are increasingly moving between rural and urban areas to secure resources from kin and gain access to parallel markets. Two recent social research projects have noted that sexual exchanges often play a central role in these processes. A study of the Luapula Valley–Copperbelt fish trading industry has indicated that undercapitalized women and girls routinely use sexual favors to buy fish and secure transport and accommodation, and research conducted on a commercial farm in rural Chiawa has also indicated that many women see their ability to sell sex for gifts as essential to their efforts to achieve economic security. Both studies also note that many women brew and sell alcohol in conjunction with their sexual services, and it is possible that increased alcohol consumption contributes to risky sexual behavior. STD and HIV incidence are on the rise in both areas, and there also appears to be an increase in unwanted pregnancies and induced abortions.[68]

Other factors associated with increased STD and HIV susceptibility are the difficulties that women face in refusing sex with infected husbands and partners, as well as with members of the husband's family in cases of widow inheritance. Condoms also remain unpopular for reasons that revolve around ideas of trust, female fecundity, and male potency.[69]

The rise in overall mortality may be hindering Zambia's movement toward economic recovery. AIDS-related mortality appears to be highest among the most productive members of society. One review of 33 businesses showed a dramatic increase in average annual mortality from 0.25 percent in 1987 to 1.6 percent by 1992,[70] and another business study showed that 96 percent of recorded deaths had occurred among persons in the normally robust 15–40-year age group.[71] HIV infection also appears to strike at a high rate among the skilled and well educated. Employers in both the public and private sectors are finding it hard to replace skilled labor even though low cost labor is still abundant. The HIV epidemic in industry is thus creating a different kind of labor problem than that of the pre-colonial period. Medical expenses and training costs have risen, and absenteeism has increased because of increases in chronic illness and obligatory funeral attendances. The process of replacing skilled workers through the state education system has also been seriously undermined by illness and absenteeism among teachers.[72] By all appearances, commercial agriculture has suffered less than the industrial and service sectors, but smaller farmers, who rely more directly on access to household labor, appear more vulnerable to labor loss and may shift their production from higher paying non-staple foods to maize production in response to such losses. The death of adult men in a household also appears to seriously affect produce marketing in the formal agricultural sector.[73]

In regard to HIV's impact on the health care sector, mortality among nurses rose during the late 1980s from 2 per 1,000 to 26.7 per 1,000, a thirteen-fold increase that was largely because of HIV.[74] The annual cost of clinical care for patients with full-blown AIDS was calculated in 1993 at $27.1 million, and the annual cost of HIV-related diseases was estimated at an additional $27.3 million.[75] Zambia's hospitals also estimate that AIDS patients occupy 50 percent of their available beds at an average cost of $1.70 per day.[76] Overall cost demands imposed on hospitals and clinics by HIV-positive patients are substantially higher than costs associated with treating HIV-negative patients.[77]

The micro-economies of individual Zambian households have borne the greatest measure of burden in coping with the pressures of structural adjustment and with the socioeconomic dislocations caused by HIV-related mortality among family members. A research study in Monze District recently estimated that one in every four local households has experienced an HIV-related death, and in 1996 Zambia's National AIDS Control Program calculated that 6.5 percent of all Zambian households were caring for chronically ill family members.[78] There is also a tendency for afflicted households to experience chronic illness and death more than once, and research shows that anywhere between 40 and 72 percent of Zambian households are caring for an orphan.[79] There are now an estimated 500,000 orphans in Zambia, and it is believed that 20 percent of all children under age 18 have lost one or both parents.[80] These child dependents are largely cared for within extended family networks, and it is women, usually older sisters and surviving mothers, who are the primary caregivers. Research indicates that orphans do not normally suffer a lack of nutrition or emotional support, but they are less likely to attend school and more likely to be sent back to live with relatives in rural areas.[81] Widows also must contend with numerous burdens, including property grabbing by their husband's kin, high costs attached to funerals, and lengthy negotiations over the proper division of household assets among survivors. Households have begun to channel precious time and resources into seeking help for their afflicted members, with members moving back and forth between a variety of healers and treatment options.[82]

People who know their HIV status are often isolated because of the stigma associated with the disease.[83] An analysis of people tested for HIV in a Lusaka counseling center found that less than half of those surveyed felt capable of informing other persons about their test result. Women especially felt a need to conceal their infections.[84] Out of personal considerations for surviving family members, doctors still rarely list AIDS as a cause of death (technically it is listed as a secondary cause), and there is little incentive to be forthright about the illness in an environment where health care options remain limited and where strong social biases are attached to the afflicted. The population-based survey revealed that only 3.6 percent of all patients had undergone voluntary testing and counseling.[85]

Witchcraft accusations also appear to play an important role in configuring popular approaches to the social dynamics that surround HIV transmission. At a certain level they have provided a measure of psychological relief by placing responsibility for affliction within an intelligible social matrix, but they have also introduced serious tensions within households and communities. In a rural community south of Lusaka, a study of households that have lost at least one member to AIDS revealed that close relatives of the dead often listed witchcraft as a cause of death. Informants described AIDS as a "sent" affliction that was motivated either by jealousy or by a desire for personal retribution.[86]

For most of the 1980s the Zambian government's response to the AIDS epidemic was characterized by relative silence, but the state began to take a more active approach in 1989, when Kaunda publicly admitted that his own son had died of an AIDS-related illness.[87] The new government has since taken active measures to intervene against AIDS, and it recently integrated its AIDS, STD, TB, and leprosy control programs. In regard to AIDS control specifically, the Ministry of Health has emphasized STD control, blood bank screening, home-based care for people with AIDS, counseling programs, and a publicity campaign targeted at children under 15. STD control includes prenatal blood exams (screening for women in Lusaka has recently risen from an estimated 25 percent of pregnant women to 80 percent), educational projects, and the distribution of condoms.[88] To reduce the heavy costs associated with STD diagnosis, a syndromic case management approach has been adopted, which identifies a consistent group of clinical symptoms and the drug therapies that should be used to treat them.[89] There have also been attempts to improve contact tracing methods, and training courses on improved STD management are conducted annually for health workers.[90] The government does not promote HIV counseling and testing nationally, however, because of the high cost of serological exams. At a broader social level, the government has also supported the establishment of the Children in Need program to address the needs of orphans, and the Health Ministry has recruited traditional healers into AIDS care and prevention through workshops and training. Another significant measure was the government's passage in 1989 of legislation to increase women's legal powers to resist property grabbing.

The problems associated with these interventions have been numerous. Most of the interventions are almost entirely supported by donor funds, so their sustainability is in question. Blood safety and STD control programs have suffered from inadequate equipment, supply shortages, rapid staff changes, problems associated with increased resistance to less expensive antibiotic therapies, and general financial difficulties.[91] Home-based AIDS care, adopted as an alternative to costly hospital stays, still remains prohibitively expensive for many patients, and condom promotion appears to have increased prophylactic distribution without dramatically increasing condom use.[92] Many Zambians have resisted counseling efforts, and counselors are now trying to develop more culturally appropriate methods. Cultural objections to AIDS education in schools have also limited the popular circulation of information on prevention methods. Finally, the problem of orphans appears to be so universal that it is difficult to know where to start, although most interested parties agree that food supplements and increased educational opportunities should be provided and institutionalization avoided.[93]

Nongovernmental organizations and churches have played a critical role in managing AIDS prevention and care and addressing some of the limitations of government intervention. Some of the more outstanding and innovative interventions have been: the deployment of people with AIDS in AIDS education and the development of income-generating projects for HIV-positive people; anti-AIDS clubs for school children; a drop-in center for widows at the Young Women's Christian Association; spiritual counseling and pastoral care for home-based patients; peer education programs in workplaces (including commercial farms); participatory AIDS dramas on radio, television, and in theater presentations; and free counseling and HIV testing. In recent years AIDS intervention efforts in the public sector have sought to adjust their approaches to prevention and care by working within popular frameworks of social meaning and within specific contexts.

CONCLUSION

It is difficult to evaluate what impact these interventions will have on HIV prevalence and incidence. Popular awareness of HIV and AIDS in Zambia is now high, and there are some indications that people are taking more preventive measures. However, economic hardships still limit the possibilities of effective state and nongovernmental intervention at both a social and biomedical level, and this means that Zambian households and parallel economies will continue to shoulder the greatest burden in addressing the socioeconomic impact of AIDS-related morbidity and mortality. It appears that STD and HIV prevalence are strongly associated with economic instability, a situation that decreases access to health services and promotes increased mobility as well as the exchange of sexual services for social and material benefits. The long-term solution to Zambia's current HIV/AIDS crisis may thus reside in the restoration of relative prosperity and the creation of broad based opportunities for access to emerging markets and production sectors.

In the short term, improvements in clinical services may help to control the spread of HIV by reducing the overall incidence of gonorrhea, syphilis, chancroid, and other STDs that facilitate contraction of the virus through open lesions and abcesses. It is unlikely that Zambia will soon benefit from recent developments in HIV/AIDS chemotherapy. Protease inhibitors are still too expensive for mass application within current treatment programs. Cost-effective reinvestments in public health programs and clinical services may help to reduce HIV transmission, however, by making antibiotic treatment for other STDs widely available once again.[94] Indeed, the widespread availability of antibiotics between the early 1950s and the mid-1970s lowered STD rates dramatically despite high concurrent rates of labor migration and urbanization. Antibiotics have enjoyed widespread popularity since their introduction, and historical evidence suggests that people will actively seek them out if they are affordable and accessible.

The development of effective interventions against HIV/AIDS will also depend on an honest evaluation of the numerous social, economic, and cultural factors that have shaped the epidemic's course. During the colonial period, British officials employed decontextualized interpretations of African sexual behavior to explain the epidemiology of STDs. Medical authorities commonly assumed that African migrant workers were predisposed toward promiscuity, and they labeled town women as primary vectors of disease transmission without commenting on the economic constraints that drove many women to practice prostitution. These easy stereotypes have little explanatory value, but they continue to play an important role in the social marginalization of both recent urban immigrants and women in contemporary Zambia. As this chapter has noted, STD incidence has been historically linked to broad economic trends, and effective responses to the HIV/AIDS epidemic will need to account for this linkage.

NOTES

1. Knut Fylkesnes, Moses Sichone, and Kalvin Kasumba, "Population-Based HIV Study using Saliva Specimens: Socio-Demographic Determinants of Infection in Zambia," Dissemination seminar, Epidemiology and Research Unit, Zambia National AIDS/STD/TB Program, Lusaka, Zambia, February 1997.

2.   Karen Hansen, *Distant Companions: Servants and Employers in Zambia, 1900–1985* (Ithaca, N.Y.: Cornell University Press, 1989), p. 89.

3.   Michael Gelfand, *Northern Rhodesia in the Days of the Charter: A Medical and Social Study, 1878–1924* (Oxford: Basil Blackwell, 1961), pp. 212–46.

4.   Andrew Roberts, *A History of Zambia* (London: Heinemann: 1976), pp. 174–94.

5.   Charles van Onselen, *Chibaro: African Mine Labor in Southern Rhodesia, 1900–1933* (London: Pluto, 1976), pp. 48–57; Ian Phimister and Charles van Onselen, *Studies in the History of African Mine Labor in Colonial Zimbabwe* (Gwelo: Mambo Press, 1978), pp. 102–50.

6.   Gelfand, *Northern Rhodesia in the Days of the Charter*, pp. 96–99; Bill Paton, *Labor Export Policy in the Development of Southern Africa* (Harare: University of Zambia Press, 1995), pp. 72–73, 75.

7.   Paton, *Labor Export Policy*, pp. 72–82.

8.   The term "Line of Rail" is used in Zambia to describe the narrow belt of commercial farms, mining towns, and commercial centers that emerged along the territory's rail line following its construction in the 1900s and 1910s. In Zambia the term connotes ideas of modernization, urbanization, and Europeanization.

9.   *Northern Rhodesia. Annual Report of the Health Department for the Years 1912–13* (unpaginated typescript).

10.   *Northern Rhodesia. Medical Report on Health and Sanitary Conditions for the Years 1925 and 1926*, p. 13; Mark Lowenthal, "The Yaws Notebook of Dr. Acheson," *Transactions of the Royal Society of Tropical Medicine and Hygiene* 76 (1982): 627–29.

11.   Paton, *Labor Export Policy*, pp. 72–82.

12.   Randall Packard, "The Invention of the 'Tropical Worker': Medical Research and the Quest for Central African Labour on the South African Gold Mines, 1903–36," *Journal of African History* 34 (1993): 271–79.

13.   Ibid.

14.   Lewis Gann, *A History of Northern Rhodesia: Early Days to 1953* (New York: Humanities Press, 1969), p. 164; *Northern Rhodesia. Annual Report of the Health Department for the Years 1918–19*. Indeed, oral historical narratives from Zambia's Eastern Province corroborate this claim. Several elderly Chewa and Ngoni informants, interviewed in Lusaka in 1995–96, attributed the origin of STDs in their home areas to returning war veterans, and the names of various illnesses reflect this belief. Two Nyanja disease terms, *chinzonono* (usually associated with gonorrhea symptoms) and *kaswende* (usually associated with venereal syphilis symptoms) are close adaptations of Swahili terms from Tanganyika. Another disease term, *songeya* (usually a gonorrhea reference), is derived from the name of a Tanganyikan district where several military actions against the Germans occurred during World War I. This information is based on 70 life-history interviews conducted by Bryan Callahan in Lusaka between November 1995 and January 1996. The authors are indebted to Luise White for providing the original Swahili disease names.

15.   National Archives of Zambia (hereafter, NAZ) BS3/303, Native Commissioner, Mumbwa, to Magistrate, Mumbwa, February 18, 1923.

16.   NAZ BS3/303, G. D. Clough, Legal Adviser, Public Prosecutor's Office, Livingstone, November 19, 1923.

17. Gann, *A History of Northern Rhodesia*, pp. 204–8.

18. George Chauncey, Jr., "The Locus of Reproduction: Women's Labor in the Zambian Copperbelt," *Journal of Southern African Studies* 7 (1981): 136–42.

19. Ibid., pp. 136–42.

20. Jane Parpart, "'Where is Your Mother?': Gender, Urban Marriage, and Colonial Discourse on the Zambian Copperbelt, 1924–1945," *International Journal of African Historical Studies* 27 (1994): 247–54.

21. For discussions of the importance of women's work in the Copperbelt, see Hansen, *Distant Companions*; Chauncey, "The Locus of Production"; and Parpart, "'Where is Your Mother?'" For a Kenya comparison, see Luise White, *The Comforts of Home: Prostitution in Colonial Nairobi* (Chicago, Ill.: University of Chicago Press, 1990).

22. Parpart, "'Where is Your Mother?'" pp. 254–57.

23. Ibid., pp. 257–71.

24. Ibid.

25. Chauncey, "The Locus of Reproduction," pp. 136–42.

26. For commentary on mine policy toward VD in South Africa, see Karen Jochelson, "The Colour of Disease: Syphilis and Racism in South Africa, 1910–1950," doctoral dissertation, Oxford University, 1993. For commentary on mine policy in Southern Rhodesia, see Phimister and van Onselen, *Studies in the History of African Mine Labor*, pp. 102–50; NAZ, H2/3/8/1, Secretary, Rhodesia Chamber of Mines, to Howard Moffat, Department of Mines and Works, January 28, 1924; NAZ, S2803/858, General Secretary, Associated Mine Workers of Rhodesia, to Minister of Native Affairs, March 17, 1942.

27. See correspondence in Zambia Consolidated Copper Mines Archives (hereafter, ZCCM) 19.1.6F, which cites labor stabilization and medical intervention as factors responsible for lower VD rates on mines north of the Zambezi.

28. NAZ, MH1/1/1, Director of Medical Services to Colonial Secretary, January 30, 1937.

29. NAZ, MH1/5/2, Director of Medical Services to Chief Medical Officer, Roan Antelope Mine, Luanshya, February 26, 1937.

30. Monica Fisher, *Nswana — The Heir: The Life and Times of Charles Fisher* (Ndola: Mission Press, 1991), pp. 89–127.

31. ZCCM, 11.3.3D, Annual Report of the Chief Medical Officer, Roan Antelope Mine for 1937, 1956, 1957.

32. ZCCM, 11.3.3D, Annual Report of the Chief Medical Officer, Roan Antelope Mine, for 1956.

33. For an outline of the role of medical policy in Anglo-American's recruiting program see ZCCM, 11.1.5A, Birt, Chief Medical Officer, Anglo-American, to General Manager, Anglo-American, December 2, 1949.

34. Paton, *Labor Export Policy*, p. 71.

35. For a general discussion of colonial concerns with rural development in the 1930s, see Henrietta Moore and Megan Vaughan, *Cutting Down Trees: Gender, Nutrition, and Agricultural Change in the Northern Province of Zambia, 1890–1990* (Portsmouth: Heinemann, 1994), pp. 1–19.

36. Great Britain. *Report of the Commission Appointed to Enquire into the Financial and Economic Position of Northern Rhodesia* (London: Her Majesty's Stationery Office, 1938), pp. 292–95.

37.   Speech by John F. C. Haslam, Director of Medical Services, in Northern Rhodesia, Legislative Council Debates, First Session (Resumed) of the Eighth Council, August 23–31, 1945, pp. 507–13.

38.   NAZ, MH1/3/54, Annual Report of the Namwala VD Campaign, 1947.

39.   NAZ, MH1/4/50, Monthly Reports of the Namwala VD Campaign, 1952–58.

40.   Cecil Hackett, "On the Origin of the Human Treponematoses," *Bulletin of the World Health Organization* 29 (1963): 7–41; Don Brothwell, "Yaws" in *The Cambridge World History of Human Disease*, edited by Kenneth Kiple (New York: Cambridge University Press, 1993), pp. 1096–2000.

41.   NAZ, KSF 3/2/3, Namwala Annual Report, 1925.

42.   For a detailed discussion of the limitations of neosalvarsan and bismuth treatment in colonial Africa, see Marc Dawson, "The 1920s Anti-Yaws Campaigns and Colonial Medical Policy in Kenya," *International Journal of African Historical Studies* 20 (1987): 417–35.

43.   NAZ, MH1/3/54, Annual Report of the Namwala VD Campaign, 1947.

44.   NAZ, MH1/4/50, Monthly Reports of the Namwala VD Campaign, 1952–58.

45.   For a detailed discussion of Ila historical demography and its relationship to the anti-VD campaign of 1946–58, see Bryan Callahan, "'Veni, V.D., Vici'?: Reassessing the Ila Syphilis Epidemic, 1900–63," *The Journal of Southern African Studies* 23 (1997): 421–40.

46.   Ibid., pp. 435–38.

47.   Ibid., pp. 433–34.

48.   The term *Wiko*, a pejorative reference meaning "westerner," refers to immigrants from Angola and northwestern areas of Northern Rhodesia who were incorporated into the Lozi polity as slaves and dependent laborers in the nineteenth and early twentieth centuries. Following their emancipation in the 1910s, many Wiko broke off their ties of fealty to the Lozi elite by migrating to Southern Rhodesia and South Africa for employment.

49.   For a discussion of changes in Lozi land settlement patterns during the colonial period, see Max Gluckman, *Economy of the Central Barotse Plain* (Livingstone: Rhodes-Livingstone Institute, 1941), pp. 37–38; Laurel Van Horn, "The Agricultural History of Barotseland, 1890–1964" in *The Roots of Rural Poverty in Central and Southern Africa*, edited by Robin Palmer and Neil Parsons (Berkeley: University of California Press, 1978), pp. 144–65.

50.   NAZ, MH1/4/62, A. J. Evans, Venereologist, "Report on Venereal Diseases on the Line-of-Rail: (January 1956 - Lusaka)," pp. 1–7.

51.   Ibid.

52.   *Northern Rhodesia. Health Department Annual Report for the Year 1958* (Lusaka: Government Printer, 1959).

53.   For a discussion of the impact of antibiotic therapy on the relative incidence of syphilis and yaws, see Dawson, "The 1920s Anti-Yaws Campaigns."

54.   *Republic of Zambia. Ministry of Health Report for the Year 1979* (Lusaka: Government Printer, 1984), p. 21.

55.   Douglas Webb, "The Socio-Economic Impact of HIV/AIDS in Zambia" *South Africa AIDS News* 4 (1996): 2–10.

56. *Republic of Zambia. Ministry of Health Report for the Year 1967* (Lusaka: Government Printer, 1969).

57. *Republic of Zambia. Ministry of Health Report for the Year 1978* (Lusaka: Government Printer, 1981).

58. Anne Bayley, "Aggressive Kaposi's Sarcoma in Zambia" *Lancet* 1 (1984): 1318–20.

59. Anne Bayley and R. G. Downing, "HTLV-III Serology Distinguishes Atypical and Endemic Kaposi's Sarcoma in Africa," *Lancet* 1 (1985): 359–61.

60. Knut Fylkesnes, Roland Msiska, and Helge Brunborg, *Zambia: The Current HIV/AIDS Situation and Future Demographic Impact* (Lusaka: Ministry of Health, 1994), p. 5.

61. Subash Hira, Joseph Kamanga, G. Bhat, C. Mwale, George Tembo, Nkandu Luo, and P. L. Perine, "Perinatal Transmission of HIV-1 in Zambia," *British Medical Journal* 2 (1989): 1250–52.

62. Peter Godfrey-Fausett, Rachel Baggaley, Guy Scott, and Moses Sichone, "HIV in Zambia: Myth or Monster?" *Nature* 368 (1994): 183–84.

63. Fylkenses, Msiska, and Brunborg, *Zambia: The Current HIV/AIDS Situation*, p. 21; "Prevalence of HIV in Children in an Urban Community" in *Viral Infections in Zambia*, Vol. 2: *Activities of the Virology Laboratory* (Lusaka: University Teaching Hospital, Virology Laboratory, 1995), pp. 45–46.

64. Webb, "The Socio-Economic Impact of HIV/AIDS in Zambia," pp. 2–10.

65. Kumbutso Dzekedzeke, "Population Dynamics: Actual Observations and Projections of Future Demographic Implications of the HIV Epidemic," Dissemination seminar, Epidemiology and Research Unit, Zambia National AIDS/STD/TB Program, Lusaka, Zambia, February 1997.

66. Fylkesnes, Sichone, and Kasumba, "Population-based HIV Study Using Saliva Specimens."

67. Rosemary Musonda, Zacchaeus Ndholovu, Kalvin Kasumba, and Knut Fylkesnes, "Trends of HIV Infection and the Representivity of the Key Sentinel Population (CBW) Using the Population-Based Data as Reference," Dissemination seminar, Epidemiology and Research Unit, Zambia National AIDS/STD/TB Program, Lusaka, Zambia, February 1997.

68. Andrew Mushingeh, William Chama, and D. Mulikelela, "An Investigation of High Risk Situations and Environments and Their Potential Role in the Transmission of HIV in Zambia: The Case of the Copperbelt and Luapula Provinces," unpublished study for the Population Council of Zambia 1990–91; Virginia Bond, "Expectations of Partnership amongst Women in a Migrant Labor Context," paper presented at the Fifth National AIDS Conference, Lusaka, Zambia, 1995.

69. Virginia Bond and P. Dover, "Men, Women and the Trouble with Condoms: Problems Associated with Condom Use by Migrant Workers in Zambia," *Health Transition Review* 7 (1996): 377–91.

70. Rachel Baggaley, Peter Godfrey-Fausett, Roland Msiska, David Chilangwa, and E. Chitu, "Impact of HIV on Zambian Businesses," *British Medical Journal* 309 (1994): 1549–50.

71. Lloyd Chingambo, *Zambia: The Impact of HIV/AIDS on a Productive Labour Force* (Lusaka: International Labor Organization, 1993).

72. Webb, "The Socio-Economic Impact of HIV/AIDS in Zambia," pp. 5–6.

73.   Mike Drinkwater, *The Effects of HIV/AIDS on Agricultural Production Systems in Zambia* (Lusaka: UN Food and Agriculture Organization, 1993); Tony Barnett, *The Effect of HIV/AIDS on Farming Systems and Rural Livelihoods in Uganda, Tanzania, and Zambia* (Lusaka: UN Food and Agriculture Organization, 1994); Webb, "The Socio-Economic Impact of HIV/AIDS in Zambia," pp. 5–6.

74.   Anne Buve, Susan Foster, C. Mbwili, E. Mungo, and N. Tollenare, "Mortality among Female Nurses in the Face of the AIDS Epidemic: A Pilot Study in Zambia," *AIDS* 8 (1994): 396.

75.   Subash Hira, Rosemary Sunkutu, D. Wadhawan, and H. Mamtani, "Direct Cost of AIDS Case Management in Zambia," Ninth International AIDS Conference, Berlin, 1993.

76.   Webb, "The Socio-Economic Impact of HIV/AIDS in Zambia," p. 7.

77.   Fylkesnes, Sichone, and Kasumba, "Population-based HIV Study using Saliva Specimens."

78.   Susan Foster, *Study of Adult Disease in Lusaka* (Lusaka: UN Overseas Development Agency, 1995), p. 4; Webb, "The Socio-Economic Impact of HIV/AIDS in Zambia," p. 7.

79.   Virginia Bond, "Death, Dysentery, and Drought: Household Coping Capacities in Chiawa," IHCAR/Hull/IAS Working Paper No. 7, 1993, pp. 47–48; Virginia Bond, "AIDS and the Family," proceedings of the Fourth National AIDS Conference, Lusaka, 1994; Webb, "The Socio-Economic Impact of HIV/AIDS in Zambia," pp. 8–9.

80.   Webb, "The Socio-Economic Impact of HIV/AIDS in Zambia," p. 7.

81.   Cathy Poulter, "Orphans and Their Foster Families," unpublished report for CARE International, 1996; Webb, "The Socio-Economic Impact of HIV/AIDS in Zambia," p. 8; Virginia Bond and Phillimon Ndubani, "Indications of Health in Chiawa," IHCAR/Hull/IAS Working Paper No. 3, 1992.

82.   Bond, "Death, Dysentery, and Drought," pp. 12–16; Bond, "AIDS and the Family," pp. 16–18.

83.   Bond, "AIDS and the Family," pp. 16–18.

84.   M. Kelly, "Voluntary HIV Counseling and Testing (C&T) in Lusaka: Who Comes, Why, and Does it Help?" Tenth International Conference on AIDS, Yokohama, 1994; Rachel Baggaley, "Barriers to HIV Counseling and Testing (C&T) in Chawama, Lusaka, Zambia," Ninth International Conference on AIDS in Africa, Kampala, 1995.

85.   Knut Fylkesnes, Pascal Kwapa, Catherine Rosenvard, and Alan Haworth, "Readiness of HIV Counseling and Testing in a Country with Extremely High Prevalence," Dissemination seminar, Epidemiology and Research Unit, Zambia National AIDS/STD/TB Program, Lusaka, 1997.

86.   Bond, "Death, Dysentery, and Drought," pp. 12–16.

87.   Interview with Alan Haworth, University Teaching Hospital, Lusaka, January 1996.

88.   Roland Msiska, Vincent Musowe, and A. Sampule, "How We Made Short-Term Projections of HIV/AIDS Cases in Zambia 1990–1995, and What They Imply for Planning," *AIDS Analysis Africa* 3 (September–October 1993): 8–10.

89.   Stefan Hanson, Rosemary Sukutu, Eric Sandstrom, Bengt Hojer, and Subash Hira, "Evaluation of the Guidelines for Case Management and Genital

Ulcer Disease and Genital Discharge," Ninth International Conference on AIDS, Berlin, 1993.

90.   Elizabeth Faxelid, "Partner Notifications in Context: Swedish and Zambian Experiences," *Social Science & Medicine* 44 (1997): 1239–44.

91.   L. Chipuka, D. Chama, and C. Tembo, "Quality of Blood Transfusion Laboratory Practice in District Hospitals in Zambia," paper presented at the Eighth International Conference on AIDS in Africa, Marrakech, 1993 (Abstract); Faxelid, "Partner Notifications in Context," pp. 1241–42.

92.   Bond and Dover, "Men, Women and the Trouble with Condoms"; the condoms are labeled "Maximum," and people quip that "Maximum condoms offer Minimum pleasure."

93.   Bond, "AIDS and the Family," pp. 99–103; Douglas Webb, in a review of research on HIV/AIDS in Zambia, notes that although much research is underway, much of it has a strong urban and Lusaka bias. Researchers have largely neglected rural areas and have paid little attention to coping strategies. See Douglas Webb, *HIV/AIDS Bibliography: An Annotated Review of Research on HIV/AIDS in Zambia* (Lusaka: UNICEF, 1996).

94.   Bacterial resistance to low-cost antibiotics may limit the effectiveness of such an intervention, however. In Lusaka, gonorrhea resistance to penicillin rose from 3 percent of surveyed patients in 1980 to 58 percent in 1996. See Doreen Mulenga, "Antibiotic Sensitivity Patterns and Prevalence of PPNG in Neisseria Gonorrhoea Isolates in Lusaka," Dissemination seminar, Epidemiology and Research Unit, Zambia National AIDS/STD/TB Program, Lusaka, Zambia, February 1997.

9

The Management of Venereal Disease in a Settler Society: Colonial Zimbabwe, 1900–30

Jock McCulloch

Sexual relations between Europeans and Africans were one of the most problematic features of colonial life. Colonial states took an active interest in protecting white women from the predations of black males especially in Southern Rhodesia, which in the period from 1900 to 1925 was swept by a series of moral panics. What was known colloquially as Black Peril, the fear of black on white sexual violence, was also important in South Africa and formed a significant element in the region's history. On occasions it was sufficient for an African man to break into a house where a white woman was alone for him to be charged with attempted rape. In incidents of criminal injury and those cases brought under the Immorality and Indecency Suppression Ordinance of 1916, the slightest indiscretion by a black man could have serious consequences.[1] Such assaults were perceived not just as an attack upon the body or person of a white woman but as an attack upon the body of the white community itself.[2] Black Peril cases were, however, uncommon, and cases of actual rape were rare. In the period from 1899 to 1906, for example, there were 53 sexual assaults reported in Bulawayo but only two cases of rape. In Salisbury in the period from 1907 to 1914 there were 63 assaults.[3] However, because of the extravagant definition of sexual crime used by victims, the police, and the courts, many of those incidents would in another context have been treated at worst as common assault. It is significant that no such threat was felt, for example, on those rare occasions on which an African killed a white man. Such murders, no matter how brutal or senseless, never provoked the same degree of anxiety.[4] They also did not have the same influence in shaping public policy.

The men who framed health policy in Southern Rhodesia had no professional interest in Black Peril or in theories about the sexuality of colonial subjects, but their perceptions of African sexuality did influence their response to the management of venereal disease. Among the lay community by 1900 an explanation for the transmission of syphilis among Africans had been established; it was supposedly the result of the sexual immorality of the Matabele and Shona, and was spread by African prostitutes and miners returning from the Kimberley.[5] It was also widely believed by the white public that venereal disease was so common that it threatened the supply of labor. Over the next 30 years those assumptions were rarely challenged.

With the exceptions of South Africa and Algeria, white settler communities in Africa were small.[6] Faced as they were with armed resistance, drought, disease, and fluctuations in world markets for their produce, they were also fragile. Where white minorities were largest the transition to political independence was most violent: Almost one-tenth of Algeria's population of 10 million was killed during the war of national liberation. Settler societies differed in terms of their histories, composition, and size but were united by their opposition to majority rule and by their ambivalence toward metropolitan governments.

The white communities of Kenya and Southern Rhodesia were minuscule. At the turn of the century there were perhaps as few as 30 whites living in the Kenyan Highlands, and at the outbreak of World War II there were only 21,000 whites in the whole of the colony. At that time there were 63,000 Europeans in Southern Rhodesia (now Zimbabwe). In 1939 blacks outnumbered whites in Southern Rhodesia by 25:1 and in Kenya there was 1 white for each 175 Africans.[7] Southern Rhodesia had a large South African-born minority, and its proximity to the Union of South Africa was reflected in its civil service and its legal system, both modelled on South African precedent. In Kenya there was no white artisan class, and restrictive immigration generally kept out poor whites; where that failed, deportation was used. Southern Rhodesia, in contrast, attracted lower middle and working class Europeans like the doomed farming couple of Doris Lessing's *The Grass Is Singing*. Despite such differences those settler societies had much in common. Both were driven by a desire for the segregation of the black majority, a desire that was compromised by a dependence upon black labor. In Southern Rhodesia in 1936, when the white population numbered 56,000, there were almost as many registered domestic servants.[8] To control that black majority, both necessary and feared, an elaborate structure of pass laws and masters and servants ordinances was erected. That structure was augmented by a system of petty apartheid, which was well developed in both colonies.

One of the major effects of colonialism in sub-Saharan Africa was to encourage migrant labor, which shifted native populations across the southern half of the continent. Besides generating wealth for settlers, those migrations helped to spread diseases, such as syphilis and gonorrhea. It was a fear of disease and the need for labor that gave whites an interest in the health of Africans, and a phobia about syphilis fostered a direct interest in their sexuality.[9]

Infectious disease was one of the main hazards facing white settlement in Rhodesia. Although by the turn of the century housing and sanitation had improved, the threat remained.[10] In 1902 rabies broke out in Matabeleland. In response the Bulawayo council ordered the destruction of 60,000 dogs. Despite such measures outbreaks of rabies were intermittent, and Pierre Loir, a nephew of Pasteur, was appointed to head an infectious diseases institute.[11] Each year with the rains came dysentery and gastroenteritis, and in 1904 there was typhoid. It was presumed that Africans spread the disease, but proposals made in council to provide latrines for blacks were rejected as being too expensive.[12] Between 1900 and 1904 bubonic plague threatened a number of major South African centers including the port cities of Cape Town and Port Elizabeth, and the hasty removal of Africans to special urban locations was deemed necessary to protect whites from infection. Those locations became a permanent feature of colonial geography and in the hands of the state a prototype for apartheid. The same policy was used throughout southern Africa, and the threat of plague in Salisbury in 1905 encouraged the establishment of an urban location.[13]

The major infectious diseases had economic significance because they discouraged white settlement; they also threatened the generation of wealth upon which colonization rested. The two main causes of premature death among adult whites were malaria and black water fever, but the event that did most to foster settler anxiety was the Spanish influenza pandemic that spread from the cape, reaching Rhodesia in October 1918.[14] However, within the cluster of anxieties shared by settlers, syphilis had particular significance.

Epidemic diseases have their own iconography, and among fearful populations they provoke metaphors. However, not all epidemics arouse the kind of dread associated with syphilis and leprosy. The Spanish influenza, for example, which within 15 months had killed almost 20 million people worldwide, never evoked the metaphor of plague. Conversely, AIDS had killed relatively few when it acquired the morbid associations of a phobic disease. It is not a disease's capacity to kill so much as its effects upon the body and its means of transmission that arouse fear. According to Susan Sontag, the most feared diseases are those that transform the body into something alienating; "Leprosy and syphilis were the first illnesses to be consistently described as repulsive."[15] The human face is supposed to mirror character and its ruin suggests the dissolution of the person.[16] For that reason, among Victorians the leper's lion face and the ulceration seen in some syphilitics aroused particular dread.

The syphilis pathogen is in fact a fragile organism that cannot survive long outside the body, and at least 95 percent of infections are transmitted through sexual contact.[17] The tropical disease yaws or framboesia is very similar to syphilis, and blood tests for syphilis are also positive for yaws. Unlike syphilis the means of transmission are non-sexual, and the primary symptom is a pimple that occurs at the site of contact. As the disease progresses, multiple blisters will appear on the skin including the face, and, if left untreated, yaws can be disfiguring. As with syphilis, infection is compatible with good general health. During the colonial period yaws and syphilis were often confused and it was difficult for even an experienced physician to distinguish between them.

Settlers in Southern Rhodesia brought with them from Britain and South Africa a fear of venereal disease. They believed syphilis so contagious and so common among blacks that the handling of cutlery, crockery, or even sheets by domestic servants was sufficient to infect an entire white household. Those fears were present from the beginning of colonization, but during the 1920s there was a perceptible shift between Black Peril and syphilis as the principal focus for anxiety among settlers; as one faded the other became more prominent. That shift occurred at a time when the tide of medical evidence showed venereal disease was not a threat and when the availability of Salvarsan had provided the first effective treatment for syphilis.

CONTROLLING INFECTION

During the first 25 years of white settlement one man, Andrew Fleming, dominated the public health department. The son of a Scottish clergyman, Fleming, who became medical director in 1897, was a forceful and independent thinker who was never afraid of speaking his mind. Despite his strengths and his obvious clinical skills in regard to venereal disease, Fleming was overwhelmed by the sheer force of public opinion and in particular by the prejudices of town councils and farming and mining interests. During Fleming's tenure the issue of venereal disease became a tussle between central and local authorities about who was responsible and who should pay for the treatment of Africans. Those two questions dominated policy making and fueled the constant stream of complaints from councils and concerned citizens. Most importantly the question of venereal disease affected the management of locations and reserves and the regulation of labor. To whites venereal disease had two distinct settings: an urban context of domestic servants and a rural setting of farm and mine labor. Each had a different white constituency, and each provoked a different imagery. The intensity of debate was such that it brought into conflict the Departments of Public Health and Native Affairs and the offices of the president and high commissioners. On at least one occasion it also involved the Colonial Office.

The Countryside

In November 1906 Fleming attended a conference of principal medical officers in Cape Town at which the issue of venereal disease was discussed. It was suggested that syphilis was spread principally from mining centers, such as the Kimberley, and on occasions from servants to the members of white families.[18] Fleming wanted all cases to be treated locally rather than taken into towns, and he favored educating Africans about how to prevent infection. However, he changed his mind several times about the best approach to use and it took some years for a firm policy to be established.

By 1907 the spread of syphilis in the Victoria, Belingwe, and Charter districts was believed to be so rapid as to threaten the supply of labor, and during August and September of that year Fleming made an extended tour of Victoria. He rejected suggestions that the rate of infection was 60 percent, believing that it was probably closer to 10 percent. Even so syphilis was more common than elsewhere, and according to Fleming its prevalence was caused by the conditions under which Africans lived; "The spread among the native population cannot be ascribed to immorality but is rather direct infection from one member of a family to another; a mother infecting a child, and a child a brother or sister or playmate."[19] Fleming found that some adult males were being prevented from entering the labor market, and there was also evidence of a loss of infant life. Because of expense, the use of lock hospitals, the ideal method to halt the spread of infection, was out of the question, and Fleming held out little hope of completely suppressing the disease.

Later in his career Fleming observed that there were two schools of opinion on the best way to control syphilis. A command system was, he believed, inefficient, and he favored a decentralized approach in which the role of the department was largely advisory.[20] In arriving at that policy Fleming had to reconcile the pleas for protection from a fearful public, the demands of employers and churches for assistance, and his department's lack of staff and resources.

Missions made frequent requests for drugs, claiming the treatment they provided to their congregations imposed a burden they could ill afford. Fleming, however, was also concerned that most missionaries were unskilled, and initially he opposed supporting medical stations on reserves under mission control.[21] If one such station were established, so he argued, then other missions would demand assistance because offering medical care was one of the ways they used to attract converts.[22] Circumstances eventually forced Fleming to change his mind because there were simply no resources to appoint more officers in native districts, and in 1912 he agreed to fund posts and dispensaries utilizing the services of missions and municipalities.[23]

The scheme was attractive to both parties. It allowed missions to do good works and thereby attract Africans to their churches; for the medical department it was a cheap means of providing care and assuaged the fears of the white community. As medical director, Fleming was under considerable pressure to respond to the perceived threat of venereal disease, but his department lacked the funds and the staff to do what the white community demanded: to place the entire African labor force under medical surveillance and to quarantine those infected in lock wards. The dispensaries were a compromise.

District surgeons treated syphilis with mercury, and in those areas where there was no surgeon drugs were supplied free of charge to missionaries, native commissioners, and in a few cases to settlers.[24] There are no records as to the success of the scheme, but we do know that some employers had little medical knowledge. In October 1927, for example, a farmer named Cooper wrote to Fleming seeking advice on prophylactic treatment for his African workers. Cooper recalled from his war service an ointment given to troops to apply after intercourse, which greatly reduced the rate of infection. He was concerned at the loss of African labor because of sickness and the effects upon the health of the white community; "It is not pleasant to think that infected natives are milking one's cows especially when the milk is sold in Bulawayo."[25] The acting medical director recommended a mixture of calomel and lanolin, and he sent Cooper a sample pot, which was to be applied before intercourse. Cooper's workers tried the ointment, and he was pleased with the results.[26]

Although missions clamored for Fleming's support, it was mine managers and owners who were most vocal in their demands. During the autumn sitting of the Legislative Council in 1923 a motion was proposed on behalf of the Rhodesian Chamber of Mines that a system of compulsory medical checks of mine employees be introduced. The chamber was worried about the prevalence of syphilis among workers, which it blamed on the travelling female prostitutes who visited mine compounds.[27] Under existing regulations resident medical officers were obliged to examine African employees every 14 days. They were also required to submit a monthly report to the compound inspector, and failure to comply could result in a fine of 20 pounds or three months in jail.[28] The chamber was aggrieved that infected Africans were treated at the expense of employers, whereas in the Transvaal the cost was born by public authorities.[29] Although it is doubtful that such procedures were followed, they did involve some expense especially for the larger mines and the chamber wanted the cost shifted to the state. It also wanted all women who visited compounds to be obliged to carry a health certificate.[30] Although some members of the legislative council were willing to second the motion, there were obstacles; it would have been expensive and it would have had to be supported by a contagious diseases act. The matter had been previously addressed by the medical director who opposed the government's taking over the cost of such a program. Government medical officers already serviced the small mines, but the larger mines were responsible for the care of their own employees.[31] Fleming told the council that although the subject aroused high feeling such concerns were not justified. The average African could not afford the cost of treatment, and he further suggested that if a contagious diseases act were introduced, it should apply also to whites, a notion he knew was abhorrent to members. The debate collapsed when Fleming presented the returns for mines, which showed a rate of infection of less than 0.5 percent.[32]

Estimates of the incidence of syphilis and gonorrhea in rural areas varied greatly. Much of the evidence was anecdotal and suggested extraordinarily high rates of infection. To provide reliable data, in November 1923 native commissioners were asked to file returns. Although the information covered all districts and was intended to be comprehensive, without credible estimates of the size of the African population and some certainty that distinctions were being made between syphilis and yaws, the figures in themselves meant little, a fact acknowledged by several informants. Among those who were willing to make a guess, the figures ranged from less than 1 percent to 15 percent.[33]

In contrast to Fleming the Department of Native Affairs believed that syphilis was a major problem, and in 1926 native commissioners at Salisbury, Bulawayo, and Victoria held conferences on the subject. Commissioners agreed that all cases should receive free treatment and, where necessary, accommodation at government expense. At the superintendents of natives' and native commissioners' conference of 1927 a number of resolutions were passed including a demand that government provide adequate funds for the segregation of African lepers and syphilitics.[34] In December I. Alexander, who worked at a mine in the Penhalonga Valley, wrote a report on venereal disease in the district. In that year he treated 52 cases, which included Africans working at the Rezende Mine, women living at the mine compound, and men and women resident at the village of Penhalonga. He was certain that the rate of infection was far higher than the official figures suggested. The district was close to the Portuguese border, and prostitutes from that territory were a potent source of infection. The situation was so serious that, "The question of the control of venereal disease is important from the economic point of view. Besides the risk of breeding up a race of congenital syphilitics there is also the serious interference with the working capacity of the native to be considered."[35] Alexander's claims about African women were endorsed by the native commissioner and encouraged settler groups to press for further government action.[36]

In January 1928 a meeting of the Bulawayo Landowners and Farmers Association was held to discuss the shortage of African labor. One member named Mitchell commented that the country was reeking with syphilis. He had raised the matter with the government but had been told the rate of infection was less than 1 percent. "Anyone who would believe that would believe anything. It did not help persons who were suffering from this horrible disease and who were spreading it throughout the country." The African laborer "was often nothing less than a walking reservoir of disease."[37] In May Fleming sought the opinion of district medical officers. At Sinoia G. Barratt judged that although venereal disease was not prevalent and did not appear to be increasing, native brothels and prostitutes in mine compounds were the main sources of infection.[38] The officer at Rusape was sure that infection originated in the towns and mine settlements.[39] According to J. S. Liptz of Enkeldoorn there were 100,000 Africans in his area, and in a two-year period he had seen only 17 cases, every one of which he could trace to the towns and mining camps. He cautioned, however, that many Africans would claim a history of syphilis to avoid having to meet payments under the native tax ordinance.[40] P. Wallace of Filabusi believed that initially the disease spread from the native reserves but had become concentrated in mine compounds. Local blacks worked in mines for a few months, contracted the disease, then returned to kraals infected. Local Matabele women who worked as prostitutes also spread infection.[41]

Such views were entirely conventional, and those who clamored for government intervention could always cite figures that suggested there was a pandemic in rural areas. Those figures, however, were compromised by the high incidence of yaws and the department's policy of using untrained mission staff and laymen within its treatment program, which increased the likelihood of misdiagnosis.

The Towns

Debate about the control of infection in urban locations was even more dramatic. Although syphilis threatened the capital of farm managers and miners, in the towns it was seen to threaten the survival of white society itself. In speaking of the danger, settlers drew upon an imagery of pollution, sexual debauchery, and social disintegration, and only Fleming and a minority of the members of his department doubted that disaster was imminent. In December 1911 a conference of native superintendents found that "the presence of syphilis among natives in European centres is not receiving adequate attention and that it is a matter calling for immediate action."[42] Its recommendation that a lock ward be established at hospitals in each of the major townships was rejected because of the cost and Fleming's initial doubts as to the extent of the problem.

During 1917 the Salisbury council made several representations to the administrator's office, and in May of that year it passed a resolution that all Africans entering the town be detained for medical inspection.[43] The council pointed out that although there were inspections at mines there were none at urban centers; "The consequence is that many natives suffering from loathsome and contagious diseases are allowed to go about towns possibly spreading the germs among European families."[44] The council proposed "That all natives should on arrival in town to seek work be obliged to go to a Central depot where they would be vaccinated, obliged to have baths, wash their clothes etc and undergo a medical examination."[45] Because government already collected taxes from employers and from Africans it should bear the cost, which the council estimated at around £700 per annum. In August the Bulawayo municipality made a similar demand. The administator's office was sympathetic to such proposals but was concerned about who should pay for the scheme.[46] The issue of medical certificates also came into conflict with existing legislation controlling the movement of African labor.[47] Legal opinion suggested that new legislation would have to be introduced, and, because it would discriminate between natives and settlers, it would have to be ratified by imperial authorities.[48]

The council supported its case with testimony from F. Appelyard, who for 15 years had worked in Salisbury. Appelyard commented that there had been several outbreaks of smallpox in the city, which in each case had been transmitted from Africans to Europeans. He had often treated Africans for syphilis, and, although he could not recall infection passing from an African to an employer, that did not mean such infection had not occurred. In his experience most Shona including a large proportion of servants suffered from scabies, but his most frightening evidence was anecdotal. He referred to a case he had heard from a Cape Town physician in which an African nurse infected a white infant with syphilis. The baby in turn infected its mother and another child.[49] Appelyard was certain that many such cases had occurred in South Africa, and he was sure the same risk existed in Salisbury.[50] His testimony was supported by the Criminal Investigation Department, which documented four cases of male servants who were found to be suffering from venereal disease.[51] The council demanded that medical inspections be comprehensive because "a great deal of disease might be carried in a natives clothing and blankets and it is our intention to provide a steam disinfector and baths where natives should cleanse themselves before medical examinations."[52] Like the white community as a whole, the council had little interest in distinguishing between syphilis and yaws, and it was impervious to evidence that showed that its fears were groundless.

Pressure on government was such that the attorney general, at the request of the administrator, prepared a draft ordinance titled the Medical Examination of Native Servants (Urban) Ordinance of 1918.[53] The draft allowed for the compulsory medical examination and treatment by local authorities of all prospective servants. Although the ordinance contained everything the Salisbury and Bulawayo councils wanted, it was never debated, being replaced by the Natives Registration Ordinance Amendment Ordinance. The amendment enabled the administrator to make regulations for the compulsory examination and vaccination of Africans applying for certificates of registration or those employed and found to be suffering from a contagious disease. Significantly the amendment made no mention of urban areas or of municipal authorities; it merely gave greater powers of discretion to the administrator, to whom municipalities could in turn appeal. After clamoring for such a scheme the council then announced that it would not bear the cost of treating those who failed a medical test.[54]

PREVENTING DISEASE: THE PUBLIC HEALTH ACT OF 1924

The fears of local councils were shaped by a number of factors, some of which were external to Southern Rhodesia. In particular they were heightened by the influenza epidemic, which arrived in central Africa in the final months of World War I. The first case of Spanish Flu occurred at Bulawayo on October 12, 1918, and within two weeks it had spread throughout the territory.[55] In a matter of days economic activity was brought to a standstill and the administration instituted a massive operation involving the native and medical departments, missions, and traditional authorities. An order forbade Africans from travelling by train and chiefs were instructed to keep their people confined to their kraals. Many Africans deserted the mines and fled north, and cattle and petrol supplies were requisitioned by the state.

The impact of the epidemic was uneven. In some kraals most people survived, but in others many perished. The flu killed almost ten times as many whites as had died in the rebellion or *Chimurenga* of 1896, and it cast a shadow over the whole community. As quickly as it had begun, by mid-November the epidemic had abated, but the effects were to be felt for many years. The infection had come from South Africa and it was assumed, without evidence, to have been spread by African laborers. The flu struck at families killing children and adults, reminding whites of their vulnerability and fueling their fears of being surrounded by a immense but invisible pool of infection. It was proof that the settlers' resources were fragile, and it provided a model for catastrophe, which like the *Chimurenga* haunted the imagination of whites.

Before the epidemic Fleming had rejected claims that venereal disease was a threat, but by the beginning of 1919 he had come to believe that many domestic servants were infected, thereby exposing European families to risk. There were no special hospital facilities, and such patients were unsuited for general wards, which moreover were under the charge of European nurses. (It was policy that such staff should not treat black males).

During the 1920s the main problem in monitoring and treating infected Africans was money.[56] A single treatment for syphilis cost 6 shillings and the cost per patient was around £1.[57] Because of distance, in many cases inpatient care was necessary, thereby increasing the expense. Fleming frequently questioned the free treatment given to African patients and demanded proof that those so treated were in fact paupers.[58] Although in his public pronouncements Fleming was sympathetic to settler fears, he was often annoyed by their hysteria. In October 1922 he told the police commissioner, "I know it is popular opinion that our natives suffer greatly from venereal disease, and therefore it may interest some people to know that in the many years I have been in medical charge of the British South Africa Police and the Native Police, I am sorry to say that a far higher proportion of venereal disease occurs amongst the white trooper as compared with the native."[59] In 1923 department estimates for male Africans resident at Salisbury, Belingwe, and at mine compounds showed the rate of infection to be less than 0.6 percent, which was probably only slightly above the rate for the African adult male population as a whole.[60] During 1924 there were reports from missionaries, some medical officers, and native commissioners of high levels of infection, but there was no evidence to support claims of an epidemic. The authors of the annual report for that year looked to the new Public Health Act to provide a remedy.

The department's annual report for 1923 noted that there was no systematic policy of treatment or prevention because of a lack of funds and an appropriate legislative framework. It was in part to provide such a framework that the Public Health Act of 1924 was introduced. The act, which was cast in the shadow of the influenza pandemic, included an entire chapter devoted to venereal disease and was designed to protect the white community from infection emanating from blacks.[61] Although whites welcomed the legislation, the provision of compulsory vaccinations caused controversy and forced some changes, with exemptions (for white citizens) on the grounds of conscientious objection being allowed.[62] The legislation gave a wide range of powers to physicians and local authorities in regulating the movement of Africans in and out of urban areas. It empowered officers to examine forcibly any African, to disinfect his or her clothes, and under certain circumstances to destroy domiciles.[63]

It also obliged schoolteachers, employers, and heads of families to give notice of any contagious disease. The definition of risk was left in the hands of medical officers and in effect allowed for the removal, isolation, or internment of any African seeking employment. The act also stipulated that any person with a venereal disease who continued in employment in a shop, domestic service, factory, hotel, or restaurant was, like his employer, guilty of an offence; it made treatment compulsory and the failure to seek treatment a crime. The minister was given the authority to designate an area as one with a high prevalence in venereal disease and thereby to order the medical examination of all inhabitants. What was most notable about the act was the extent to which it appeared to have been motivated by the threat of syphilis and the lack of reference to such disease in the correspondence that surrounded its drafting.[64] Why that should have been so is unclear.

The immediate effect of the act was to increase the amount of time and money spent in identifying and treating syphilis.[65] Within 12 months the municipal medical officer at Salisbury reported a rise of almost 100 percent in the number of cases treated. However, because many of those had come to the town specifically for treatment, the increase was not in itself significant.[66] The department also attributed a similar increase among mine workers to that cause. Health officers noted that Africans would readily present for treatment and were impressed by the speed with which lesions could be healed. The main problem faced by medical officers was in gaining access to those early cases that were most infectious.

After the passing of the act the fears of whites were if anything greater, because it was not designed to provide the kind of surveillance of black labor they demanded. The white community wanted disease among blacks controlled; it also wanted disease rendered invisible, and the provision of clinics only made whites more anxious. In October 1928 Fleming met with a delegation from the Bulawayo Landowners and Farmers Association. The association demanded reform of the Bulawayo hospital and increased funding for health care. It also wanted a bacteriological laboratory established in the town. However, more important than each of those issues were the association's fears of venereal disease, and to that end it wanted the Department to conduct a comprehensive survey of the African population.

The association was a powerful group that Fleming could not ignore no matter how fanciful he found its claims. He patiently explained that syphilis was prevalent among Africans who worked in towns because they were young adult males who, while employed, were divorced from family life and among whom promiscuity was common.[67] According to the 1926 census there were 110,041 African males employed and only 2,908 females resident in urban or mining centers. Fleming told the delegation that much nonsense was talked on the subject and he objected to

ed to end the

agged on for
esolved with
a small clinic
pital. Within
h four rooms
demand by
hose treated
barrassed to
nces in scale
the fact that
e, and, there-

ghlights one
re whites so
rse for such
nobia about
the sexual
urses about
en were, for
ed by Euro-
contamina-
behavior of
debate, and
uppression
tlers.

r need for
heir desire
Those best
g Africans
ndations of
d the dis-
ne patterns
er wealth.
ted in the

tion rose.
oth were
their ori-
men. The
of cheap
epressive
out their

claims made by the association that Africans were riddled with syphilis. Although no general survey had been conducted, statistics were available for Africans in urban areas and jails, for members of the Native Police Force, for patients under treatment at government hospitals, and for Africans working in mines and railways. The rate of infection among those groups was between 2 percent and 3 percent, and figures for those seeking employment as servants in Bulawayo during 1926 were even lower.[68] As Fleming pointed out, the figures were in fact far lower than for the British armed services.[69]

In April 1929 the Chambers of Commerce held a congress at Bulawayo at which the issue of syphilis was prominent. According to one participant the matter was raised because "all delegates employed blacks and therefore such health matters had commercial significance."[70] The meeting passed a number of resolutions demanding greater control and surveillance of African workers. It wanted more clinics and a guarantee that no black female would be allowed employment as a servant without a medical certificate. There was strong feeling that the government was not doing enough and that as a result white women and children were coming into contact with infected Africans. The Rhodesian Women's League, which had supported previous council initiatives, wrote to the colonial secretary demanding that a clinic be set up in a Salisbury location to examine African women as well as those males seeking domestic work.[71] The colonial secretary responded by referring them in turn to their municipalities.

Throughout his struggles with Salisbury and Bulawayo councils, Fleming sought to minimize the costs imposed on his department. His position was made more difficult because there were many within the administration who believed that syphilis was a major threat.[72] Finally in 1930 the government agreed to fund a lock hospital in Salisbury and the Native Isolation Hospital (later called the Native Venereal Diseases, Fever, and Isolation Hospital) was established.[73] The facility was small, and no attempt was made to provide comprehensive treatment for urban Africans.

KENYA: A PARALLEL

In assessing the history of venereal disease in Southern Rhodesia, it is useful to make a comparison with another settler colony in which the rates of infection were comparable. Kenya and Rhodesia were in many ways similar, and one would expect their administrations to have displayed similar attitudes toward public health.[74] In the instance of venereal disease that was not so. In Kenya, as in Southern Rhodesia, health care for Africans was provided because the economic welfare of the colony depended upon their labor.[75] In the shadow of the Spanish influenza epidemic, it was also motivated by a desire to protect the white community

from infection. Howev(
ed upon a more realisti
ing the 1920s there w(
plague and, although t
special attention was
there was no suggestic

In the period from
number of Africans t
that changed dramat
patients in 1925 two
is not clear why a sud
reason lay in the prov
the greater willingne
time a dramatic rise
al report for 1921 th
overestimated.[78] To
willingness (or abili
between yaws and
ease. There was n(
about the prevalen
labor shortages cau
Rhodesia could no

In the Zimbabv
dealing with vener
tion for Kenya. In
erences to syphili
in the annual rep(
ments show that
plague, or malari
of Health no c(
syphilis, and the
posed a threat to
to interest group
whites in Rhode
Kenya did not. S
by black men u
ous than any tha
Black Peril pani
phobic disease.

Although th
Kenya and Sou
differences bet
in terms of the
Kenyan white

Low rates of infection and the high cost of treatment combi
suppression campaign.

Although the issue of venereal disease among blacks d
years, the question of provision for the care of whites was
ease. In October 1927 the Salisbury Council requested that
for Europeans be established as part of the government ho
two months a ward for whites was operating at Salisbury w;
for male patients and four for female patients.[85] Because c
December Fleming had agreed to extend facilities. Most of
were private patients who because of the stigma were too er
go to a special clinic.[86] There were of course major differe
between the black and white communities; there was also
among whites venereal disease had little political significanc
fore, the provision of care was merely a technical matter.

The history of venereal disease in colonial Zimbabwe h;
major question; why, in the absence of any proof of threat, w
afraid of infection from blacks? There were precedents of co
a reaction, as settlers brought with them from Europe a p
syphilis; there were also repressed elements emanating fro
conduct of white males that helped to shape colonial disc(
infection. Sexual relations between white men and black won
example, common. In terms of the models of infection favor
peans, such miscegenation provided a perfect conduit for the
tion of white households. Although knowledge of the sexual
white men was widespread, it was rarely admitted in public
it was never admitted in discussion of venereal disease. The
of that knowledge probably contributed to the anxieties of se

Whites sought to reconcile two incompatible needs: the
access to black labor as a means to generate wealth and
through segregation to render black populations invisible.
informed, like Fleming, knew that the source of infection amo
lay in the migrant labor and segregation, which were the fou
the colonial economy. Therefore, to eradicate syphilis requi:
mantling of settler capitalism; the fear of infection was fed by
of urbanization and wage labor, which were the sources of set
In Southern Rhodesia Black Peril and the fear of syphilis eru
space between those conflicting wishes.

As fears of Black Peril subsided, the fear of venereal inf(
Both phobias relied upon the same imagery of pollution,
believed to threaten the survival of white society, and both ha
gins in settlers' perceptions of the sexuality of black men and w
success of the white economy depended upon a ready suppl
black labor, which could only be guaranteed through the use of
labor practices, practices that in turn heightened settlers' fears :

own physical safety. It was the resonance of such factors for white men in particular that allowed the panics over syphilis to become so widespread and to survive for so long.

NOTES

1. In December 1924 an African named Joseph was charged with *Criminal Injuria*. His crime was having written a letter to a white woman named Johanna du Plessis saying that he loved her and suggesting they have sexual relations. He was found guilty in Salisbury High Court and sentenced to two years hard labor and 15 cuts with the cane. S628 No. 1863 Criminal Cases Salisbury High Court. In another case heard under *The Immorality and Indecency Suppression Ordinance* of 1916 a man named Akutizwi was sentenced to two years hard labor and ten cuts with the cane. In resting his bicycle against the Hessian door of a privy he lifted the flap thereby exposing a young white woman who was inside. Although such cases were uncommon the heavy penalties handed down to those found guilty were not. See S628 No. 1690 Criminal Cases.

2. According to a confidential Criminal Investigation Division report on Black Peril written during World War I, Black Peril was defined as any actual rape of white females or any assault with intent to commit rape on white females. It also included indecent assault, acts, or overtures or molesting white females for the purpose of exciting or satisfying bestial needs. The author admitted that there was a problem of a lack of statistics on such crimes. He also commented that police records were incomplete and that the most serious cases did not appear to have come to prosecution. *Black and White Peril in Southern Rhodesia*, Special File CID, 1916, S1227/2.

3. *Black and White Peril in Southern Rhodesia*, S1227/2.

4. Such a case is that of the murder of the three van Rensberg children. In October 1924 the children were killed by a farm laborer named Chakawa. Chakawa, who was employed by the children's father, became disturbed after a prolonged quarrel over the payment of his wages. Having killed the children with an axe he made little attempt to escape; he was tried in Salisbury High Court, found guilty of murder, and hanged. See 15/10/1924 S628 Case No. 1731.

5. See the individual files contained in *Venereal Disease Among Natives June/July 1900*, Native Department N1/2/4.

6. For example, in 1940 the European population of Angola was 44,000, of Mozambique 27,000, and of Tanganyika 10,000. See L. H. Gann and P. Duignan, *White Settlers in Tropical Africa* (Westport, Conn.: Greenwood Press, 1977), p. 65.

7. Dane Kennedy, *Islands of White: Settler Society and Culture in Kenya and Southern Rhodesia 1890–1939* (Durham, N.C.: Duke University Press, 1987), p. 4.

8. Colin Leys, *European Politics in Southern Rhodesia* (London: Oxford University Press, 1959), pp. 14, 17.

9. See Megan Vaughan, *Curing Their Ills: Colonial Power and African Illness* (London: Polity Press, 1991), pp. 129–54.

10. For a medical history of white settlement, see Michael Gelfand, *Tropical Victory: An Account of the Influence of Medicine on the History of Southern Rhodesia, 1890–1923* (Cape Town: Juta Press, 1953); Michael Gelfand, *A Service to the Sick: A*

History of the Health Services for Africans in Southern Rhodesia 1890 to 1953 (Salisbury: Mambo Press, 1967).

11.   G. H. Tanser, *A Sequence of Time: The Story of Salisbury, Rhodesia 1900 to 1914* (Salisbury: Pioneer Head, 1974), p. 78.

12.   Ibid., p. 96.

13.   M. W. Swanson, "The Sanitation Syndrome: Bubonic Plague and Urban Native Policy in the Cape Colony," *Journal of African History* 3 (1977): 388.

14.   In 1923 black water fever resulted in 85 deaths among whites. In addition there were in that year 70 deaths among white children under one year of age from malaria and influenza. See *Annual Report, Public Health Department for the Year 1923* (Salisbury: Government Printer), p. 23.

15.   S. Sontag, *Aids and Its Metaphors* (New York: Farrar, Straus and Giroux, 1989), p. 45.

16.   Ibid., pp. 39–42.

17.   C. Quetel, *History of Syphilis* (Cambridge: Polity Press, 1987), p. 255.

18.   Letter from the Medical Director to the Chief Secretary, Salisbury, March 22, 1907, Public Health H2/3/8/1.

19.   Spread of VD Among Natives in the Victoria District, Memo Dr. Fleming Medical Director July 9, 1907, Public Health H2/3/8/1, p. 3.

20.   Transcript of Meeting held at Municipal Offices, Bulawayo October 6, 1928 S 1173/220, Public Health Department, p. 15.

21.   Letter from Fleming to the Secretary, Department of Administrator, November 30, 1909, Public Health: General 1909–1919, H 2/10/1.

22.   Letter from Fleming to the Secretary, Department of Administrator, December 15, 1909, Public Health: General 1909–1919, H 2/10/1.

23.   Estimates: Fleming, the Medical Director January 29, 1912 for 1912–1913, H 2/10/1 Public Health: General 1909–1919, p. 3.

24.   The average supply provided for district surgeons per month was 5,000 Mercury Calk and Dovers powder pills, 1 gram each: 1,000 Mercury and Calk pills, 1/2 gram each; 7 pounds of mercurial ointment; 5 pounds of vaseline; 1 gall blackwash; 1 pound blue stone; 5 pounds calomel and starch dusting powder; and 1 gross chip boxes (nested). Letter from Dr. Eaton, Acting Medical Director to Dr. J. Mitchell, Assistant Medical Officer, August 17, 1916, Public Health H2/3/8/1.

25.   Letter from S. Cooper, "Chambrecy" to the Medical Director, November 29, 1927, Public Health Department Syphilis, S1173/214.

26.   See letter from S. Cooper to the Medical Director, November 29, 1917, Public Health Deppartment Syphilis, S1173/214.

27.   Legislative Council Debates, Vol. 7, May 30, 1923, p. 56.

28.   Mines and Works regulations: Government Notice No. 447 of 1914, Public Health H 2/3/8/2.

29.   Letter from the Secretary, Rhodesia Chamber of Mines to the Secretary, Department of Administrator, May 4, 1923, Public Health H2/3/8/1. See also letter from the Rhodesian Small Workers and Tributors Association to the Mining Commission, Gatooma, December 12, 1922, Public Health H 2/3/8/2.

30.   Mines and Works regulations: Government Notice No. 447 of 1914, Public Health H 2/3/8/2.

31.   Letter from the Medical Director to the Secretary, Department of Administrator, April 28, 1923, Public Health H2/3/8/1.

32. Legislative Council Debates, May 30, 1923, p. 64.

33. Returns from Offices of Native Commissioners: Incidence of VD, November 27, 1923, Public Health H2/3/8/1.

34. Letter from the Chief Native Commissioner to the Secretary of the Premier, January 23, 1928, Public Health Department Syphilis, S1173/214.

35. Report from Dr. I. Alexander, Rezende Mines Ltd., December 15, 1927, Public Health Department February to June 1927 Syphilis, S1173/214, p. 4.

36. See letter from the Clerk in charge, Native Department, Penhalonga to the Native Commissioner, Umtali, June 25, 1927 and letter from the Native Commissioner, Umtali to the Chief Native Commissioner, June 30, 1927, S1173/214.

37. "Landowners Meeting," *The Rhodesian Herald*, January 14, 1928.

38. Letter from G. Barratt, Medical Officer, Sinoia to the Medical Director, Salisbury, May 30, 1928, S246/534.

39. Letter from Vernon Vickers, Medical Officer, Rusape to the Medical Director, April 25, 1928, S246/534.

40. Letter from J. S. Liptz, Medical Officer, Enkeldoorn to Medical Director, Salisbury, April 18, 1928, S246/534.

41. Letter from P. Wallace, Filabusi to the Medical Director, April 23, 1928, S246/534.

42. Minutes of the Conference of Superintendents of Natives, Salisbury October 31–November 3, 1911, H 2/10/1, Public Health: General 1909–1919, p. 18.

43. Letter from the Town Clerk, Salisbury to Department of Administrator, May 11, 1917, Medical Inspections of Urban Natives 1917–1920, H 2/9/2.

44. Memo Town Clerk from Salisbury Council Meeting to Secretary, Office of Administrator, April 19, 1917, Public Health H 2/9/2.

45. Memo Town Clerk from Salisbury Council Meeting, April 19, 1917, Public Health H 2/9/2.

46. Letter from the Secretary, Office of Administrator to the Medical Director, June 18, 1917, Public Health H 2/9/2.

47. For example, Ordinance No. 16 of 1902 provided for the registration of African servants and the issue of passes to urban areas. It contained, however, no provision for the refusal of such a pass. See letter from Office of Chief Native Commissioner to the Secretary, Department of Administrator August 7, 1917, Public Health H 2/9/2.

48. Letter from J. Robertson, Secretary, Department of Administrator to the Town Clerk, Salisbury, August 21, 1917, Public Health H 2/9/2.

49. Report from F. E. Appelyard, Medical Officer, Salisbury to W. Jenkins, Town Clerk, September 2, 1917, Public Health H 2/9/2.

50. For further testimony on the extent of that risk, see letter from W. Jenkins, Town Clerk to the Office of Administrator, September 26, 1917, Public Health H 2/9/2.

51. Letter from the CID, Bulawayo, British South Africa Police to the Secretary, Office of Administrator, December 12, 1917, Public Health H 2/9/2.

52. Memo from the Town Clerk, Salisbury to the Secretary, Office of Administrator, undated, Public Health H 2/9/2.

53. Draft for the Medical Examination of Native Servants (Urban) Ordinance, 1918, Public Health H 2/9/2.

54. See letter from the Town Clerk, Salisbury to the Medical Director, March 6, 1919, Public Health H 2/9/2.

55. For an account of the epidemic, see letter from the Chief Native Commissioner to the Secretary, Department of Administrator, November 11, 1918, Administrator Spanish Influenza A 3/12/30/1.

56. See letter from Father Butler, Chimanza Mission to the Medical Director, September 15, 1921, Public Health H2/3/8/1. The total outlay on anti-venereal disease measures for 1929 was £4,700. *Report on the Public Health for 1932*, p. 12.

57. *Report on the Public Health for 1932*, p. 12.

58. See letter from Fleming to the Assistant Magistrate, Que Que, April 26, 1923, Public Health H2/3/8/1.

59. Letter from Fleming to the Acting Commissioner, British South Africa Police, Salisbury, October 13, 1922, Public Health H2/3/8/1.

60. That rate was estimated at around 0.5 percent. The numbers identified as being infected with venereal disease were as follow: 14,369 for Salisbury; 37,482 for mine compounds; and 6,577 at Belingwe. See *Annual Report, Public Health Department for the Year 1923*, S2419 Public Health Department, p. 23.

61. See Public Health Act File, 1922–1924, S1173/357.

62. See "The Health Act," *The Bulawayo Chronicle*, May 24, 1924.

63. For example, article 27 states: "Where a cleansing station is provided within the district of a local authority or within a reasonable distance therefrom, any person within that district certified by the medical officer of health, school medical inspector or other medical practitioner or by any certified sanitary inspector to be dirty or verminous may on order of the medical officer of health be removed together with his clothing and bedding to such cleansing station and be cleansed within." *The Public Health Act 1924*, p. 10.

64. See Public Health Act File, 1922–1924, S1173/357.

65. Public Health Department files Venereal Disease, 1928–1933, S1173/221.

66. *Annual Report Public Health Department for the Year 1925*, p. 19.

67. Transcript of meeting held at Municipal Offices, Bulawayo, October 6, 1928, Public Health Department, S 1173/220, p. 4.

68. Ibid., p. 6.

69. Ibid., p. 8. The 1926 figure for the Royal Navy for a population of 90,000 men was almost 7 percent; for the Army just over 4 percent; and for the Royal Air Force it was 1.7 percent. During 1926 the figure for the total population of New South Wales was 2.6 percent.

70. Letter from Association of Chambers of Commerce of Rhodesia to the Colonial Secretary, April 22, 1929, S246/531. This was accompanied by a transcript of the proceedings of the chambers' congress.

71. Letter from the Rhodesian Women's League, Salisbury to the Colonial Secretary, April 27, 1929, S246/531.

72. For example, at the government medical officers' conferences held in 1929 when there was some comment that existing facilities were inadequate and that the problem was serious. See Proceedings, Government Medical Officers' Conferences, 1925–1929, S1173/27-29.

73. Letter from Department of Colonial Secretary to the Town Clerk, Salisbury, June 19, 1930, S246/531.

74. See John A. Carman, *A Medical History of Kenya: A Personal Memoir* (London: Rex Collings, 1976).

75. According to the annual report for 1921 it was also a recognition of the debt owed Africans for the taxation they paid and for their role during the war against Germany. See *Annual Medical Report for The Colony and Protectorate of Kenya for the year ending 31/12/1921*, p.18.

76. Ibid.

77. The following table shows that until 1920 there was a steady decline in the number of cases treated:

TABLE 9.1
Numbers of Cases of Yaws and Syphilis Treated at
Hospitals and Dispensaries, Selected Years, 1907–22

Year	Yaws	Syphilis
1907	215	1,861
1910	164	1,413
1914	112	1,043
1917	344	782
1920	657	1,614
1921	7,401	1,914
1922	21,733	2,896

Source: Annual Medical Report Year Ending 1922 (Salisbury: Government Printer, 1923), p. 31. See also Annual Reports for 1925 and 1926.

78. See *Annual Report, 1921* (Salisbury: Government Printer, 1922), p. 90.

79. The lack of importance attached to venereal disease is also apparent in the attitude toward African fertility and infant mortality rates. In 1922 a study was carried out in the central Kavirondo district into infant mortality and fecundity rates. The high infant morality rate was attributed to poor methods of infant feeding, malaria, and diarrhea rather than to venereal disease. See *Annual Medical Report Year Ending 1922* (Salisbury: Government Printer, 1923), p. 20.

80. Susan Sontag writes: "Even more than comparing society to a family, comparing it to a body makes an authoritarian ordering of society seem inevitable, immutable." Sontag, *Aids and Its Metaphors*, p. 6.

81. Native Labor Committee Report and Transcripts, 1906 ZAA 1/1.

82. *Report of the Native Affairs Committee of Enquiry 1910–1911* (Salisbury: Government Printer, 1991), pp. 1–75 in *Southern Rhodesia Miscellaneous Reports 1909–1916* (Salsibury: Government Printer, 1916), p. 3.

83. This figure is representative for all but purely anecdotal estimates made in the period between 1910 and 1930. See *Annual Medical Report for 1927* (Salsibury: Government Printer, 1928), p. 21.

84. The Contagious Diseases Act of 1895 allowed for the detention of any person suspected of having a contagious disease under order of a magistrate. See letter from W. Eaton, Acting Medical Director to GMO Hartley, September 28, 1921, Public Health H2/3/8/1. Also, under Section 18 of the Mines and Works

regulations (Government Notice 350 of 1911) any case of infectious disease had to be reported to a district magistrate, and in December 1915 the Medical Director sent a memo to all medical officers reminding them of the regulations. See Circular from the Medical Director to all Government Medical Officers, December 1915, Public Health H2/3/8/1.

85.   Letter from the Senior Government Medical Officer to the Medical Director, December 23, 1927, S246/531.

86.   Letter from the Medical Director to the Secretary, Department of Colonial Secretary, February 20, 1928, S246/531.

10

Sexually Transmitted Diseases in Nineteenth- and Twentieth-Century South Africa

Karen Jochelson

The history of sexually transmitted diseases (STDs) in South Africa has been shaped by the broader processes of landlessness, poverty, migrancy, proletarianization, urbanization and consequent changes in family relationships and sexual mores. High morbidity rates of preventable diseases, including STDs, have been the toll exacted as a precapitalist, rural, and agricultural society was transformed into a capitalist, industrial economy dependent largely on male, migrant labor.[1] White and African women, socially and economically marginalized in rural and urban areas, regarded prostitution as the means to financial independence and survival. Both whites and Africans contracted STDs, but from the turn of the century they received very different treatment. The schemes that emerged to detect and treat STDs in the twentieth century were not simply shaped by advances in medical therapeutics, but complemented government efforts to shape a racially segregated society.

HISTORICAL EPIDEMIOLOGY AND POLITICAL ECONOMY OF SEXUALLY TRANSMITTED DISEASES

From the earliest days of European settlement and as British administrators replaced the Dutch, prostitution and STDs were evident in coastal, port, and garrison towns as slave and, later, free poor women prostituted themselves to soldiers, sailors, and local townsmen.[2] In 1866 more than 13 percent of British troops at the cape were hospitalized for STDs, and the War Office warned that the troops were being "more than decimated" by these diseases.[3] Prostitutes now were mainly colored women and local white English and Dutch speakers who were orphans or came from families where the male breadwinner had died. By the 1890s the women were mostly migrants from the cape hinterland, the daughters of farm laborers who came to Cape Town to enter domestic service.[4]

From the 1880s, however, a rash of medical reports warned that syphilis was occurring extensively in the rural African population in the central and northern cape. In Barkly West the district surgeon treated 1,140 patients in 1883 following the establishment of a free dispensary and out-stations in the reserves.[5] In Oudtshoorn the district surgeon treated 1,074 patients in 1882 and 1,003 in 1883.[6] In Bedford the district surgeon had examined 2,044 Africans of whom 1,122 were syphilitic in 1887.[7] Doctors explained that the disease spread from district to district as infected people sought work with other white families or became thieves and vagrants.[8] The disease also affected whites living in rural areas, and in some communities fear of contagion was so great that people refused to attend church or take communion.[9]

In the Transvaal the government set up a commission in 1906 to investigate the extent of syphilis in the country. It concluded that syphilis was very common in northern and northwestern districts and very seriously prevalent among the Basotho and Ndebele tribes. Cases of syphilis appeared to be more frequent in rural than urban areas.[10] Doctors' evidence to the commission about the extent of syphilis in their districts was again startling. The district surgeon of Pietersburg thought that "8 out of 10 natives who consult me come in regard to syphilis." K.H.R. Franz, a German missionary in the worst affected area of the Zoutpansberg, stated "not less than 75 percent of the western tribes (Basuthos and Matabeles) were syphilitic." He treated 5,000 cases between 1902 and 1906.[11] Other STDs seemed uncommon. Max Mehliss, medical superintendent of the Rietfontein Lazaretto, which cared for STD patients, stated "compared with syphilis, soft chancre and gonorrhea are of comparatively infrequent occurrence," but a district surgeon in Middelburg maintained that there was "practically no venereal disease other than syphilis" in his district.[12]

The high incidence of syphilis in the northern cape and northern and northwestern Transvaal was probably because of indigenous endemic syphilis or yaws rather than venereal syphilis. Today four treponemal infections are recognized: venereal syphilis, yaws, pinta, and endemic syphilis. The agent of venereal syphilis, *T. pallidum*, is virtually identical to that causing endemic syphilis, but although the diseases are clinically similar, endemic syphilis is epidemiologically closer to yaws. An initial lesion is rare in endemic syphilis, although common in yaws; lesions are of limited extent in intertriginous areas in endemic syphilis, and widespread on skin and bone in yaws; constitutional symptoms are rare in both. Late complications occur in 25–50 percent of endemic cases usually

in bone lesions, but in only 10 percent of yaws cases; neurological, cardiovascular, and congenital complications do not occur. Non-sexual contact is typical of endemic syphilis and yaws where direct lesion-to-skin
contact or indirect contact with fingers or objects contaminated with saliva containing treponemes is a significant mode of transmission especially in poor, overcrowded communities lacking sanitation. The reservoir of
infection in endemic syphilis and yaws is latent cases and children
between the ages of 2 and 15.[13] Venereal syphilis can coexist with endemic syphilis or yaws, although the latter give cross-immunity to venereal
syphilis.[14]

Most doctors in the cape attributed the strange symptoms of syphilis to
the peculiar nature of diseases in the African body, rather than an indication that the disease was not venereal syphilis. District surgeons constantly remarked on the absence of primary, tertiary, and congenital
cases. They most frequently described cases of lesions in the throat,
mouth, under the armpits, and in the groin, and, in advanced cases,
destruction of the nasopharyngeal tract — symptoms typical of endemic
syphilis. Doctors also described how the disease seemed to spread
through non-sexual contact: children playing together and families sharing eating utensils and bed linen or clothing. In case after case of syphilis,
district surgeons agreed, the source of contagion was never "immoral
practices,"[15] that is, sexual intercourse, as occurred with venereal syphilis.
Knysna's district surgeon commented that children and adults seemed to
contract the disease "quite innocently" as "quite a third of those brought
under treatment are virgins, girls whose innocence is beyond doubt and
children, some of whom are only a few months old."[16] Many doctors
recounted cases of how infection of one child quickly spread to other children in the family and to the parents.[17] They also reported that healthy
children were born to parents who were known to have had syphilis.[18]
Contemporary medical surveys also offer corroborating evidence for the
existence of indigenous endemic syphilis,[19] and archaeological evidence
similarly suggests that a yaws-like treponemal disease was present in
South Africa from 1000–1300 A.D.[20]

The opening of the diamond fields in 1869, the discovery of substantial
gold deposits on the Witwatersrand in 1886, the construction of railway
networks into the hinterland, and the enormous influx of people into mining towns heralded the spread of STDs and endemic syphilis into the interior. Many prostitutes from Cape Town and Port Elizabeth left for the
richer pickings in the mainly male digger camps in Kimberley and on the
Rand.[21] In areas characterized by endemic syphilis, doctors associated the
introduction of syphilis with the mineral discoveries, thus implying that
the disease was spread by migrants. African headmen from various locations in the Zoutpansberg (an area characterized by endemic syphilis) tes-
tified to the Contagious Diseases Commission in a similar vein. The 1906

commission thus concluded that the introduction of syphilis in the Transvaal was "of comparatively recent date, having usually been brought to the kraals by natives who had been to work at some mining centre, especially Kimberley, where . . . the disease is very prevalent."[22]

Sexually transmitted syphilis was also spread through migrancy, although more slowly. In Natal, doctors thought that syphilis occurred infrequently. A survey of 37 magistrates and district surgeons in Natal and Zululand in early 1899 showed that 18 thought syphilis was uncommon among Africans, 7 thought it was increasing, although they personally had not seen many cases, and 12 stated that they treated cases frequently, although not on the scale of the Transvaal. A practioner in Ingwavuma, for example, had found only one case among 7,000 Africans he had examined and vaccinated for smallpox.[23] In almost every case, the district surgeons associated the disease with migrancy and contact with the urban centers. The resident magistrate of Nkandla recalled that "about two years ago a native who had been working in Johannesburg was reported to have come home infected with the disease and to have conveyed it to his wives and he and the women, three in number, were said to be very bad with it." The district surgeon of Ngutu had treated very few cases, but in each one "the disease [was] from either Johannesburg or Natal."[24] That this was venereal syphilis is evident from several reports describing the treatment of the initial chancre of primary syphilis, the wives of infected men, and mention of stillbirths or deaths of infants with congenital syphilis.[25]

The mineral discoveries marked South Africa's transition from a precapitalist, rural backwater to an industrial, capitalist economy shaped by the mining industry and its dependence on cheap migrant labor. From 1871 to 1875 between 50,000 and 80,000 Africans worked in Kimberley each year.[26] The rapid expansion of the gold industry resulted in the growth of Johannesburg from a tented mining town of 3,000 people in 1887 to a city of 100,000 in 1896, and more than 250,000 inhabitants by 1914.[27] The mainly African, male, migrant mine workforce increased from 78,000 in 1903–4 to 208,000 by 1910 and continued to expand.[28] The white population was also predominately male. In 1897 only 12 percent of Rand gold mine employees were married and lived with their families, although the proportion increased gradually to 20 percent in 1902 and had reached 42 percent by 1912.[29]

Prostitution became a profitable business in mainly male towns and became the domain of organized crime. From the mid-1890s locally born women began to be replaced by continental women, victims of the white slave trade and of female unemployment and underemployment following an economic depression in Europe.[30] Health officials reported that syphilis and gonorrhea were well entrenched in the white and African working class by 1895.[31] The Transvaal government finally broke the crime rings in 1909 and 1910 and deported hundreds of foreign-born pimps and prostitutes from the Transvaal. However, already there was a decreasing demand for commercial sex in the white population as more men were able to marry, and women immigrated to the colony. During this time the prostitute population had changed, and in 1907 the first brothels appeared in Fordsburg and Vrededorp, the white working class slums of Johannesburg.[32] The women were now mainly Afrikaans-speaking, the first representatives of the poor white problem. The upheavals following the Anglo-Boer War, the beginning of capitalist agriculture, white landlessness, locusts, intermittent drought, and cattle diseases had fostered the influx of Afrikaans speakers into the towns. As mechanization forced Afrikaner men out of the entrepreneurial niches they had established in the towns as transport riders, cab drivers, and brick manufacturers, for example, families sent their daughters out to work.[33] By the 1920s white Afrikaans-speaking women who were frequently new to Johannesburg, unskilled, and lacking social or kin support networks and, thus, economically and socially marginal, became dependent on prostitution.

From the onset of World War I doctors began to voice concern about the effects of STDs on South Africa's white population. *The Medical Journal of South Africa* stated in July 1916 that although no accurate statistics on STDs existed "there is nevertheless, reason to believe that this prevalence is very real and alarming, and also that it is increasing, especially amongst whites."[34] One doctor estimated in 1917 that 30 percent of whites had syphilis.[35] However, these fears seem exaggerated. After five years' practice between 1914 and 1919 and the examination of 80,000 white, Transvaal school children, a school medical inspector discovered only 45 (0.06 percent) with syphilis.[36] From the 1920s local authorities expanded their free STD treatment services, and on the basis of patient records, the Department of Public Health (DPH) suggested in 1928 that only 5 percent of the white population living in inland towns had STDs.[37]

The estimates about the extent of STDs in the African population were even wilder. Press reports in the early 1920s alleged that between 50 and 60 percent or even 80–90 percent of Africans had syphilis. These estimates were rejected by the DPH, which thought that 10 percent was a more likely figure.[38] Doctors continued to make wild estimates in the 1940s. The medical officer of health for Pretoria, for example, suggested that probably more than half the African population had STDs.[39]

The confusion over the extent of syphilis among Africans may have resulted from the presence of the still unrecognized endemic syphilis. A similar distribution of high and low prevalence areas seems to have existed in the 1920s and 1930s as in the late nineteenth century. However, in the relatively lower prevalence rural areas, such as the eastern cape and in urban areas, the clinical descriptions of primary, tertiary, and congenital syphilis seemed to indicate that sexually transmitted venereal syphilis was increasingly common. A doctor describing symptoms of syphilis in the Transkei in the 1940s noted that the primary stage was often seen, particularly among men, and it was seldom extragenital. He had also seen tertiary symptoms, such as cardiovascular disease and neurosyphilis. Tertiary symptoms also appeared among mental asylum inmates where 7 percent of African inmates in 1936–40 suffered from cerebral syphilis.[40] A six-month study of postmortems on natural deaths revealed that 12 percent were because of syphilitic aortitis.[41] Congenital syphilis occurred in urban and rural populations. In Alexandra, a freehold township near Johannesburg, of 506 infants who died in 1940 during their first year, 19 deaths (3.8 percent) were attributed to congenital syphilis.[42] Records from King Edward VIII Hospital in Durban in 1941 showed that 22 percent of infantile deaths resulted directly from syphilis.[43] Figures were also high in rural areas. Between 1941 and 1946 in Polela, Zululand, 20.6 percent of newly born infants had congenital syphilis.[44] District surgeons also frequently reported on sterility and miscarriages among women associated with STDs.[45]

The spread of sexually transmitted syphilis was again related to the impact of migrancy. In 1925 the DPH reported that syphilis was increasing in areas where it had formerly been rare, such as Pondoland and the eastern Transvaal.[46] This seemed associated with migrancy: The assistant health officer of the Union of South Africa commented in 1922 that "syphilis was practically non-existent in Pondoland thirty or even twenty years ago, and has only become so terribly prevalent since the M'Pondo went to Durban, Johannesburg and Kimberley."[47] In Sibasa in the eastern Transvaal STD cases were still infrequent by 1936, but the district surgeon reported that "in nearly every case it was possible to trace the infection to an individual who had recently returned from town."[48] Syphilis also seemed to be increasing in Natal. Park Ross, reminiscing in 1931 about his medical experience as a district surgeon in Ngutu, Natal, recalled "there was very little venereal disease" in the past, whereas the current district surgeon reported that he saw "a great deal."[49] A study tracing the sources of venereal infection in Polela in Zululand in the 1940s showed that most married and single women were infected in their rural homes by their husbands or lovers who had recently returned from work in a town or on a farm. Only 2 out of 20 male patients were infected by their wives, who were assumed by the researchers to have been adulterous.[50] The reports of Native Affairs Department (NAD) officials, government doctors, and the mining industry during the 1920s and 1930s certainly suggest that male migrants contracted STDs from the African women in urban slums, peri-urban settlements, or farms surrounding mines, who depended on prostitution and brewing beer for a living. Only in the late 1930s did missionaries and some doctors begin to point to prostitution in rural areas as a source of STDs.

The association between STDs, prostitution, and migrancy reflected the consequences of the broader processes of landlessness, poverty, proletarianization, and urbanization on family relationships and sexual mores for men and women. The institutionaliation of the migrant labor system and urbanization reflected the gradual collapse of rural agricultural economies. The Land Act of 1913 had defined the restricted boundaries of African reserves and, together with antisquatting legislation, facilitated the demise of an independent African peasantry.[51] Increasing population density and land degradation meant that by the 1920s the reserves produced less than half the subsistence needs of their populations, and some homesteads no longer had access to land or owned cattle, although the pattern varied in different areas.[52] As reserve conditions worsened, dependence on migrancy began to dominate rural economies. Through the nineteenth century migrants were predominantly young, unmarried men, but now older men as well as women entered the migrant labor market. In relatively conservative areas, such as Pondoland, the proportion of economically active men aged 15–45 away from home increased from 24 percent in 1911 to 43 percent by 1936. Other districts were more heavily involved in migrancy, and overall for the total Transkeian Territories the proportion steadily rose from 41 percent in 1911 to 57 percent in 1936.[53] In Basotholand the number of men absent from home rose steadily from 10 percent of the total male population in 1911 to 28 percent by 1946.[54] Migrant men spent longer periods on contract and shorter periods at home, gradually losing contact with their rural homes. Worsening conditions in rural areas and migrants' attenuated contact resulted in some men abandoning their rural families and settling in urban areas with town women, although others brought along their families to settle permanently in urban areas.[55]

The long absences of men from their homes, wives' dependence on inadequate remittances, and fear of abandonment imposed great strains on marital relationships. For women abandoned by their husbands or lovers, brewing and selling beer and sexual relationships with returned migrants were the means to survival.[56] Other young women chose to leave the rural areas for the towns. Those most likely to migrate were women who, under the strains of rural pauperization and the migrant labor system, had become socially and economically marginal in rural society. The largest number of migrants, suggests Philip Bonner in his study of Basotho women migrants, were in fact women who had been properly married with the alliance cemented through *lobola* (a gift of cattle from the family of the bride to that of the groom) and were living with their children in monogamous homes.[57] Within a few months of marriage husbands returned to an urban-based job and remained away for long periods, returned infrequently, sent home remittances intermittently, and sometimes abandoned their families. Wives had to deal not only with insecurity and poverty, but as new wives they lived in their in-laws' homesteads and had to cope with conflict over the allocation and distribution of their husband's remittances, strict restrictions on their own behavior and etiquette toward their in-laws, and conflicts over the allocation of work.[58]

Women who went in search of their husbands often found their men had disappeared or refused to renew contact, so they had to establish themselves independently in town. There they were excluded from the formal sector of employment by a rigid sexual and racial division of labor. For many women beer brewing was the only way to establish an independent livelihood.[59] Beer brewing was often associated with what was seen by administrators and anthropologists as prostitution, although the relationships ranged from prostitution to cohabitation. Administrators regarded any sexual relationship outside of marriage as prostitution, yet many informal relationships seem to have been long-term and stable.[60] The trend toward informal relationships rather than marriage, the decline in traditional communal and peer controls over adolescent sexuality, and the growing acceptance of illegitimate births reflected changes in marriage customs and sexual mores caused by proletarianization and poverty.[61] Involvement in numerous sexual relationships exposed individuals to greater likelihood of contracting STDs. Transient sexual relationships in urban and rural areas and the constant traffic of men between rural and urban areas probably contributed to the high prevalence of STDs in the African population.

CONTROLLING SEXUALLY TRANSMITTED DISEASES

Government attempts to control the spread of STDs in South Africa from the late nineteenth century to the mid-twentieth century, although shaped by international trends in schemes for intervention, also reflected the gradual development of a segregationist state.

Until 1868 the British colonial authorities at the cape did little to control widespread prostitution, believing it was inevitable in port and garrison towns. The Contagious Diseases Act of 1868, modelled on the earlier British acts of 1864 and 1866,[62] was forced on the colonial legislature by the British War Office anxious about the extent of STDs in the troops, then withdrawn in 1872 after vigorous local opposition. The discovery in the 1880s that syphilis seemed epidemic in the colony meant that the act was reintroduced in 1885 as the Contagious Diseases Prevention Act (CDPA). This time it was divided into two sections: Part 1 allowed for the registration and regulation of prostitutes, and part 2 tried to deal with syphilis in rural areas by giving district surgeons authority to place anyone, male or female, suffering from STDs under medical treatment. Although the most serious threat was seen as lying in the country districts, the act

finally was promulgated only in the seaports of Cape Town, Port Elizabeth, East London, and Kingwilliamstown in 1888, and a lock hospital
was built in Cape Town next to the jail. Intervention in the country districts and large-scale hospitalization was too expensive, prostitutes an
easier group to control, and the act was regarded as successful once military doctors noted a decline in the percentage of soldiers with STDs.[63] The
Natal legislature tried unsuccessfully to introduce a similar bill in the late
1880s, but by the early twentieth century authorities still had no statutory
powers to compel any syphilitic to submit to treatment in a hospital.

The Contagious diseases legislation in the Transvaal, in contrast, was
linked to pass controls reflecting the significance of the enormous labor
market centered on the mining industry. As the African work-seeking
population increased there was a greater need to exert some control over
its health status to prevent the transmission of infectious diseases, such as
smallpox, tuberculosis, and STDs, between urban and rural areas. The
Contagious Diseases Law (No. 12 of 1895) compelled farm owners and
headmen to report the appearance of syphilis to a government official,
and compelled all Transvaal residents, regardless of skin color, to have
themselves treated and healed by a doctor. The pass laws of 1895 (Law
No. 22 of 1895), which introduced rudimentary efflux and influx control
in agricultural and mining districts, also prohibited the issue of a travelling or working pass to any applicant obviously suffering from an infectious disease, and thus marked out Africans as different from whites. In
practice the state did not have the financial or administrative power to
enforce the provisions of the law.[64] However, the 1895 laws had laid the
foundation for detecting STDs in the African and white populations in
different ways and for the assumption that all Africans were potentially
diseased. Subsequent legislation was based on this premise.

The Urban Areas Native Pass Act (No. 18 of 1909) seems to have been
the first legislation requiring that African work-seekers in urban areas in
the Transvaal be vaccinated against smallpox and medically examined at
the pass office for infectious diseases, including syphilis and tuberculosis,
before their service contracts were registered. To monitor the African
population more thoroughly, the government also instructed district surgeons to accompany local magistrates on their tax collection tours, to
inspect Africans for STDs, and vaccinate them against smallpox.[65] Syphilitics, when detected, were either isolated in their homesteads or brought
to the local jail for isolation and treatment. A chronic sick home was
opened in 1895 at Rietfontein, 7 miles northeast of Johannesburg, for
African and white pauper patients with incurable diseases. After the
Anglo-Boer War it was used for infectious diseases, such as smallpox,
scarlet fever, and measles, and increasingly for people with syphilis. As at
the Cape Town lock hospital, the intention was to remove morally and
physically contaminating people from healthy and respectable society. In

the Orange Free State local authorities were responsible for treating infectious diseases, but because most did not have the resources to provide hospital facilities the law was ineffectual.[66]

Even after union, the control and treatment of people with STDs remained regulated by different legislation in each province. However, the government, in consultation with medical officers of health and the medical association, began to discuss an appropriate form of control to be applied nationally. The terms of the debate were influenced by developments in Europe, where from the turn of the century the medical profession, enthused by a new chemotherapy and urged on by feminist organizations, had begun to reject the regulation of prostitution in favor of free, state-funded treatment and moral education for all men and women.[67] Similarly, in South Africa the debate revolved around whether the CDPA was still the appropriate way to deal with STDs and what degree of coercive monitoring of the population was warranted.

Doctors in favor of continuing the CDPA argued that STDs were a punishment for a moral failing in individuals and that offenders should be excluded from society in isolated hospitals. They regarded prostitutes as the source of STDs, whose health should thus be regulated. The lobby against the CDPA was an alliance of doctors, who viewed STDs from a secular stance, and philanthropic and suffragette organizations, which also included doctors among their members. They considered STDs a threat to the national health necessitating state provision of voluntary treatment based on newly discovered scientific therapies. They believed the CDPA punished women for male promiscuity and believed STDs were caused by ignorance rather than just moral failing. They supported scientific and moral education to complement accessible treatment for men as well as women.

The anti-CDPA lobby was particularly influenced by the findings of the English Royal Commission on Venereal Disease, which had reported in 1916. The medical officer of health of Johannesburg, Charles Porter, an extremely influential figure in urban and health planning, drew up an STDs scheme for Johannesburg modelled directly on the recommendations of the English commission. His proposal was duplicated by several other large municipalities, publicized in the medical journal, and presented before the public health conference debating the Public Health Bill in 1918.[68]

The assumptions of the anti-CDPA lobby shaped the Public Health Act of 1919, which repealed pre-union legislation and introduced uniform legislation for the union. The state now defined STDs as a contagious disease deserving of modern, voluntary treatment in general hospitals. The act made the government responsible for providing free laboratory diagnosis to ascertain if a person had an STD; free treatment, including hospitalization if necessary; and for refunding two-thirds of the costs of local authorities' STD schemes. General hospitals could now offer treatment for STDs, which formerly they had refused to do. The act instructed any person suffering or suspecting infection with STDs to consult a medical practitioner and place himself under treatment until no longer infectious or be guilty of an offense.

The Public Health Act reflected a new welfarist approach to white health. This secular medical approach argued that moral condemnation of individuals with STDs and the punishment of STD carriers by their removal from society and criminalization were outdated. The state was now obliged to provide accessible medical services and educational propaganda so citizens recognized their national obligations to avoid STDs and, if necessary, sought treatment without fear of judicial sanction. Only people who failed to take these responsibilities seriously were subject to penalties. The welfarism was also tied to a new political project. In a period in which a new South African nationalism began to emerge, uniting English and Afrikaans speakers, STDs and promiscuous sexuality were viewed as public matters, because they affected the health, virility, and future of a new South African nation. Administrators believed that free, accessible treatment and health propaganda would complement social welfare for poor whites (including racially segregated housing and job reservation). This would clearly elevate poor whites above Africans and, doctors and administrators hoped, halt the moral and physical decline of the white race and thus help protect white political supremacy.

Until the 1919 Public Health Act, Africans and whites had been treated in the same lock hospitals, in prison hospitals, or suffered similar neglect. Now this was seen as demeaning for the white population, and there were calls for segregated facilities. By 1922 clinics for whites existed in Johannesburg, East London, Pretoria, Pietermaritzburg, Barberton, Stellenbosch, and several other centers. By 1928 the government supported 26 local authority clinics.[69] The cape lock hospital was closed in 1925.[70] The number of white inpatients at Rietfontein declined during the 1920s, because the emphasis was on outpatient treatment, and only a few severely infected white cases continued to be committed to Rietfontein.[71]

The Public Health Act was not overtly racially discriminatory, but the government treated STDs in the African population very differently. In debates preceding the act, medical and administrative officials often called for compulsory STD examinations of the African population. This was not without precedent and had been implemented in Windhoek, then under South African martial law, in 1917, 1918, and 1920.[72]

After union, the central government had attempted to consolidate the pass laws through the Native Labor Regulation Act of 1911. This had made similar provisions to the 1909 law for the examination of work seekers on their arrival, but was concerned mainly with ensuring that Africans were vaccinated against smallpox. Inspection for STDs could not be made compulsory, and pass offices also did not have sufficient personnel to ensure that each work seeker was examined or to monitor Africans coming from areas where syphilis (probably endemic syphilis) was known to be widespread.[73] South African municipalities frequently demanded regular, compulsory examinations to detect syphilis, if not in the male and female African work-seeking population, then at least in the male. Public health officials also declared that Africans, but not whites, should be subject to notification and compulsory treatment. The government, however, opposed blatant racial legislation that might unnecessarily arouse the hostility of the African elite or undermine their sense of economic and social privilege.[74] Therefore, the Public Health Act of 1919 made free and voluntary treatment applicable to all races.

The Native Urban Areas Act (NUAA) (No. 15 of 1923), rather than the Public Health Act of 1919, proved to be the crucial legislation shaping the government's approach to African health and the control of STDs, as well as underpinning policy on African influx and settlement in urban areas. It was also a means to monitor STDs in the African population in a more coercive way than permissible in the white population without introducing blatantly racially discriminatory health legislation.

The administration was increasingly concerned about the need to control the growing numbers of Africans in the cities that it feared, through force of numbers and miscegenation, might lead to the swamping of whites in urban areas.[75] The growth of inner-city slums, regarded as the incarnation of immorality and disease, was also seen as a threat to the health of the white population.

The NUAA was premised on the continuation of the migrant labor system and sought to restrict the influx of African male work seekers according to the labor needs of white urban areas. The act intended to select only healthy workers and prevent unhealthy workers from entering the town. Before being registered as a work seeker, a man had to submit to a vaccination and medical examination for syphilis, tuberculosis, or any other disease considered dangerous to public health. If free from infectious diseases, the medical officer endorsed his permit to seek work or his service contract with the words "medically examined and vaccinated." The registering officer would not register a service contract of an African who had not been examined or failed the examination. If a work seeker was found to suffer from an infectious disease, his service contract was cancelled by the registering officer.[76] The antecedents of this provision clearly lay in earlier pass medical examination legislation. The NUAA also went beyond this. It tried to protect the health and welfare of Africans who were resident or working in towns by cleansing urban areas of redundant, criminal, and immoral Africans, especially women, and moving Africans with rights to reside or work in towns from unregulated slums to approved, racially segregated housing. Section 17 of the act allowed municipalities to send to labor colonies or repatriate to rural areas men and women deemed "habitually unemployed," "without honest livelihood," and "leading an idle or dissolute life." The administration considered independent women, newly settled in urban areas, as prime malefactors under section 17. J. A. Mitchell, the minister of public health, promised optimistically that the NUAA would prove "a valuable adjunct in safeguarding the natives in the towns against venereal infection," because section 17 meant that "the diseased native prostitute" could now be controlled.[77]

Local authorities were dissatisfied with these provisions, especially their lack of control over the influx, health, and activities of women in urban areas. They regularly urged the government to introduce compulsory examination on arrival and periodic examinations thereafter for men and women. This the government refused to do, fearing not only widespread protest by Africans about such a measure but also because it pointed out that only daily examinations would effectively ensure that a worker was free of disease, and this was impractical and expensive.[78]

The process of detecting and treating STDs among Africans was coercive and authoritarian. The authorities tended to hospitalize Africans with STDs or deport them to rural areas, in a very literal sense cleansing white society of its contaminating elements. In Johannesburg, for example, Africans detected through the pass inspection, and especially domestic workers, were sent to Rietfontein for treatment. Although the hospital offered outpatient treatment, it was too inaccessible to be practical. Africans were not permitted to travel on the tram line in that direction and so had to walk, and workers who took time off to seek treatment risked losing their jobs. Employers tended to dismiss servants with STDs, and without a health certificate a worker was ineligible for a pass and lost his right to live and work in the urban area.[79] Thus, the pass system criminalized Africans with STDs. Most rural districts and small towns had no accommodation for syphilitics, and even voluntary patients were housed in or near the local jail, which similarly connoted that contracting STDs was a criminal offence.[80]

In many country districts, magistrates advocated compulsory treatment and "a proper system of rounding up patients" in the belief that Africans were indifferent to their own health.[81] In Pondoland, for example, police rounded up suspects in raids and then prosecuted the prisoners for failing to comply with the provisions of the Public Health Act.[82] Offenders were sentenced to a fine of £25 or more and usually imprisonment because the intention was to "enable the District Surgeon to treat, house and control patients (prisoners) whilst under treatment for a month or six weeks." The only drawbacks, the magistrates reckoned, were that this scheme was expensive and the districts occasionally ran out of prison accommodation. When Africans under treatment absconded to Johannesburg to look for work, the director of native labor also alerted all pass offices to keep watch for the offenders, so they could be tried under the Public Health Act for avoiding treatment, which was a criminal offence.[83] Urban local authorities relied on the NUAA to detect, deport, or consign for treatment single, economically independent women whom they believed to be prostitutes.

Government health services for Africans were premised on the assumption that Africans were primarily migrants whose health was only important insofar as it determined their fitness to labor and suitability for contact with the white population. Thus, medical services were concentrated in urban areas to ensure that the current workforce was healthy, and services were exceptionally meager in rural areas where the bulk of the African population resided. Africans also did not benefit from advances in chemotherapy. The DPH and the mining industry considered too expensive the newer arsenical treatments, which rendered patients non-infective more quickly and with long, intensive treatment offered a better chance of a cure than mercury treatments. Africans were given just sufficient medication by district surgeons so that they were no longer infectious but not completely cured.[84] The mining industry argued similarly that it would not reap the results of expensive but complete cures, because its contract workers were all short term.[85] This inadequate treatment made a worker fit for work in the short term, but could make syphilis latent and lead to tertiary complications many years later. By then, however, a worker might have ended his migrant career, so his health was of little concern to employers.[86]

By the mid-1930s some doctors had begun to criticize coercive practices in health policy for Africans, arguing that health programs had to be based on public trust, not induced by pass laws and raids.[87] Some doctors tied their call for noncoercive treatment to the merits of preventive medicine and argued that STDs could not be controlled simply by building more hospitals, but only by changing the socioeconomic system dependent on migrant labor.[88] The new welfarism that emerged in health programs for Africans in the 1940s was restricted to the urban African population. This reflected official recognition that a permanent urban population was irreversible and had to be protected from undercutting by migrants through stricter influx control and measures such as higher wages and better housing.[89] The government began to encourage urban local authorities to establish voluntary outpatient clinics that the central government would partly subsidize and for which it would provide free drugs as it had for white STD clinics.

DPH beneficence did not extend to rural areas, where it also insisted on outpatient treatment despite doctors' complaints that long distances from the clinic made regular attendance by patients impossible. The department argued that its funds were limited, and it now refused to subsidize the treatment of tertiary and congenital syphilitic cases admitted to hospital, because these were not infectious, and it would only approve of inpatient treatment for grossly infectious cases or patients who lived excessive distances from a clinic.[90] In some rural areas, even in the 1940s, the DPH continued to supply mercury treatment, and its policy was still to render patients noninfectious rather than cured.[91]

Despite the reformist ethos of the new urban STDs services, Africans were still subject to coercive regulation by the state. The new STDs service introduced more extensive surveillance and control of the urban, resident, and working African population, which was more thorough than simply pass examinations of Africans at their point of entry to the city. Thus, as well as expanding health services, some health departments tried to ensure that outpatients attended regularly for a full course of treatment. Pietermaritzburg was the first town to use native health assistants to follow up patients who did not attend the clinic regularly and for contact-tracing to bring in for treatment the person identified as the original source of infection. As a result attendances jumped from 1,884 in 1932–33, to 4,334 in 1933–34 and reached 10,111 in 1934–35.[92] Durban introduced a similar system in 1939 and also tried to survey its resident African population to detect cases of STDs. By 1946 the city health department frequently received requests from industrial firms and schools to conduct mass blood-testing surveys, and it organized a mobile injection team.[93]

The contact and defaulter tracing and screening programs made eminent medical sense as a way of ensuring that patients completed a full course of treatment, and similar programs were in place in the United States and the United Kingdom.[94] However, in South Africa more effective monitoring of the health of urban Africans was still linked to the pass system, and, thus, tied to a more inquisitorial and authoritarian state. Being labelled a venereal disease patient or defaulter could result in an African losing his job and right to seek work in an urban area. In Durban a defaulting patient who could not be traced was blacklisted by the NAD and when he sought registration again, he was detained and sent to hospital.[95] Hospitalized patients who absconded were tracked down by police.[96] The calls by local authorities and white residents' associations for medical examinations and pass laws for women were renewed in the late 1930s and again rejected by the government. However, possibly reflecting the growing numbers of women entering domestic service, from the late 1930s the DPH and NAD began to recommend that employers encourage their servants to seek an examination as a condition of service.[97]

By the 1950s a racially segregated system of detecting and treating STDs in the white and African population was in place. For whites free, nonpunitive treatment was part of a social welfare ethos upgrading their physical and moral environment. For Africans the continued association between pass controls and STDs treatment can only have reinforced the idea that disease was a crime.

FROM SEXUALLY TRANSMITTED DISEASE TO HIV

Official concern about STDs in the African population seems to have declined during the 1950s, possibly because of the widespread use of penicillin, which was very effective. However, STDs remained a serious problem. The mining industry noted increasing morbidity among migrant mineworkers from the mid-1970s. STD morbidity in the gold mines in the Transvaal rose from 51.19 per 1,000 employees per year in 1978 to 104.41 per 1,000 in 1985, and in the Orange Free State from 39.61 to 76.11 per 1,000.[98] The true statistics may be even higher, because many workers consulted private practioners rather than mine doctors.[99] Other small-scale studies of the general population also revealed an extremely high incidence of STDs. A sample of 587 men and women attending a Johannesburg hospital between 1969 and 1970 showed that 17 percent had syphilis.[100] Of 232 women attending an antenatal clinic in Durban in 1981, 10 percent had gonorrhea.[101] In rural areas the incidence was similarly high: Of 193 women attending a rural antenatal clinic in KwaZulu, 12 percent had syphilis and 6 percent had gonorrhea.[102] A study of women in the Orange Free State in 1994 revealed that 12 percent of rural women and 16 percent of urban women tested positive for syphilis.[103]

The disruption wrought by migrant labor on social relationships was as significant as earlier in the century. In 1986 2.6 million workers were officially registered as migrants from areas within South Africa, 2.2 million from the independent homelands, and a further 378,000 migrants from Lesotho, Mozambique, Malawi, Botswana, Swaziland, Zimbabwe, and Zambia.[104] Migrants' frequent and lengthy absences from their homes disrupted stable familial and sexual relationships. Living in lonely and hostile single-sex hostels, some men assuaged loneliness and anxieties about home and work by engaging in relationships with many partners.[105] A study of 240 migrant mineworkers attending an STD clinic in a Transvaal mining town in 1986 showed that 49 percent had contracted an infection from a regular girlfriend, 33 percent from casual sexual contacts, and 15 percent from local prostitutes. Ten percent of the men had had more than one sexual partner in the previous month.[106] A study conducted for the Chamber of Mines showed that only 2.6 percent of migrants had more than one girlfriend, and 2.1 percent claimed sexual contact with a bar girl or prostitute in the preceding month.[107] These studies imply that STDs are widespread in the general population. Attitude surveys showed that condoms were seldom used, because they were associated with infidelity and distrust of a partner.[108]

The migrant labor system also continues to ensure rapid distribution of infections within urban areas from urban to rural areas, within rural areas, and across national boundaries. In the study of 240 migrants mentioned above, 55 percent of the men acquired their STD infections locally, 20 percent in Lesotho, 10 percent in Botswana, 5 percent in KwaZulu, and 3 percent in Transkei. The remaining 7 percent contracted infections in Ciskei, Malawi, Swaziland, and Johannesburg.[109] Another study of 429 mine workers found that 36.5 percent had picked up an infection in neighboring townships and 24.8 percent in Transkei.[110]

The extent of STDs in the general population is a somber warning about the future spread of HIV and AIDS. The first two AIDS cases in South Africa were diagnosed in December 1982.[111] The number of cases escalated rapidly, reaching 8,784 reported cases by November 1995, made up of 3,941 adult males, 3,873 adult females, and 909 children.[112] The cases of HIV infection were higher. Annual, national surveys of women attending antenatal clinics revealed that the prevalence among women had increased from 0.73 percent in 1990 to 10.44 percent by 1995. Based on this survey it was estimated that probably just more than 1.8 million people were infected with HIV by the end of 1995, of which 719,862 were male, 986,113 were female, and 40,557 were infants.[113] Two patterns of transmission became apparent. In the white population, HIV was initially concentrated in the homosexual male population, although gradually cases were found in the heterosexual population; in the African population, HIV had been contracted predominantly through heterosexual intercourse.

The low number of AIDS cases probably reflects the early stages of the epidemic in South Africa, underdiagnosis, and inconsistent case reporting. HIV prevalence rates in countries to the north of South Africa are far higher, a sign that the disease has moved southward. One study of the projected demographic impact of HIV and AIDS in South Africa estimates that by the year 2000, between 3.7 and 4.1 million people will be infected with HIV and about 600,000 may have died of AIDS.[114] An indication of the future magnitude of HIV in South Africa and the significance of heterosexual transmission among whites and blacks is evident from studies of STD patients, blood donor, and antenatal groups. These show that the incidence of HIV in white and black, male and female populations is increasing.[115] HIV still appears to be a predominanely urban disease, and surveys in rural areas have revealed very few cases.[116]

AIDS proved a powerful image for social disorder in the 1980s, metaphorically evoking white fears about escalating black political protest and the disintegration of apartheid. Through the 1970s and 1980s as the country slipped into recession, the currency devalued, and the union movement consolidated its strength, the country's economic vulnerability was of prime public concern. AIDS heightened the country's sense of economic crisis and anxieties about dependence on a volatile African labor force. Some newspaper reports warned that as the epidemic took hold, it would curtail African population growth by 1995 and that by the year 2000, 50–70 percent of Africans would have HIV or be dying of AIDS. This, it was prophesized, would lead to labor shortages, a fall in demand for consumer goods, and an enormous medical burden that white taxpayers would have to fund. South Africa was already in the midst of recession, and AIDS would hasten the decline of the economy.[117]

Other images associated with AIDS embraced current political tensions. The African National Congress (ANC) and South African Communist Party were still banned in the 1980s, but their insignia, symbols, and songs were part of the popular uprising led from within the country during the mid-1980s. Stayaways, boycotts, and strikes became part of daily existence in large cities and small country towns. Umkhonto we Siswe, the guerilla army of the ANC, began to infiltrate the country more successfully, and the discovery of arms caches or bomb blasts in major cities were regularly featured on national news. The revolt was followed by severe state repression. In an attempt to discredit the ANC the government characterized HIV as the new *swart gevaar* (black peril) sweeping down from the north in the form of ANC guerillas.[118] A popular book warned that "infected terrorists" could "establish themselves in townships and infect prostitutes" leading to a serious spread of AIDS. Soweto, the largest township adjacent to Johannesburg was an "obvious danger area."[119] Smear pamphlets distributed in Johannesburg in 1988 warned "socialize with the ANC freedom fighters and cry and die from AIDS," in a crude attempt to discredit the ANC and scare potential supporters.[120] The association between AIDS and the ANC implied that the organization and political protest were a disease spreading across the country, which unless rooted out and destroyed, could lead to an ugly and violent death. In 1990 when the ANC was unbanned another smear pamphlet, in the name of a prominent ANC leader, was distributed warning the parents of ANC exiles that returnees would be quarantined and tested for AIDS.[121] Again the intention was to discredit the organization.

White unease about racial desegregation also fed off myths about AIDS. From the early 1980s the government gradually removed social segregation measures, for example, allowing blacks and whites to enter by the same entrances in liquor stores or visit cinemas and restaurants. By the late 1980s the extreme housing shortage had forced increasing numbers of blacks to seek accommodation illegally in the white cities. Certain areas of Johannesburg became informal grey areas, that is, racially mixed. These changes were clear indications that apartheid was crumbling. Other smear pamphlets, aimed at a white audience, claimed that all blacks would be infected with AIDS by 1992 and that the disease was spread by informal social contact, such as sneezing and coughing, or by mosquitoes. The pamphlet warned that "to save the white race from extinction," whites should avoid visiting multiracial hotels, restaurants, and churches and should regularly test their black domestic servants "to safeguard your family."[122] The Conservative Party insisted that AIDS could be spread by informal social contact in its effort to reinforce the fears among its supporters about social integration.[123]

As in the 1920s, the government's and industry's main concern was maintaining a healthy, productive workforce. Foreign migrants seeking work in South Africa were blamed for importing the disease into the country. The mining industry initially intended to screen all prospective African mine employees routinely, although it eventually abandoned this plan. It planned to repatriate only HIV-positive workers or those with AIDS who were no longer fit for work.[124] In 1987 the government introduced health regulations for the compulsory testing of foreign labor recruits and repatriation of all HIV-positive foreign workers.[125] Recruitment from Malawi, where HIV prevalence was higher than in South Africa, came to a halt. This action was short-sighted as a preventive measure; it failed to deal with cases already existing in the local population and, by demonstrating that job loss and repatriation would follow detection, effectively forced cases underground and undermined the potential impact of any educational or outreach programs. The government also embarked on education programs, but these, too, were limited in outlook and impact. Educational material for whites emphasized that long-term monogamous relationships were more significant than promiscuity, while material aimed at the black population focused on debilitation and death. Many people were left more confused than informed about the causes and prevention of HIV.[126] The government was also reluctant to promote condoms, believing this would encourage promiscuity, and only from 1993 did it allow limited advertising for condoms on late night television.[127]

The most creative preventive responses came from community groups. In 1987 the director-general of the Department of Health stated publicly that the department would do nothing to help the homosexual community because "homosexuality is not accepted by the majority of the population" and it was the community's "own affair." The gay community took matters into its own hands and modelled its network of education and support structures on the U.S. movement.[128] In the townships and workplaces progressive groups tried to develop appropriate community-based educational and counselling services aimed at workers, residents, and health workers.[129] There were also attempts to draw traditional healers into the formal health education system in recognition of their importance in dealing with a range of health problems, including STDs.[130]

In 1994 the ANC assumed power in a new, democratically elected government. Its election platform was tied to its vision of reconstruction and development, and the health service was seen as a prime target for restructuring. The government drew up a National AIDS Plan, called on the resources of international donors and health agencies, and in 1994 allotted a budget of R256.77 million to deal with AIDS, compared to the previous government's R21 million in the two years previous.[131] In 1996 new billboard posters tied HIV prevention to health for all, but the reality of the task is immense. The government faces not only escalating cases of HIV and AIDS with their attendant medical and social costs but also a broad range of preventable diseases that are endemic in the country because of poverty. Thus, it will have to decide on its priorities. The problem with HIV, as with many other diseases, is that its causes are as much social as natural. The spread of HIV, like that of syphilis earlier this century, will be shaped by the economic and social disruption accompanying institutionalized migrancy, urban and rural poverty, and massive unemployment. These problems, although easy to pinpoint, are difficult to solve.

NOTES

The author was funded by a two-year research fellowship from the Wellcome Trust during the research for and writing of this article.

1.   S. Marks and N. Andersson, "Diseases of Apartheid," in *South Africa in Question*, edited by J. Lonsdale (London: Cambridge African Studies Centre with James Currey, 1985), pp. 172–99.

2.   P. W. Laidler, *South Africa Its Medical History, 1652–1898: A Medical and Social Study* (Cape Town: C. Struik, 1971), pp. 22, 93; E. B. van Heyningen, "Public Health and Society in Cape Town 1880–1910," doctoral dissertation, University of Cape Town, 1989, pp. 351–52; C. P. Anning, "History of Venereal Diseases in South Africa," *The Leech* 19 (1988): 9–13.

3.   E. B. van Heyningen, "'The Social Evil in the Cape Colony 1868–1902': Prostitution and the Contagious Diseases Acts," *Journal of Southern African Studies* 10 (1984): 173.

4.   van Heyningen, "The Social Evil in the Cape Colony," pp. 180–83.

5.   G67-84, "Cape of Good Hope, Reports of District Surgeons for 1883," p. 7.

6.   Ibid., p. 23.

7.   G13-88, "Cape of Good Hope, Reports of District Surgeons for 1887," p. 9.

8.   G67-84, "Cape of Good Hope, Reports of District Surgeons for 1883," pp. 12, 16, 32, 40.

9.   A13-88, "Cape of Good Hope, Report of District Surgeons on Public Health and Special Reports on the Prevalence of Contagious Diseases, 1889," p. 46.

10.   "Report of the Contagious Diseases Amongst Natives Commission, 1907," paras 4, 5, 29–32 (hereafter CDC).

11. CDC, paras 25, 26, 37.

12. CDC, para 11.

13. P. L. Perine, D. R. Hopkins, R. K. St John, P.L.A. Niemel, G. Causse, and G. M. Antal, *Handbook of Endemic Treponematoses: Yaws, Endemic Syphilis and Pinta* (Geneva: World Health Organisation, 1984), pp. 2, 14.

14. Perine et al, *Handbook of Endemic Treponematoses*, p. 13.

15. G67-84, "Cape of Good Hope, Reports of District Surgeons for 1883," p. 41.

16. G3-86, "Cape of Good Hope, Reports of District Surgeons for 1885", p. 17.

17. G19-85, "Cape of Good Hope, Reports of District Surgeons for 1884", p. 14.

18. For a more detailed discussion see K. Jochelson, "HIV and Syphilis in the Republic of South Africa: The Creation of an Epidemic," *African Urban Quarterly* 6 (1991): 20–34; K. Jochelson, "Tracking Down the Treponema: Patterns of Syphilis in South Africa, 1880–1940," History Workshop Conference, University of the Witwatersrand, February 6–10, 1990.

19. W. N. Taylor, "Endemic Syphilis in a South African Coloured Community," *South African Medical Journal* 28 (1954): 176–78; J. A. van Beukering, "Endemic Extravenereal Treponematosis in the North of the Cape Province," *Tropical and Geographical Medicine* 17 (1965): 40–44; J. A. du Toit, "Endemic Syphilis in the Karoo," *South African Medical Journal* 43 (1969): 355–58; F. P. Scott and J.G.H. Lups, "Endemiese Sifilis," *South African Medical Journal* 47 (1973): 1347–50.

20. M. Steyn and M. Haciej, "Pre-Columbian Presence of Treponemal Disease: A Possible Case from Iron Age Southern Africa," *Current Anthropology* 36 (1995): 869–73.

21. C. van Onselen, *Studies in the Social and Economic History of the Witwatersrand 1886–1914. Vol. 1. New Babylon* (Johannesburg: Ravan Press, 1982), pp. 106–7.

22. CDC, para 12.

23. TAB, CS 965, 19784, 9149/1898, "Synopsis of Opinions of Magistrates, District Surgeons and City Health Officers re Prevalence of Syphilis, 1899"; TAB, CS 965 19784 1344/1899, district surgeon to magistrate, Ingwavuma, December 30, 1898.

24. TAB, CS 965 19784 1344/1899, resident magistrate to chief magistrate and civil commissioner, Eshowe, January 4, 1899; district surgeon to magistrate, Ngutu, January 2, 1899.

25. TAB, CS 965 19784 1344/1899, district surgeon to resident magistrate, Ndwandwe, December 23, 1898; TAB, CS 965, 19784, 9149/1898, district surgeon to resident magistrate, Ixopo, January 20, 1899; district surgeon to chief magistrate, Estcourt, January 21, 1899.

26. R. Turrel, *Capital and Labor on the Kimberley Diamond Fields 1871–1890* (Cambridge: Cambridge University Press, 1987), p. 19.

27. van Onselen, *Studies in the Social and Economic History of the Witwatersrand 1886–1914*, vol. 1, p. 2.

28. A. H. Jeeves, *Migrant Labour in South Africa's Mining Economy: The Struggle for the Gold Mines Labour Supply 1880–1920* (Johannesburg: Witwatersrand University Press, 1985), pp. 265–67.

29. van Onselen, *Studies in the Social and Economic History of the Witwatersrand*

1886–1914. vol. 1, p. 147; C. van Onselen, *Studies in the Social and Economic History of the Witwatersrand 1886–1914*, vol. 2. *New Nineveh* (Johannesburg: Ravan Press, 1982), pp. 9–12.

30.   van Onselen, *Studies in the Social and Economic History of the Witwatersrand 1886–1914*, vol. 1, pp. 108–9.

31.   Ibid., p. 114.

32.   Ibid., p. 146.

33.   van Onselen, *Studies in the Social and Economic History of the Witwatersrand 1886–1914*, vol. 2, pp. 111–70; T. Keegan, *Rural Transformations in Industrialising South Africa: The Southern Highveld to 1914* (Basingstoke: Macmillan, 1987), chaps. 2–3.

34.   "The National Prevention and Treatment of Venereal Disease," *Medical Journal of South Africa* 11 (1916): 211.

35.   B. G. Brock, "Syphilis and the Commonweal," *South African Medical Record* 15 (1917): 20.

36.   C. L. Leipoldt, "Venereal Disease in Transvaal School Children," *Medical Journal of South Africa* 16 (1920): 27.

37.   Leipoldt, "Venereal Disease in Transvaal School Children," p. 25; UG 47-28, Annual Report of the Department of Public Health, Year Ending 30 June 1928, p. 47.

38.   UG 14-23, "Department of Public Health Report for the Year Ended 30 June 1922 in Annual Departmental Reports (Abridged) No. 2 Covering the Period 1921–22," p. 212; UG 09-24, "Department of Public Health Report for the Year Ended 30 June 1923 in Annual Departmental Reports (Abridged) No. 3 Covering the Period 1922–23," p. 254.

39.   IADJ, SGJ Box 201 File 59/5, "Disease Prevalent in Union," *The Star*, June 20, 1946.

40.   Becker cited in I. J. Grek, "Venereal Disease in the Bantu," *The Leech* 21 (1950): 70.

41.   G. A. Elliot, "The Future of Disease and Health in the Bantu," *The Leech* 21 (1950): 96.

42.   HPW, AD843 B2.1.1, "Alexandra Health Committee. Medical Officer of Health's Report for the Year ended 30 June 1940," p. 3.

43.   Department of Native Affairs (1942), "Report of the Interdepartmental Committee on the Social, Health and Economic Conditions of Urban Natives," (Chairman: D. L. Smit), para 10, p. 120.

44.   S. L. Kark, "The Social Pathology of Syphilis in Africans," *South African Medical Journal* 23 (1949): 78.

45.   SAB, NTS 5760 15/315, P. Targett Adams to the Secretary for Public Health, March 22, 1922.

46.   UG 21-26, "Annual Report of the Department of Public Health for the Year Ended 30 June 1925," p. 31; see also HPW, A1212/Caf. Dr. Mitchell, "Venereal Diseases in South Africa," (undated), pp. 4-5.

47.   SAB, NTS 5760 15/315, Assistant Health Officer for the Union to the Secretary for Public Health, March 22, 1922, pp. 1–2; see also UG 14-23, p. 212.

48.   SAB, NTS 5761 15/315 Part III, "Annual Health Report: 1935–36, Additional District Surgeoncy of Sibasa," July 22, 1936.

49.   HPW, AD1438 Box 6, evidence of Dr. Park Ross, 6123–24; see also SAB,

98.　K. Jochelson, M. Mothibeli, and J. Leger, "Human Immunodeficiency Virus and Migrant Labour in South Africa," *International Journal of Health Services* 21 (1991): 159.

99.　C. B. Ijsselmuiden, G. N. Padayachee, W. Mashaba, O. Martiny, and H. P. van Staden, "Knowledge, Beliefs and Practices among Black Gold Miners Relating to the Transmission of Human Immunodeficiency Virus and Other Sexually Transmitted Diseases," *South African Medical Journal* 78 (1990): 521.

100.　M. Dogliotti, "The Incidence of Syphilis in the Bantu: Survey of 587 Cases from Baragwanath Hospital," *South African Medical Journal* 45 (1971): 9.

101.　A. A. Hoosen, S. M. Ross, and M. Patel, "The Incidence of Selected Vaginal Infections Among Pregnant Urban Blacks," *South African Medical Journal* 59 (1981): 828.

102.　N. O. Farrell, A. A. Hoosen, A.B.M. Kharsany, and J. van den Ende, "Sexually Transmitted Pathogens in Pregnant Women in a Rural South African Community," *Genitourinary Medicine* 65 (1989): 277.

103.　H. S. Cronje, G. Joubert, A. Muir, R. D. Chapman, P. Divall, and R. H. Bam, "Prevalence of Vaginitis, Syphilis and HIV Infection in Women in the Orange Free State," *South African Medical Journal* 84 (1994): 602.

104.　South African Institute of Race Relations, *Race Relations Survey 1987/88* (Johannesburg: South African Institute of Race Relations, 1988), pp. 17, 312–13.

105.　T. Dunbar Moodie, "Mine Culture and Miners' Identity on the South African Gold Mines," in *Town and Countryside in the Transvaal*, edited by B. Bozzoli (Johannesburg: Ravan Press, 1983), pp. 181, 187–88; Jochelson, Mothibeli, and Leger, "HIV and Migrant Labour in South Africa," pp. 163–66.

106.　Y. Dangor, G. Fehler, F. da L.M.P.P. Exposto, and H. J. Koornhof, "Causes and Treatment of Sexually Acquired Genital Ulceration in Southern Africa," *South African Medical Journal* 76 (1989): 339.

107.　Ijsselmuiden et al., "Knowledge, Beliefs and Practices among Black Gold Miners," p. 522.

108.　C. R. Evian, C. B. Ijsselmuiden, G. N. Padayachee, and H. S. Hurwitz, "Qualitative Evaluation of an AIDS Health Education Poster," *South African Medical Journal* 78 (1990): 518; C. Mathews, L. Kuhn, C. A. Metcalf, G. Joubert, and N. A. Cameron, "Knowledge, Attitudes and Beliefs about AIDS in Township School Students in Cape Town," *South African Medical Journal* 78 (1990): 513–14.

109.　Dangor et al, "Causes and Treatment of Sexually Acquired Genital Ulceration in Southern Africa," p. 339.

110.　Ijsselmuiden et al, "Knowledge, Beliefs and Practices among Black Gold Miners," p. 521.

111.　C. B. Ijsselmuiden, M. H. Steinberg, G. N. Padayachee, B. D. Schoub, S. A. Strauss, E. Buch, J.C.A. Davies, C. de Beer, J.S.S. Gear, and H. S. Hurwitz, "AIDS and South Africa — Towards a Comprehensive Strategy. Part 1," *South African Medical Journal* 73 (1988): 457.

112.　Department of National Population Health and Development, Republic of South Africa, "AIDS in South Africa. Reported AIDS Cases as on 30 November 1995," *Epidemiological Comments* 22 (1995): 233.

113.　Department of National Population Health and Development, Republic of South Africa, "Sixth National HIV Survey of Women Attending Antenatal Clinics of the Public Health Services in the Republic of South Africa,

NTS 5761 15/315, acting Chief Native Commissioner, Natal to Secretary for Native Affairs, March 18, 1930.

50.　Kark, "The Social Pathology of Syphilis in Africans," p. 823; UG 08-45, "Annual Report of the Department of Public Health, Year Ended 30 June 1944," p. 17.

51.　On decline of the peasantry, see C. Bundy, *The Rise and Fall of the South African Peasantry* (London: Heinemann, 1979) and on the creation of a labor supply for the mining industry, see Jeeves, *Migrant Labour in South Africa's Mining Economy.*

52.　C. Simkins, "Agricultural Production in the African Reserves of South Africa, 1918–69," *Journal of Southern African Studies* 7 (1981): 264, 266, 275.

53.　Calculated from Table 4 in W. Beinart, *The Political Economy of Pondoland 1860–1930* (Johannesburg: Ravan Press, 1982), p. 172.

54.　C. Murray, *Families Divided: The Impact of Migrant Labour in Lesotho* (Cambridge: Cambridge University Press, 1981), p. 4.

55.　I. Schapera, *Migrant Labour and Tribal Life* (London: Oxford University Press, 1947), pp. 61–63.

56.　I. Schapera, "Premarital Pregnancy and Native Opinion: A Note on Social Change," *Africa* 6 (1933): 70; HPW, AD843/RJ/Aa12.14.1, "Evidence of the South African Institute of Race Relations to the Native Laws Commission of Enquiry [Fagan Commission (1946–48)], no date," p. 65.

57.　P. L. Bonner, "'Desirable or Undesirable Basotho Women?' Liquor, Prostitution and the Migration of Basotho Women to the Rand, 1920–1945," in *Women and Gender in Southern Africa to 1945*, edited by C. Walker (Cape Town: David Phillip, 1990), pp. 235–40; C. Walker, "Gender and the Development of the Migrant Labour System c. 1850–1930" in *Women and Gender in Southern Africa to 1945*, edited by C. Walker (Cape Town: David Phillip, 1990), pp. 187, 189, 192–93.

58.　M. Hunter, *Reaction to Conquest: Effects of Contact with Europeans on the Pondo of South Africa* (London: Oxford University Press, 1961), pp. 203–8.

59.　Walker, "Gender and the Development of the Migrant Labour System," p. 190; Bonner, "Desirable or Undesirable Basotho Women?" pp. 228–29; M. Janisch, "Some Administrative Aspects of Native Marriage Problems in an Urban Area," *Bantu Studies* 15 (1941): 4; E. Hellmann, "The Importance of Beer Brewing in an Urban Native Yard," *Bantu Studies* 8 (1934): 39–60.

60.　Janisch, "Some Administrative Aspects of Native Marriage Problems in an Urban Area," pp. 2, 8–9; P. L. Bonner, "Family Crime and Political Consciousness on the East Rand, 1939–1955," *Journal of Southern African Studies* 14 (1988): 395.

61.　D. Gaitskell, "'Wailing for Purity': Prayer Unions, African Mothers and Adolescent Daughters 1912–1940" in *Industrialisation and Social Change in South Africa: African Class Formation, Culture and Consciousness, 1870–1930*, edited by S. Marks and R. Rathbone (London: Longman, 1982), pp. 338–57.

62.　See for example, R. Davenport-Hines, *Sex, Death and Punishment: Attitudes to Sex and Sexuality in Britain Since the Renaissance* (London: Fontana Press, 1991), pp. 168–70; J. Walkowitz, *Prostitution and Victorian Society: Women, Class and the State* (Cambridge: Cambridge University Press, 1980).

63.　van Heyningen, "The Social Evil in The Cape Colony."

64.　S. Marks and S. Trapido, "Lord Milner and the South African State" in

Working Papers in Southern African Studies, vol. 2, edited by P. Bonner (Johannesburg: Ravan Press, 1981), p. 68.

65.   TAB, CS 908 17850, "Control and Treatment of Syphilitic Natives, circular No. 1 (CSA 3/18524), January 15, 1910, Annexure 1: Regulations under the Urban Areas Native Pass Act 1909. Part II. Medical Examination and Vaccination," paras. 14–20; TAB, CS 908 17843, Circular Minute CSO 42/18524, April 8, 1910.

66.   K. Jochelson, "Moralising Treatment: Medical Policy and Education on VD for Whites, 1880s–1940s," unpublished paper, 1992, pp. 7–8, 13–14.

67.   D. Evans, "'Tackling the Hideous Scourge': The Creation of the Venereal Disease Centres in Early Twentieth Century Britain," *Social History of Medicine* 5 (1992): 413–35; P. Weindling, "The Politics of International Co-ordination to Combat Sexually Transmitted Diseases, 1900–1980s," in *AIDS and Contemporary History*, edited by V. Berridge and P. Strong (Cambridge: Cambridge University Press, 1993), pp. 93–107; Davenport-Hines, *Sex, Death and Punishment*, pp. 156–209.

68.   IADJ, SJG Box 149 File 9728, "Municipal Council of Johannesburg. Special Report by the Medical Officer of Health on the Prevention and Treatment of Venereal Diseases, 28 August 1916," p. 6; Evidence of C. Porter on Public Health Bill in parliament, session 1919.

69.   UG 47-28, p. 47.

70.   UG 21-26, "Annual Report of the Department of Public Health for the Year Ended 30 June 1925," p. 31.

71.   IADJ, SGJ Box 2 File A6340, Minutes of committee meeting, November 25, 1927.

72.   M. Wallace, "Urban Control and the Compulsory Examination of Women in Windhoek, 1915–1940," Institute of Commonwealth Studies Postgraduate Seminar: Health and Empire, March 12, 1993, p. 1.

73.   For the provisions of the Native Labour Regulation Act of 1911 see D. Hindson, *Pass Controls and the Urban African Proletariat* (Johannesburg: Ravan Press, 1987), pp. 24–25; Jeeves, *Migrant Labor in South Africa's Mining Economy*, p. 122. On shortcomings of the act see SAB, NTS 5760 15/315. Acting Secretary for the Interior to Secretary for Native Affairs, July 29, 1911; Memo to Minister of Native Affairs, "Syphilis among Natives on the Rand: Resolutions of the Public Health Committee (Johannesburg)," August 16, 1911; "Report of Acting Chief Pass Officer, Johannesburg, 21 January 1911," in Johannesburg Council Minutes, April 26, 1911, p. 1918.

74.   S. Dubow, *Racial Segregation and the Origins of Apartheid in South Africa, 1919–36* (London: Macmillan, 1989), p. 44.

75.   SAB, GES 49/33, J. A. Mitchell, "Venereal Diseases in South Africa," address to Imperial Social Hygiene Congress, September 7, 1925.

76.   For details on other provisions of the NUAA see Hindson, "Pass Controls," pp. 41–42.

77.   HPW, A1212/Caf. Mitchell, (undated), p. 4.

78.   K. Jochelson, *The Colour of Disease: Syphilis and Racism in South Africa, 1910–1950*, doctoral dissertation, University of Oxford, 1993, pp. 121–66.

79.   Johannesburg City Council Minutes, June 24, 1930, p. 478.

80.   See for example, HPW, AD1438 Box 2, "Health and Child Welfare, Transkei, 2524-3960." Port St John's sitting, November 10, 1930: evidence of E.J.P.

Almon (for local Village Management Board), p. 55.

81.   SAB, NTS 5760 15/315, Klipdam Magistrate to Secretary of Public Health, December 9, 1924.

82.   A person who knew or believed he suffered from venereal disease could be prosecuted under the Public Health Act if he failed to consult a doctor and place himself under treatment until cured.

83.   SAB, NTS 5760 15/315, Adams, Assistant Health Officer for the Union to the Secretary for Public Health, March 22, 1922, pp. 2, 4; SAB, NTS 5761 15/315, C. H. Blaine, magistrate Groot Marico, July 10, 1930; TAB, GNLB 149 136/14, H. G. Falwasser, for Director of Native Labour to Native Sub-Commissioners and Pass Officers, Witwatersrand, April 12, 1927; SAB, GES 376 4/5B, Extract from minutes of Council of Public Health held at Cape Town on January 26, 1939.

84.   SAB, NTS 5761 15/315, Secretary for Public Health to Native Commissioner, Ubombo, November 18, 1932; GNLB 388 33/58, E. H. Cluver, Assistant Health Officer to Secretary for Public Health, February 18, 1931.

85.   "General Discussion on Venereal Diseases," *proceedings of the Transvaal Mine Medical Officers Association* 4 (1924): 3, 6.

86.   UG 28-48, "Department of Native Affairs, Report of the Native Laws Commission, 1946–48," (Chairman: H. A. Fagan), evidence of Gale, 39, para 54.

87.   SAB, GES 375 4/5A, "The Medical Examination of Male Natives at the Pass Offices on the Witwatersrand: Report of the Inspection Undertaken by Dr. H. S. Gear on the Instructions of the Secretary for Public Health, May 1937," p. 2.

88.   HPW, AD843 B8.1.6, Dr. G. W. Gale, "Health Services in the Union" (undated).

89.   Hindson, "Pass Controls," p. 44.

90.   SAB, GES 1233 53/19A, Under Secretary for Public Health to Secretary, Jane Furse Hospital, May 2, 1939, and September 8, 1939.

91.   S. V. Humphries, "Syphilis — A Major Cause of Ill Health in Native Labourers and Suggestions for Mass Treatment," *Proceedings of the Transvaal Mine Medical Officers' Association* 17 (1938): 124; F.W.F. Purcell, "Syphilis in South Africa," *South African Medical Journal* 14 (1940): 455–56; E. H. Cluver, "Syphilis and the Public Health," *South African Medical Journal* 14 (1940): 457.

92.   HPW, AD843/RJ/Na.10, Pietermaritzburg Public Health Department to Mayor, Pietermaritzburg, April 28, 1936, pp. 1–2.

93.   City of Durban, Mayor's Minutes, 1946, pp. 150–51.

94.   A. Brandt, *No Magic Bullet: A Social History of Venereal Disease in the United States Since 1880* (Oxford: Oxford University Press, 1987), pp. 149–54; R. Davidson, "'A Scourge to be Firmly Gripped': The Campaign for VD Controls in Interwar Scotland," *Social History of Medicine* 6 (1993): 213–36.

95.   SAB, GES 455 47/9B, City Medical Officer of Health to Under Secretary for Public Health, June 24, 1940, p. 4.

96.   City of Durban, Annual Report of Borough Medical Officer of Health, the Year ending 30 June 1939, p. 15.

97.   SAB, GES 376 4/5B, Secretary for Public Health to Secretary for Native Affairs, January 23, 1939; Secretary for Public Health to Municipal Association, the Transvaal, January 31, 1941; NAB, 3/DBN 4/1/3/1625, 359c, Extract, City Council minutes, November 10, 1943; Secretary for Native Affairs to Town Clerk, Durban, December 2, 1943.

October/November 1995," *Epidemiological Comments* 23 (1996): 9, 11.

114. P. Doyle, "The Demographic Impact of AIDS on the South African Population" in *Facing Up To AIDS: The Socio-Economic Impact in Southern Africa*, edited by S. Cross and A. Whiteside (London: Macmillan, 1993), p. 103.

115. B. D. Schoub, A. N. Smith, S. Johnson, P. J. Martin, S. F. Lyons, G. N. Padayachee, and H. S. Hurwitz, "Considerations on the Further Expansion of the AIDS Epidemic in South Africa — 1990," *South African Medical Journal* 77 (1990): 615; M. Shapiro, R. L. Crookes, and E. O'Sullivan, "Screening Ante-Natal Blood Samples for Anti-Human Immunodeficiency Virus Antibodies by a Large Pool Enzyme Linked Immunoabsorbent Assay System," *South African Medical Journal* 76 (1989): 245–47.

116. Schoub et al, "Considerations on the Further Expansion of the AIDS Epidemic in South Africa — 1990," p. 617.

117. "AIDS a Hazard 'Beyond Concept'," *Business Day*, June 6, 1989; "It Will Kill One in Four Blacks in SA — Sanlam," *Saturday Star*, June 10, 1989; "AIDS Is Wiping Out SA Workers," *Saturday Star*, January 21, 1990; M. Crewe, *AIDS in South Africa: The Myth and the Reality* (London: Penguin, 1992), pp. 58, 65.

118. *The Star*, August 9, 1988.

119. K. Edelston, *AIDS: Countdown to Doomsday* (Johannesburg: Media House, 1988), p. 186.

120. "Anti-AIDS Campaign AIDS from Freedom Fighters," pamphlet, 1988.

121. "Sisulu's Name on Fake 'AIDS' Leaflet," *Weekly Mail*, October 5, 1990, p. 3.

122. Aids Information Distributing Society of South Africa, "FACTS ON AIDS: Press Won't Print!! AIDS Hushed — Why???" (Johannesburg: no publisher, 1989), pamphlet; West Gossip, "AIDS — Hushed — Why?? The Origins of AIDS," (Johannesburg: no publisher, 1989), pamphlet.

123. "AIDS Rising Fast Among Black South Africans," *New York Times International*, September 27, 1990, p. 27; Crewe, *AIDS in South Africa*, p. 73.

124. A. Zwi and D. Bachmayer, "HIV and AIDS in South Africa: What Is an Appropriate Public Health Response," *Health Policy Planning* 5 (1990): 320–23.

125. Government Gazette No. 11014, Reg. No. 2438 and Reg. No. 2439, Pretoria, October 30, 1987.

126. Crewe, "AIDS in South Africa," pp. 63, 75. M. Crewe, "AIDS in South Africa — Progressive Perspectives," *Critical Health* 22 (1988): 20.

127. D. Webb, "The Social Epidemiology of HIV and the Development of AIDS Prevention in Southern Africa," doctoral dissertation, University of London, 1995, pp. 82, 84.

128. Quoted in Zwi and Bachmayer, "HIV and AIDS in South Africa: What Is an Appropriate Public Health Response," p. 321.

129. Zwi and Bachmayer, "HIV and AIDS in South Africa: What Is an Appropriate Public Health Response," pp. 323–24; Webb, *The Social Epidemiology of HIV and the Development of AIDS Prevention in Southern Africa*, pp. 85–87

130. S. S. Abdool Karim, "Traditional Healers and AIDS Prevention," *South African Medical Journal* 83 (1993): 423–25.

131. Webb, "The Social Epidemiology of HIV and the Development of AIDS Prevention in Southern Africa," pp. 84, 222.

Selected Bibliography

CÔTE D'IVOIRE

Amat-Roze, Jeanne-Marie. "Les inégalités géographiques de l'infection à VIH et du sida en Afrique sub-saharienne." *Social Science and Medicine* 36 (1993): 1247–56.

Amat-Roze, J-M. and G-F. Dumont. "Le sida et l'avenir de l'Afrique." *ETHIQUE* 2 (1994): 37–60.

Béchu, Nathalie, Eric Chevallier, Agnès Guillaume, and Bi Tah Nguessan. "Les conséquences socio-économiques du sida dans les familles africaines (Burundi et Côte d'Ivoire), premiers jalons, premières réflexions." In François Deniau, ed., *Jeunes et préservatifs en Abidjan, une recherche d'ethno-prévention du sida et des NST*. Bingerville: Actes de l'atelier du CRES, 1993.

De Cock, Kevin M., Bernard Barrere, Lacina Diaby, Marie-France Lafontaine, Emmanuel Gnaore, Anne Porter, Daniel Pantobe, Geoarges C. Lafontant, Augustin Dago-Akribi, Marcel Ette, Koudou Odehouri, and William L. Heyward. "AIDS, the Leading Cause of Adult Death in the West African City of Abidjan, Ivory Coast." *Science* 249 (1990): 793–96.

De Cock, Kevin M., Bernard Barrere, Marie-France Lafontaine, Lacina Dialy, Emmanuel Gnaore, Daniel Pantohe, and Koudou Odehouri. "Mortality Trends in Abidjan, Côte d'Ivoire, 1983–1988." *AIDS* 5 (1991): 393–98.

De Cock, Kevin M., Emmanuel Gnaore, Georgette Adjorlolo, Miles M. Braun, Marie-France Lafontaine, Gilberte Yesso, Geneviève Bretton, Issa M. Coulibaly, Guy-Michel Gershy-Damet, Raymond Bretton, and William L. Heyward. "Risk of Tuberculosis in Patients with HIV-I and HIV-II Infections in Abidjan, Ivory Coast." *British Medical Journal* 302 (1991): 496–99.

De Cock, Kevin M., Koudou Odehouri, Jacques Moreau, Justin C. Kouadio, Anne

Porter, Bernard Barrere, Lacina Dialy, and William L. Heyward. "Rapid Emergence of AIDS in Abidjan, Ivory Coast." *Lancet* 2 (1989): 408–11.

Dédy, Séry and Gozé Tapé. "Jeunesse, Sexualité et sida en Côte d'Ivoire." In François Deniau, ed., *Jeunes et préservatifs en Abidjan, une recherche d'ethno-prévention du sida et des NST.* Bingerville: Actes de l'atelier du CRES, 1993.

Denis, François, Françoise Barin, and Guy-Michel Damet-Gershy. "Prevalence of Human T-lymphotropic Retrovirus Type III (HIV) and Type IV in Ivory Coast." *Lancet* 1 (1987): 408–11.

Djomand, Gaston, Alan E. Greenberg, Madeleine Sassan-Morokro, Odette Tossou, Mamadou O. Diallo, Ehounou Ekpini, Peter Ghys, Benoît Soro, Kari Bratte-gaard, Achy Yapi, Koudou Odehouri, Doulhourou Coulibaly, Issa-Malick Coulibaly, Auguste Kadio, Emmanuel Gnaore, and Kevin M. De Cock. "The Epidemic of HIV/AIDS in Abidjan, Côte d'Ivoire: A Review of Data Collected by Project Retro-CI from 1987 to 1993." *Journal of AIDS* 10 (1995): 358–65.

Domergue-Cloarec, Danielle. *La santé en Côte d'Ivoire 1905–1958.* Paris: Association des publications de l'Université Toulouse-Le Mirail — Académie des Sciences d'Outre-Mer, 1986.

Gayle, Hélène D., Emmanuel Gnaore, Georgette Adjorlolo, Ehounou Ekpini, Ramata Coulibaly, Anne Porter, Miles M. Braun, Marie Louise Klein Zabban, Joseph Andou, Adjoua Timite, Jèrôme Assi-Adou, and Kevin M. De Cock. "HIV-1 and HIV-2 Infection in Children in Abidjan, Côte d'Ivoire." *Journal of Acquired Immune Deficiency Syndromes* 5 (1992): 513–17.

Ghys, Peter D., Mamadou O. Diallo, Virginie Ettiègne-Traoré, Kouadio M. Yeboué, Emmanuel Gnaore, Félix Lorougnon, Marie-Jeanne Teurquetil, Marie-Laure Adom, Alan E. Greenberg, Marie Laga, and Kevin M. De Cock. "Dual Seroreactivity to HIV-1 and HIV-2 in Female Sex Workers in Abidjan, Côte d'Ivoire." *AIDS* 9 (1995): 955–58.

Grosfillez, Jean. "Les principales maladies observées dans les colonies et les terri-toires sous mandat en 1932." *Annales de Médecine et de Pharmacie Coloniale* 32 (1934): 153–268.

"Instructions relatives au développement des services de médecine préventive, hygiène et assistance dans les colonies." *Journal Officiel de la Côte d'Ivoire 1925,* December 30, 1924, pp. 72–78.

Nguessan, Bi Tah. "Aspects économiques de la prise en charge du sida, exemple de centres antituberculeux d'Abidjan." In François Deniau, ed., *Jeunes et préservatifs en Abidjan, une recherche d'ethno-prévention du sida et des NST.* Bingerville: Actes de l'atelier du CRES, 1993.

Senoussi, Abbas. "Le sida en Côte d'Ivoire: projections démographiques et épidémiologiques, 1988–2003." In François Deniau, ed., *Jeunes et préservatifs en Abidjan, une recherche d'ethno-prévention du sida et des NST.* Bingerville: Actes de l'atelier du CRES, 1993.

GHANA

Agadzi, V. K. *AIDS: The African Perspective of the Killer Disease.* Accra: Ghana Universities Press, 1989.

Barnett, Tony and Piers Blaikie. *AIDS in Africa: Its Present and Future Impact*. New York: Guilford Press, 1992.

Herdt, Gilbert and Shirley Lindenbaum, eds. *The Time of AIDS: Social Analysis, Theory and Method*. Newbury Park, Calif.: Sage, 1992.

Inhorn, Marcia C. and Peter J. Brown. "The Anthropology of Infectious Disease." *Annual Review of Anthropology* 19 (1990): 89–117.

Latham, Michael. "AIDS in Africa: A Perspective on the Epidemic." *Africa Today* 40 (1993): 39–54.

O'Connor, Kathleen and William L. Leap, eds. "AIDS Outreach, Education, and Prevention: Anthropological Contributions." *Practicing Anthropology* 15(4) (1993).

Painter, Thomas M. *Migrations and AIDS in West Africa: A Study of Migrants from Niger and Mali to Cote d'Ivoire: Socio-Economic Context, Features of Their Sexual Comportment, and Implications for AIDS Prevention Initiatives*. New York: CARE, 1992.

Parker, R. G., G. Herdt, and M. Caballo. "Sexual Culture, HIV Transmission, and AIDS Research." *Journal of Sex Research* 28 (1991): 77–98.

Patterson, K. David. "Health in Urban Ghana: The Case of Accra 1900–1940." *Social Science and Medicine* 13B (1979): 251–68.

Porter, Robert W. "AIDS in Ghana: Priorities and Policies." In D. A. Feldman, ed., *Global AIDS Policy*. Westport, Conn.: Bergin & Garvey, 1994.

Weston, Kath. "Lesbian/Gay Studies in the House of Anthropology." *Annual Review of Anthropology* 22 (1993): 339–67.

Williams, A. Olufemi. *AIDS: An African Perspective*. Boca Raton, Fla.: CRC Press, 1992.

MALAWI

Akeroyd, Anne V. "HIV/AIDS in Eastern and Southern Africa." *Review of African Political Economy* 60 (1994): 173–84.

Azevedo, Mario J. "Epidemic Disease Among the Sara of Southern Chad, 1890–1940." In Gerald W. Hartwig and K. David Patterson, eds., *Disease in African History: An Introductory Survey and Case Studies*. Durham, N.C.: Duke University Press, 1978.

Broadhead, R. L., and J. M. Moorhouse. *Policy and Management Issues Associated with AIDS/HIV Infection*. Blantyre: Medical Association of Malawi, 1992.

Callahan, Bryan. "'Veni, V.D., Vice'?: Reassessing the Ila Syphilis Epidemic." *Journal of Southern African Studies* 22 (1997): 421–40.

Carr, C., ed. *Technical Analysis of HIV/AIDS Situation in Malawi*. Lilongwe: U.S. Agency for International Development, 1992.

Chirwa, I. "AIDS Epidemic in Malawi: Shaking Cultural Foundations." *Network* 1 (1993): 31–32.

Chirwa, Wiseman C. "Aliens and AIDS in Southern Africa: The Malawi-South Africa Debate." *African Affairs* 97 (1998): 53–79.

Chirwa, Wiseman C. "Migrancy, Sexual Networking and Multi-Partnered Sexuality in Malawi." *Health Transition Review* 7 (Supplement 3) (1997): 5–16.

Chirwa, Wiseman C. "Malawian Migrant Labour and the Politics of HIV/AIDS, 1985 to 1993." In Jonathan Crush and Wilmot James, eds., *Crossing Boundaries:*

Mine Migrancy in a Democratic South Africa. Ottawa: International Development Research Council, 1995.

Cross, David Kerr. *Health in Africa.* London: James Nisbet, 1897.

Cuddington, John, and John D. Hancock. "Assessing the Impact of AIDS on the Growth Path of the Malawian Economy." *Journal of Development Economics* 43 (1994): 363–68.

Hartwig, Gerald W., and K. David Patterson. *Disease in African History: An Introductory Survey and Case Studies.* Durham, N.C.: Duke University Press, 1978.

House, William and George Zimalirana. "Rapid Population Growth and Poverty in Malawi." *Journal of Modern African Studies* 30 (1992): 141–61.

Kamtengeni, Lillian R. "An Overview of Sexually Transmitted Diseases in Malawi." Paper prepared for Parent Education Project in the Ministry of Community Services, Lilongwe, 1991.

King, Michael and Elspeth King. *The Story of Medicine and Disease in Malawi: The 130 Years Since Livingstone.* Blantyre: Montfort Press, 1992.

Kishindo, Paul. "High Risk Behaviour in the Face of the AIDS Epidemic: The Case of Bar Girls in the Municipality of Zomba, Malawi." *Eastern Africa Social Science Research Review* 11 (1995): 35–43.

Kishindo, Paul. "Sexual Behaviour in the Face of Risk: The Case of Bar Girls in Malawi's Major Cities." *Health Transition Review* 5 (Supplement) (1995): 153–60.

Ministry of Health (Malawi). *Sexually Transmitted Diseases: A Treatment Guideline.* Lilongwe: Ministry of Health, 1989.

Packard, Randall and Paul Epstein. "Epidemiologists, Social Scientists, and the Structure of Medical Research on AIDS in Africa." In Zena Stein and Anthony Zwi, eds., *Action on AIDS in Southern Africa: Maputo Conference on Health in Transition in Southern Africa, April 1990.* New York: Columbia University, Committee for Health in Southern Africa and the HIV Center for Clinical and Behavioural Studies, 1990.

Patterson, K. David. *Health in Colonial Ghana: Disease, Medicine, and Socio-Economic Change, 1900–1955.* Waltham, Mass.: Crossroads Press, 1981.

Ransford, Oliver. *"Bid the Sickness Cease": Disease in the History of Black Africa.* London: John Murray, 1983.

The AIDS Secretariat (Malawi). *Malawi AIDS Control Programme: Medium-Term Plan II, 1994–1998.* Lilongwe: AIDS Secretariat, 1994.

Vaughan, Megan A. *Curing Their Ills: Colonial Power and African Illness.* Stanford, Calif.: Stanford University Press, 1991.

Vaughan, Megan A. "Syphilis, AIDS, and the Representation of Sexuality: The Historical Legacy." In Zena Stein and Anthony Zwi, eds., *Action on AIDS in Southern Africa: Maputo Conference on Health in Transition in Southern Africa, April 1990.* New York: Columbia University, Committee for Health in Southern Africa and the HIV Center for Clinical and Behavioural Studies, 1990.

SENEGAL

Baudet, Henri. *Extension actuelle de la syphilis dans les pays de nouvelle colonisation.* Paris: Legrand, MD thesis, 1936.

Becker, Charles. "Past Social Responses to Epidemics and the Present Outbreak of

HIV-AIDS in Senegal: Community Responses of the Past and Current Ethical Issues." In United Nations Development Programme, *African Network on Ethics Law and HIV. Proceedings of the Intercountry Consultation, Dakar, Senegal, 27 June –1 July, 1994.* Dakar: United Nations Development Programme, 1995.

Becker, Charles and René Collignon. "Épidémies et médecine coloniale en Afrique de l'ouest." *Cahiers Santé* 9 (forthcoming).

Collignon, René and Charles Becker. *Santé et population en Sénégambie des origines à 1960. Bibliographie annotée.* Paris: INED, 1989.

Coquery-Vidrovitch, Catherine, ed. *Les Africaines. Histoire des femmes d'Afrique noire du XIXe au XXe siècle.* Paris: Desjonquères, 1994.

Enel, Catherine and Gilles Pison. "Sexual Relations in the Rural Area of Mlomp (Casamance, Senegal)." In Tim Dyson, ed., *Sexual Behavior and Networking: Anthropological and Socio-Cultural Studies on the Transmission of HIV.* Liège: Editions Derouaux Ordina, 1992.

Kermorgant, A. "Aperçu sur les maladies vénériennes dans les colonies françaises."*Annales d'Hygiène et de Médecine coloniales* 6 (1903): 428–60.

Kermorgant, A. "Maladies endémiques, épidémiques et contagieuses dans les colonies françaises en 1906."*Annales d'Hygiène et de Médecine coloniales* 11 (1908): 379–80.

Le Guenno, Bernard, Gilles Pison, Catherine Enel, Emmanuel Lagarde, and Cheikh Seck. "HIV-2 Seroprevalence in Three Rural Regions of Senegal: Low Levels and Heterogeneous Distribution."*Transactions of the Royal Society of Tropical Medicine and Hygiene* 86 (1992): 301–2.

M'bokolo, Elikia. "Histoire des maladies, histoire et maladie: l'Afrique." In Marc Augé and Claudine Herzlich, eds., *Le sens du mal. Anthropologie, histoire, sociologie de la maladie.* Paris: Archives Contemporaines, 1984.

Pison, Gilles, Bernard Le Guenno, Emmanuel Lagarde, Catherine Enel, and Cheikh Seck. "Seasonal Migration: A Risk Factor for HIV Infection in Rural Senegal."*Journal of the Acquired Immune Deficiency Syndromes* 6 (1993): 196–200.

Sankalé, Marc. *Médecins et action sanitaire en Afrique Noire.* Paris: Présence Africaine, 1969.

Vaucel, Marcel Augustin. "Le pian dans les territoires africains français." *Bulletin of the World Health Organization* 8 (1953): 183–204.

Werner, Jean-François. *Marges, sexe et drogues à Dakar. Enquête ethnographique.* Paris: Karthala-Orstom, 1993.

SOUTH AFRICA

Caldwell, J. C. "Editorial: Understanding the AIDS Epidemic and Reacting Sensibly to It." *Social Science and Medicine* 41 (1995): 299–302.

Cross, S. and A. Whiteside. *Facing Up to AIDS: The Socio-Economic Impact in Southern Africa.* London: Macmillan, 1993.

Danziger, R. "The Social Impact of HIV/AIDS in Developing Countries." *Social Science and Medicine* 39 (1994): 905–17.

Green, E. "Sexually Transmitted Disease, Ethnomedicine and Health Policy in Africa." *Social Science and Medicine* 35 (1992): 121–30.

Hunt, C. "Migrant Labour and Sexually Transmitted Disease: AIDS in Africa." *Journal of Health and Social Behaviour* 30 (1989): 353–73.

Hunt, C. "Social vs Biological: Theories on the Transmission of AIDS in Africa." *Social Science and Medicine* 42 (1996): 1283–96.

Jochelson, K. *The Colour of Disease: Syphilis and Racism in South Africa, 1910–1950.* Doctoral dissertation, Oxford University, 1993.

Russell, C. "The AIDS Crisis: A Mining Industry Perspective." *Mining Survey* 2 (1991): 21–31.

Sitas, F., A. F. Fleming, and J. Morris. "Residual Risk of HIV Transmission through Blood Transfusion in South Africa." *South African Medical Journal* 84 (1994): 142–44.

South African Journal of Human Rights, HIV and South Africa — Special Edition 9 (1993).

Stein, Z. and A. Zwi, eds. *Action on AIDS in Southern Africa: Maputo Conference on Health in Transition in Southern Africa, April 1990.* New York: Columbia University, Committee for Health in Southern Africa and the HIV Center for Clinical and Behavioural Studies, 1990.

Streble, A. "'There's absolutely nothing I can do, just believe in God': South African Women with AIDS." *Agenda* (1992): 50-62.

Vaughan, M. "Syphilis in East and Central Africa: The Social Construction of an Epidemic." In T. Ranger and P. Slack, eds., *Epidemics and Ideas: Essays on the Historical Perception of Pestilence.* Cambridge: Cambridge University Press, 1992.

TANZANIA

Barongo, L. R., M. W. Borgdorff, F. F. Mosha, A. Nicoll, H. Groskurth, K. P. Senkoro, J. N. Newell, J. Changalucha, A. H. Klokke, and J. Z. Killewo. "The Epidemiology of HIV-1 Infection in Urban Areas, Roadside Settlements and Rural Villages in Mwanza Region, Tanzania." *AIDS* 6 (1992): 1521–28.

Borgdorff, M. W., L. Barongo, E. van Jaarsveld, A. H. Klokke, K. Senkoro, J. N. Newell, A. Nicoll, F. F. Mosha, H. Grosskurth, R. Swai, H. van Asten, J. Velema, R. Hayes, L. Muller, and J. Rugemalila. "Sentinel Surveillance for HIV-1 Infection: How Representative Are Blood Donors, Outpatients with Fever, Anaemia, or Sexually Transmitted Diseases, and Antenatal Clinic Attenders in Mwanza Region, Tanzania?" *AIDS* 7 (1993): 567–72.

de Zalduondo, Barbara O., Gernard I. Msamanga, and Lincoln Chen. "AIDS in Africa: Diversity in the Global Pandemic." *Daedalus* 118 (1989): 165–204.

Kaijage, Fred J. "The AIDS Crisis in Kagera Region, Tanzania, in Historical Perspective." In J. Z. Killewo and G. K. Lwihula, eds., *Behavioral and Epidemiological Aspects of AIDS Research in Tanzania: Proceedings from a Workshop in Dar es Salaam.* Dar es Salaam: Swedish Agency for Research Cooperation, 1989.

Killewo, J., K. Nyamuryekunge, A. Sandstrom, U. Bredberg-Raden, S. Wall, F. Mhalu, and G. Biberfeld. "Prevalence of HIV-1 in the Kagera Region of Tanzania: A Population-Based Study." *AIDS* 4 (1990): 1081–85.

Mnyika, Kagoma S., Knut-Inge Klepp, Gunnar Kvåle, Steinar Nilssen, Peter E. Kissila, and Naphtal Ole-King'ori. "Prevalence of HIV-1 Infection in Urban, Semi-Urban and Rural Areas in Arusha Region, Tanzania." *AIDS* 8 (1994): 1477–81.

Msamanga, Gernard I. and K. J. Pallangyo. "Characterization of Tanzanian Out-patients Presenting with Sexually Transmitted Diseases." *East African Medical Journal* 64 (1987): 30–36.

Nkya, W.M.M., S. H. Gillespie, W. Howlett, J. Elford, C. Nyamuryekunge, C. Assenga, and B. Nyombi. "Sexually Transmitted Diseases in Prostitutes in Moshi and Arusha, N Tanzania." *International Journal of STD & AIDS* 2 (1991): 432–35.

Nkya, W.M.M., William P. Howlett, C. Assenga, and B. Nyombi. "AIDS in North-ern Tanzania: An Urban Disease Model." Paper presented at the Fourth Inter-national Conference on AIDS, Stockholm, 1988.

Nkya, W.M.M., W. Howlett, C. Assenga, and B. Nyombi. "Seroepidemiology of HIV-1 Infection in the Kilimanjaro Region." In G. Giraldo, E. Beth-Giraldo, N. Clumeck, Md-R. Gharbi, S. K. Kyalwazi, and G. de The, eds., *AIDS and Asso-ciated Cancers in Africa*. Basel: Karger, 1988.

Obbo, Christine. "HIV Transmission through Social and Geographical Networks in Uganda." *Social Science and Medicine* 36 (1993): 949–55.

Schoepf, Brooke G. "Gender, Development and AIDS: A Political Economy and Cultural Framework." *Women and International Development Annual* 3 (1993): 53–85.

Schoepf, Brooke G. "Women, AIDS, and Economic Crisis in Central Africa." *Cana-dian Journal of African Studies* 22 (1988): 625–44.

Swantz, Marja-Liisa. *Women in Development: A Creative Role Denied?* London: C. Hurst, 1985.

Wallace, Roderick. "Travelling Waves of HIV Infection on a Low Dimensional 'Socio-Geographic' Network." *Social Science and Medicine* 32 (1991): 847–52.

Weiss, Brad. "'Buying Her Grave': Money, Movement, and AIDS in North-West Tanzania." *Africa* 63 (1993): 19–35.

UGANDA

Ankrah, Maxine. "AIDS and the Social Side of Health." *Social Science and Medicine* 32 (1991): 967–80.

Armstrong, Jill. *Uganda's AIDS Crisis: Its Implications for Development*. World Bank Discussion Paper No. 298. Washington, D.C.: World Bank, 1995.

Barnett, Tony, and Piers Blaikie. *AIDS in Africa: Its Present and Future Impact*. Lon-don: Belhaven Press, 1992.

Bond, George C., and Joan Vincent. "Living on the Edge: Structural Adjustment in the Context of AIDS." In Holger-Bernt Hansen and Michael Twaddle, eds., *Changing Uganda: The Dilemmas of Structural Adjustment and Revolutionary Change*. London: James Currey, 1991.

Chirimuuta, Richard C., and Rosalind J. Chirimuuta. *AIDS, Africa and Racism*. London: Free Association Books, 1989.

Farmer, Paul. *AIDS and Accusation: Haiti and the Geography of Blame*. Berkeley: Uni-versity of California Press, 1992.

Green, Edward C. "Sexually Transmitted Disease, Ethnomedicine and Health Pol-icy in Africa." *Social Science and Medicine* 35 (1992): 121–30.

Hunt, Charles W. "Social vs. Biological: Theories on the Transmission of AIDS in Africa." *Social Science & Medicine* 42 (1996): 1283–96.

Hunt, Charles W. "Africa and AIDS: Dependent Development, Sexism and Racism." *Monthly Review* 9 (February 1988): 10–22.

Kirumira, Edward, Anne Katahoire, Anthony Aboda, and Karin Edstrom. "Study on Sexual and Reproductive Health in Ugandan Women." Study supported by The World Bank and Swedish International Development Agency, Sweden, October 1993.

Larson, Ann. "Social Context of Human Immunodeficiency Virus Transmission in Africa: Historical and Cultural Bases of East and Central African Sexual Relations." *Reviews of Infectious Diseases* 2 (1989): 716–31.

Lindenbaum, Shirley. "Anthropology Rediscovers Sex: Introduction." *Social Science and Medicine* 33 (1991): 865–66.

McGrath, Janet, Charles B. Rwabukwali, Debra A. Schumann, Jonnie Pearson-Marks, Sylvia Nakayiwa, Barbara Namande, Lucy Nakyobe, and Rebecca Mukasa. "Anthropology and AIDS: The Cultural Context of Sexual Risk Behaviour among Urban Baganda Women in Kampala, Uganda." *Social Science and Medicine* 36 (1993): 429–39.

Mulder, Daan. "Two Year HIV-1 Associated Mortality in a Uganda Rural Population." *Lancet* 343 (1994): 1021–23.

Obbo, Christine. "HIV Transmission through Social and Geographical Networks in Uganda." *Social Science and Medicine* 36 (1993): 949–55.

Seidel, Gill. "The Competing Discourses of HIV/AIDS in Sub-Saharan Africa: Discourses of Rights and Empowerment vs Discourses of Control and Exclusion." *Social Science and Medicine* 36 (1993): 175–94.

ZAMBIA

Baggaley, Rachel, Peter Godfrey-Fausett, Roland Msiska, DavidChilangwa, and E. Chitu. "Impact of HIV on Zambian Businesses." *British Medical Journal* 309 (1994): 1549–50.

Barnett, T., and P. Blaikie. *AIDS in Africa — Its Present and Future Impact.* New York: Guilford Press, 1992.

Bledsoe, Caroline. "The Politics of AIDS and Condoms for Stable Heterosexual Relations in Africa: Recent Evidence from Local Print Media." *Disasters* 15 (1991): 1–11.

Bond, Virginia, and Paul Dover. "Men, Women and the Trouble with Condoms: Problems Associated with Condom Use by Migrant Workers in Zambia." *Health Transition Review* 7 (1997): 377–91.

Bond, Virginia, and Phillimon Ndubani. "The Difficulties Associated with Compiling a Glossary of Diseases Associated with Sexual Intercourse in Chiawa, Rural Zambia." *Social Science & Medicine* 44 (1997): 1211–20.

Brelsford, W. Vernon. "Analysis of African Reaction to Propaganda Film." *NADA* (1948): 7–22.

Buve, A., M. Carael, R. Hayes, and N. J. Robinson, "Variations in HIV Prevalence between Urban Areas in Sub-Saharan Africa: Do We Understand Them?" *AIDS* 9 (1995): S103–9.

Callahan, Bryan. "'Veni, V.D., Vici'?: Reassessing the Ila Syphilis Epidemic, 1900–1963." *Journal of Southern African Studies* 23 (1997): 421–40.

Evans, Arthur J. "The Ila V.D. Campaign." *Rhodes-Livingstone Institute Journal* 9 (1950): 40–47.

Faxelid, Elizabeth. "Partner Notifications in Context: Swedish and Zambian Experiences." *Social Science & Medicine* 44 (1997): 1239–44.

Godfrey-Fausett, Peter, Rachel Baggaley, Guy Scott, and Moses Sichone. "HIV in Zambia: Myth or Monster?" *Nature* 368 (1994): 183–84.

Haslam, John. *Northern Rhodesia Health Services Development Plans, 1945–55.* Lusaka: Government Printer, 1945.

Jones, John D. Rheinallt. "The Development of Central and Southern Africa — Suggestions for Research and Action on Some of the Problems Common to These Territories." *Rhodes-Livingstone Institute Journal* 7 (1949): 1–23.

Keller, Bonnie. "Marriage by Elopement." *African Social Research* 27 (1979): 565–85.

Keller, Bonnie. "Marriage and Medicine: Women's Search for Love and Luck." *African Social Research* 26 (1978): 489–505.

Kuczynski, Robert R. "Northern Rhodesia." In R. R. Kuczynski, ed., *Demographic Survey of the British Colonial Empire*, Vol. II. London: Oxford University Press, 1949.

Lal, D., and C. Kennedy. "AIDS and Heterosexuals and Africa," Discussion Paper No. 88, University College London, 1988.

Larson, Ann. "Social Context of HIV Transmission in Africa: Historical and Cultural Bases of East and Central African Sexual Relations." *Reviews of Infectious Diseases* 5 (1989): 716–31.

Mogensen, Hanne Overgaard. "The Narrative of AIDS among the Tonga of Zambia." *Social Science and Medicine* 44 (1997): 431–39.

Oppong, Joseph. Review of Tony Barnett, and Piers Blaikie. "AIDS in Africa: Its Present and Future Impact." *Social Science and Medicine* 43 (1996): 278–79.

Packard, Randall, and Paul Epstein. "Epidemiologists, Social Scientists, and the Structure of Medical Research on AIDS in Africa." *Social Science and Medicine* 33 (1991): 771–94.

Philpott, R. "The Mulobezi-Mongu Labour Route." *Rhodes-Livingstone Institute Journal* 3 (1945): 50–54.

Ranger, Terence. "Plagues of Beasts and Men: Prophetic Responses to Epidemic in Eastern and Southern Africa." In Terence Ranger and Paul Slack, eds., *Epidemics and Ideas: Essays on the Historical Perception of Pestilence.* Cambridge: Cambridge University Press, 1992.

Runganga, Agnes, Marian Pitts, and John McMaster. "The Use of Herbal and Other Agents to Enhance Sexual Experience" *Social Science and Medicine* 35 (1992): 1037–42.

Schopper, Doris, Serge Doussantousse, and John Orav. "Sexual Behaviors Relevant to HIV Transmission in a Rural African Population — How Much Can a KAP Survey Tell Us?" *Social Science and Medicine* 37 (1995): 401–12.

Siegel, Brian. "The 'Wild' and 'Lazy' Lamba: Ethnic Stereotypes on the Central African Copperbelt." In Leroy Vail, ed., *The Creation of Tribalism in Southern Africa.* Berkeley: University of California Press, 1991.

Spring, Anita. "Epidemiology of Spirit Possession among the Luvale of Zambia." In Judith Hoch-Smith and Anita Spring, eds., *Women in Ritual and Symbolic Roles.* New York: Plenum Press, 1978.

Ulin, Priscilla R. "African Women and AIDS: Negotiating Behavioral Change." *Social Science and Medicine* 34 (1992): 63–73.

Vaughan, Megan. *Curing Their Ills: Colonial Power and African Illness.* Stanford, Calif.: Stanford University Press, 1991.

White, Charles M. N. "A Preliminary Survey of Luvale Rural Economy." Rhodes-Livingstone Institute Papers No. 2, Manchester University Press, 1959.

ZIMBABWE

Aries, Philippe, and Andre Bejin, eds. *Western Sexuality: Practice and Precept in Past and Present Times.* Oxford: Basil Blackwell, 1985.

Gelfand, Michael. *A Service to the Sick: A History of the Health Services for Africans in Southern Rhodesia 1890 to 1953.* Salisbury: Mambo Press, 1967.

Gelfand, Michael. *The Sick African: A Clinical Study.* Cape Town: Juta Press, 1957.

Gelfand, Michael. *Tropical Victory: An Account of the Influence of Medicine on the History of Southern Rhodesia, 1890–1923.* Cape Town: Juta, 1953.

Gilman, Sander. *Difference and Pathology: Stereotypes of Sexuality, Race and Madness.* Ithaca, N.Y.: Cornell University Press, 1985.

Hansen, Karen. *Distant Companions: Servants and Employers in Zambia, 1900–1985.* Ithaca, N.Y.: Cornell University Press, 1989.

Hyam, Ronald. *Empire and Sexuality: The British Experience.* Manchester: Manchester University Press, 1990.

Jeater, Diana. *Marriage, Perversion and Power: The Construction of Moral Discourse in Southern Rhodesia 1894–1930.* Oxford: Clarendon Press, 1993.

Kennedy, Dane. *Islands of White: Settler Society and Culture in Kenya and Southern Rhodesia, 1890–1939.* Durham, N.C.: Duke University Press, 1987.

Laubscher, B.J.F. *Sex, Custom and Psychopathology: A Study of South African Pagan Natives.* London: George Routledge & Sons, 1937.

Macleod, Roy, and Milton Lewis, eds. *Disease, Medicine and Empire: Perspective on Western Medicine and the Experience of European Expansion.* London: Routledge, 1988.

Mandaza, Ibbo. *White Settler Ideology, African Nationalism and the "Coloured" Question in Southern Africa: Southern Rhodesia/Zimbabwe, Northern Rhodesia/Zambia and Nyasaland/Malawi 1900–1976.* Doctoral dissertation, University of York, 1979.

Mort, Frank. *Sexualities: Micro-Moral Politics in England since 1830.* London: Routledge & Kegan Paul, 1987.

Phimister, Ian. *An Economic and Social History of Zimbabwe, 1890–1948: Capital Accumulation and Class Struggle.* London: Longman, 1988.

Quetel, Claude. *History of Syphilis.* Cambridge: Polity Press, 1987.

Sontag, Susan. *Aids and Its Metaphors.* New York: Farrar, Straus and Giroux, 1989.

Strobel, Margaret. *European Women and the Second British Empire.* Bloomington: Indiana University Press, 1991.

van Onselen, Charles. *Studies in the Social and Economic History of the Witwatersrand, 1886–1914,* Vol 2. Johannesburg: Ravan Press, 1982.

van Onselen, Charles. *Chibaro: African Mine Labour in Southern Rhodesia.* Johannesburg: Ravan Press, 1980.

Index

About the Contributors

Jeanne-Marie Amat-Roze, is professor at the University of Paris-Sorbonne where she teaches the geography of health and several courses in the medical faculty. Her primary interest is in the relationship between disease, locality, and the environmental determinants of human health. Her major focus is on Africa and the spatial dynamics of HIV infection and AIDS.

Charles Becker is a researcher at the Centre National de la Recherche Scientifique in France and is attached to the Institut Français de Recherche scientifique pour le développement en Coopération in Dakar. His present fields of interest are demographic and social history and the anthropology and history of health in Senegal and West Africa. He has published numerous studies on these topics including *Santé et population en Sénégambie des origines à 1960* with René Collignon (1989).

Virginia Bond is based at the Institute for Economics and Social Research, University of Zambia. She has had recent publications in *Social Science and Medicine* and *Health Transition Review* and has conducted research on the impact of health and education fees on poor communities, refugees in southwest Uganda, and housing in London.

Bryan T. Callahan is a doctoral candidate at Johns Hopkins University. He has published excerpts of his research in the *Journal of Southern African Studies* and in various edited volumes.

Wiseman Chijere Chirwa is a sociologist and historian at Chancellor College, University of Malawi. His works have appeared in such periodicals as the *Journal of Modern African Affairs*, *Journal of Southern African Studies*, *African Affairs*, *African Rural and Urban Studies*, *International Journal of African Historical Studies*, *Health Transition Review*, and *Development in Practice* and in edited books.

René Collignon is a clinical psychologist and director of research at the Centre national de la Recherche Scientifique. His areas of research are comparative psychiatry, medical anthropology, and history of psychiatry in Africa. He is editor of *Psychopathologie africaine*.

Karen Jochelson is currently completing an MBA and consulting on human rights and business issues and on scenarios for sustainable development. She recently completed *The Colour of Disease: Syphilis and Racism in South Africa, 1870–1950*.

Milton Lewis is National Health and Medical Research Council Senior Research Fellow in the Department of Public Health and Community Medicine, University of Sydney. He has published widely on the history of medicine and public health, including the history of psychiatry, of alcohol policy, of infant and maternal health, of "imperial medicine," of sexually transmitted diseases and HIV/AIDS, and of the professionalization of medicine.

Maryinez Lyons is a research fellow at the Institute of Commonwealth Studies, University of London. She is also an Honorary Research Fellow at the London School of Hygiene & Tropical Medicine. She published *The Colonial Disease: A Social History of Sleeping Sickness in Northern Zaire, 1900–1940* (1992). She is presently beginning a new study in Uganda.

Jock McCulloch has worked as a legislative Research Specialist in foreign affairs for the Australian Parliament and has taught at various universities. His principal interest is in contemporary African history, and he has carried out research in Algeria, Zimbabwe, South Africa, and Kenya. His most recent book is a study of sexual crime in colonial Zimbabwe.

Deborah Pellow is professor of anthropology at Syracuse University. Her ongoing work in a migrant community in Accra has appeared in various journals, including *Africa* and *Ethnohistory*. She edited *Setting Boundaries: The Anthropology of Spatial and Social Organization* (1996).

Philip W. Setel is a senior research fellow at the School of Clinical Medical Sciences, University of Newcastle upon Tyne and project director of the Adult Morbidity and Mortality Project of the Ministry of Health of the United Republic of Tanzania, based in Dar es Salaam. He has published numerous papers on the social and cultural dimensions of AIDS, sexuality, gender relations, and fertility and family planning in East Africa and Papua New Guinea. His *A Plague of Paradoxes: AIDS, Culture and Demography in Northern Tanzania* will be published in 1999.